Developmental Counseling and Therapy

Promoting Wellness Over the Lifespan

ALLEN E. IVEY
University of Massachusetts, Amherst

MARY BRADFORD IVEY
Microtraining Associates, Inc.

JANE E. MYERS
University of North Carolina, Greensboro

THOMAS J. SWEENEY
Ohio University

Lahaska Press
Houghton Mifflin Company
Boston ▪ New York

To our students, who continually facilitate our development and growth

Publisher, Lahaska Press: Barry Fetterolf
Development Editor, Lahaska Press: Mary Falcon
Editorial Assistant: Lisa Littlewood
Senior Project Editor: Tracy Patruno
Manufacturing Manager: Florence Cadran
Marketing Manager: Brenda L. Bravener-Greville

Cover image: Whirling Squares © Lois Grady

Lahaska Press, a unique collaboration between the Houghton Mifflin College Division and Lawrence Erlbaum Associates, is dedicated to publishing books and offering services for the academic and professional counseling communities. The partnership of Lahaska Press was formed in late 1999. The name "Lahaska" is a Native American Lenape word meaning "source of many writings." The small eastern Pennsylvania town of Lahaska, named by the Lenape, is the home of the Lahaska Press editorial offices.

Portions of this book adapted from *Developmental Strategies for Helpers: Individual, Family, and Network Interventions* by Allen E. Ivey, originally published in 1991 by Wadsworth, Inc. and assigned in 1993 to Microtraining Associates, Inc.

Printed in the U.S.A.

Library of Congress Control Number: 2003110192

ISBN: 0-618-43988-9

23456789-MP-08 07 06 05 04

CONTENTS

PREFACE

Counseling, psychology, human services, and social work professionals are the audience for *Developmental Counseling and Therapy: Promoting Wellness Over the Lifespan*. This book is designed for the developmental or lifespan course, particularly if the focus is on taking the theory into practice. The concepts presented here have been used effectively in both basic and advanced interviewing skills courses. Students completing professional preparation programs in practica and internships will find these ideas useful in integrating their own thinking and practice in counseling and therapy. Those studying theories of counseling can benefit from the integrative theory-into-practice concepts of this book. It also might be useful as a supplemental text in a multicultural counseling course, especially in relation to interview action and treatment planning.

Developmental Counseling and Therapy: Promoting Wellness Over the Lifespan can be summarized in five major objectives:

1. Provide a theoretical/practical background in wellness theory and positive lifespan developmental psychology that will enable readers to take these ideas into concrete practice in the interview.
2. Show in specific terms how developmental theory can be integrated into the counseling and therapy interview and treatment plan.
3. Demonstrate the relationship of multicultural theory to developmental theory and interview action.
4. Present a wellness approach to *DSM-IV-TR* that makes affirmative and constructive work with severely distressed clients more possible.
5. Supply a wide range of practical applications, exercises, and practice activities that can be used by each reader in his or her next interviewing session.

Putting theory into practice is the central task of this book. Each developmental theory presented here has important practice implications. Furthermore, readers will find in the developmental models a new approach leading toward an integrated and metatheoretical practice of counseling and psychotherapy.

Key Features

This book can make a significant difference in counseling and therapy practice, whether the reader is a student or an experienced professional. We have placed a major emphasis on accountability and results-oriented interviewing, examining both client assessment and suggested actions to follow from that assessment. The following are key features oriented toward these goals:

- *Wellness and developmental theories.* Major attention is given to basic theories and their multicultural usefulness, all within a wellness and positive psychology framework. These include Bowlby's attachment theory, Erikson's lifespan concepts, and Schlossberg's transitions theory. Several cognitive-developmental theories and concepts of wellness and positive psychology are explored. Jeanne Piaget provides much of the background for taking developmental theory into practice.

- *Specifics of developmental assessment in the here and now of the interview.* The focus is on client meaning making and how clients make sense of their world. Developmental counseling and therapy (DCT) theory provides details and examples that will show readers how to match (or mismatch, as appropriate) their interviewing approach to the cognitive/emotional style of the client. Moreover, through the Confrontation Impact Scale, it becomes possible to assess immediately how clients respond to interventions.

- *Traditional theories of counseling enriched by developmental treatment planning.* The four major forces of counseling and psychotherapy (psychodynamic, cognitive-behavioral, existential-humanistic, and multicultural counseling and psychotherapy) all can benefit from more attention to a developmental view. Examples of integrated treatment planning can be found throughout the text.

- *Movement toward a culture-centered developmental counseling and therapy model.* "Psychotherapy as liberation" is based on the revolutionary ideas of the Brazilian, Paulo Freire. Multicultural counseling and therapy (MCT) is presented in a developmental framework, and readers will learn how to facilitate client cultural identity development and to help clients discover and cope with oppressive elements in their lives.

- *Developmental applications with families, bibliotherapy, early recollections, and spirituality.* The developmental and wellness models offer specific practices that can be used with many types of clients, in diverse settings, and in concert with multiple issues and interventions. Strategies and examples are provided for working with families, using bibliotherapy and early recollections as interventions, and helping clients explore their spirituality. Moreover, the reader is encouraged to discern her or his own meaning and spiritual mission through reading and exercises.

- *The portfolio of competence.* Each chapter concludes with exercises and practice activities to make theory real and useful. Readers are encouraged to develop a portfolio summarizing their knowledge and accomplishments. Important in this process is personal growth and self-assessment. The competence-building activities are also available on the Lahaska Press website (www.lahaskapress.com), where instructors can download and print out the activities for their students.

Teaching Aids

A downloadable *Instructor Resource Guide* is available through the publisher's website, http://college.hmco.com/lahaskapress. It includes chapter summaries, classroom activities, multiple-choice and essay questions, a syllabus, and supplementary resources.

Downloadable PowerPoint slides are also available through the publisher's website, http://college.hmco.com/lahaskapress. Instructors can show these overheads directly from their own computer or print them out as transparency masters.

Videotapes supporting this book are available. A video on developmental counseling and therapy (DCT) illustrates developmental assessment and practice, the impact of varying developmental questions, and ways to use the developmental model with personality style "disorders." Videos are also available on cultural identity theory, early recollections, dream analysis, and lifespan interviewing. Contact Microtraining Associates at 888-505-5576 or at www.emicrotraining.com.

Acknowledgments

Victor Frankl commented to Mary and Allen Ivey during a visit to his office in Vienna, "We all build on the shoulders of giants." This book definitely relies on some developmental and wellness giants, particularly Alfred Adler, John Bowlby, Erik Erikson, and Jeanne Piaget. We should recall that Adler, Bowlby, and Erikson were not interested only in therapy; they were all *developmentalists* who were aware of cultural differences and the importance of considering developmental history when working with clients. Piaget, the Swiss epistemologist, has received relatively little attention in relation to counseling and therapy. In this book, we suggest that Piaget's ideas have had profound implications. Multicultural counseling and therapy theorists and practitioners—especially the cultural identity frameworks of William Cross and Janet Helms—have been highly influential in the conceptualization of this book. Paulo Freire's ideas concerning psychological liberation resonate widely throughout the text.

Allen and Mary acknowledge the following: Ursula Delworth was the first person to recognize the importance and value of the developmental model, and we especially recognize her support. Dr. Machiko Fukuhara, president of the Japanese Microcounseling Association, has taken these ideas to Japan, and we have enjoyed our work with her for many years. Dr. Koji Tamase, also of Japan, has completed extensive research on the developmental model. Terry Anderson, Bruce Oldershaw, George Forman, Teresa LaFromboise, Oscar Gonçalves, Maurie and Fran Howe, and Sandra Rigazio-DiGilio have been particularly important figures in the history of this book and its concepts. More recently, John Marszalek's work on gay identity development has expanded our thinking. Lois Grady, who developed the DCT spherical model and the cover of this book, is given special thanks and recognition. We also offer particular thanks and love to our multicultural family, the National Institute of Multicultural Competence—Patricia Arredondo, Michael D'Andrea, Judy Daniels, Don Locke, Thomas Parham, Beverly O'Bryant, and Derald Wing Sue.

Jane and Tom acknowledge the following: Mel Witmer was our earliest professional partner as we joined forces to develop and revise the Wheel of Wellness model, in terms of both the theoretical/conceptual components and clinical assessment. Courtland Lee, Don C. Locke, Michael Garrett, Lisa Levers, Sandra Lopez-Baez, Rose Marie Hoffman, and Thelma Vriend were especially helpful as we defined cultural and gender identity as aspects of wellness. Many doctoral students over the years have been instrumental in expanding our views of wellness based on their research projects and in incorporating DCT into their teaching, supervision, and clinical practice.

Noteworthy for their integration of DCT and wellness concepts are Casey Barrio, Catharina Chang, Kathleen Connolly, Brian Dew, Andrea Dixon Rayle, Suzanne Degges White, Holly Hartwig Morehead, Linda Makinson, Natasha Mitchell, Keith Mobley, Anne Powers, Matthew Shurts, Stacey Sinclair, and Shawn Spurgeon. Special thanks for help with preparation of chapters of the book and instructor materials are owed to Matthew Shurts, Holly Landry, and Phil Clarke.

For all of us, it has been a pleasure to work with Barry Fetterolf, Publisher, and Mary Falcon, Senior Editor, of Houghton Mifflin/Lahaska Press. We truly appreciate the careful and thoughtful work of Patterson Lamb, our most able copy editor. Anne Draus of Scratchgravel Publishing Services remains one of the most capable and dependable people we know.

A book is only a moment in time. It may look solid and permanent, but in actuality, it is a developmental process that changes with every keystroke, word, and—later—each reading of the final text. *Developmental Counseling and Psychotherapy: Promoting Wellness Over the Lifespan* is a set of ideas, always in process. We welcome your feedback and your ideas.

Allen E. Ivey
Mary Bradford Ivey
Jane E. Myers
Thomas J. Sweeney

ABOUT THE AUTHORS

Allen E. Ivey is Distinguished University Professor (Emeritus) at the University of Massachusetts, Amherst, and is currently President of Microtraining Associates, an educational publishing firm. He earned his doctorate at Harvard University. Dr. Ivey is a past president and Fellow of the Division of Counseling Psychology of the American Psychological Association and is a life member of American Counseling Association. He is also a Diplomat of the American Board of Professional Psychology and an elected Fellow of the Society for the Psychological Study of Ethnic Minority Issues of APA. He is on the Board of Directors of the National Institute for Multicultural Competence.

The originator of microcounseling and developmental counseling and therapy (DCT), Dr. Ivey has won wide recognition and national and international awards, including the ACA Professional Development Award. Dr. Ivey is author and co-author of more than 30 books and 200 articles and chapters, and his works have been translated into at least 17 languages. He did original work on the multicultural implications of the microskills from 1968 to 1974 and has been developing his work in multicultural studies ever since. He is co-author of *A Theory of Multicultural Counseling and Therapy* (with Derald Wing Sue and Paul Pedersen) and *Theories of Counseling and Psychotherapy: A Multicultural Approach,* 5th ed. (with Michael D'Andrea, Mary Bradford Ivey, and Lynn Simek-Morgan).

Spirituality and counseling are recent extensions of Allen and Mary Ivey's work on interviewing skills combined with multicultural and developmental thinking. Their most recent writings have focused on "psychotherapy as liberation," multicultural issues, and a theoretical/practical approach to working in a positive developmental framework with so-called "pathology" and *DSM-IV.*

Mary Bradford Ivey, Vice President of Microtraining Associates, has three areas of expertise and experience: writing, independent consulting, and school guidance. She earned her master's degree in counseling at the University of Wisconsin, Madison, and her doctoral degree in organizational development at the University of Massachusetts, where she worked closely with Kenneth Blanchard, author of the well-known *One-Minute Manager.*

Dr. Ivey received national recognition in 1988 when her elementary counseling program at the Fort River School was named one of the ten best in the nation at the

Christa McAuliffe Conference. She is co-author of seven books plus numerous articles, translated into several languages. In addition, she has produced a number of videotapes illustrating counseling and therapy strategies, including the popular video, *Counseling Children*. She has just completed a new video, *Counseling Latina/o Children: Brief Interventions*, with Enedina Vazquez and Luis Vazquez. Her most recent book is *Intentional Interviewing and Counseling*, 5th ed. (with Allen Ivey).

Dr. Ivey has taught or held appointments at the University of Massachusetts in Amherst, Keene State College, the University of Hawai`i in Manoa, and Flinders University in Australia. She has lectured widely throughout the United States, Mexico, Canada, Europe, Asia, Australia, and New Zealand. She is on the Board of Directors of the National Institute for Multicultural Competence. She is a National Certified Counselor and a licensed mental health counselor. One of her specialties is applying consultation skills to school and management environments. Recently, she has applied the developmental model to the positive treatment of children with special attention to issues of child abuse.

Jane E. Myers is a Professor of Counselor Education at the University of North Carolina at Greensboro. She is a National Certified Counselor, National Certified Gerontological Counselor, and a Licensed Professional Counselor. She is a Fellow of the Gerontological Society of America, the Association for Gerontology in Higher Education, and the National Rehabilitation Counseling Association, and a Charter Fellow of the Chi Sigma Iota Academy of Leaders for Excellence.

Dr. Myers is past president of the American Counseling Association and two of its divisions, the Association for Assessment in Counseling and the Association for Adult Development and Aging, for which she was founding president. Dr. Myers also served as Chair of the Council for Accreditation of Counseling and Related Educational Programs (CACREP). In 2003, she was selected for inclusion in *Leaders and Legacies in Counseling*, a book that chronicles the contributions of 25 of the most significant leaders in the counseling profession over the past century.

Dr. Myers developed a model and curriculum resources for infusion of gerontological counseling into counselor education, and she co-authored (with Thomas J. Sweeney) the national competencies for training gerontological counselors. Together, Dr. Myers and Dr. Sweeney co-produced seven training videotapes to promote counselor competence in this specialty. Dr. Myers has written and edited numerous publications, including 16 books and monographs and over 100 refereed journal articles, and she was noted as being in the top 1 percent of contributors to the *Journal of Counseling & Development*, ACA's flagship journal. Her books include *Adult Children and Aging Parents*, *Empowerment for Later Life* and (as co-editor) *The Handbook of Counseling*. She is also co-creator of one theoretical and two evidence-based models of wellness as well as assessment instruments based on these models. Dr. Myers is an advocate for wellness lifestyles for her students and people of all ages.

Thomas J. Sweeney has more than 40 years of higher education teaching and leadership experience. He is Professor Emeritus and past Coordinator of the Counselor Education program at Ohio University where he began teaching in 1972. He has held leadership offices at state, regional, national, and international levels, including president of the American Counseling Association (ACA) and the Association for Counselor Education and Supervision (ACES). He was founding president of the International Association of Marriage and Family Counseling and served on the boards of both the National Vocational Guidance Association and the Association for Adult Development and Aging. His works include *Adlerian Counseling*, 4th ed., *Wellness* (co-author of the model and assessment instrument), and *Gerontological Counseling* (video series). His most recent book, co-authored with Dr. Myers, is *Wellness in Counseling: Theory, Research, and Practice.*

Dr. Sweeney is founder and current Executive Director of Chi Sigma Iota Counseling Academic and Professional Honor Society International (CSI). CSI was first established at Ohio University in 1985 and now has more than 250 chapters and 38,000 members worldwide. Dr. Sweeney was instrumental in starting the credentialing movement of professional counselors and advancing counselor preparation and accreditation at the national level. He authored ACA position papers on these topics and served as first chair of the respective professional initiatives (Licensure Committee and CACREP).

Dr. Sweeney has received numerous awards for leadership and service to the counseling profession. His national award-winning *Coping with Kids* telecourse was distributed on film and broadcast worldwide on public television. In 2003 he was selected for inclusion in *Leaders and Legacies in Counseling*, a book that chronicles the contributions of 25 of the most significant leaders in the profession of counseling over the past century. He also was noted as among the top 2 to5 percent of contributors to the counseling profession's *Journal of Counseling and Development,* over a recent 15-year period.

BEFORE YOU START

Lifespan Wellness, Objectives of This Book, and Ethics

CENTRAL PRACTICE OBJECTIVE

Developmental Counseling and Therapy: Promoting Wellness Over the Lifespan focuses on how you can integrate developmental theory into four major areas of clinical practice. This book provides theory and strategies that will enable you to

- Utilize key developmental theories in the here and now of the interview.
- Relate theories of counseling and treatment planning to developmental concepts.
- Understand and master a wellness approach to working with clients who face normal issues and those who face severe and complex problems, such as the ones outlined in the *Diagnostic and Statistical Manual of Mental Disorders* (DSM-IV) (American Psychiatric Association, 2000).
- Integrate multicultural thought and practice into your daily interviewing practice.

The Council for Accreditation of Counseling and Related Educational Programs (CACREP) specifies required coursework in eight core curricular areas (CACREP, 2001). These include professional identity, social and cultural diversity, human growth and development, career development, helping relationships, group work, assessment, and research and program evaluation. Studies in the area of human growth and development "provide an understanding of the nature and needs of individuals at all developmental levels, including all of the following: (a) theories of individual and family development and transitions across the life-span, (b) theories of learning and personality development; (c) human behavior including an understanding of developmental crises, disability, exceptional behavior, addictive behavior, psychopathology, and situational and environmental factors that affect both normal and abnormal behavior; (d) strategies for facilitating optimum development over the life-span; and (e) ethical and legal considerations" (pp. 61–62).

The information in this book provides an in-depth orientation to the human growth and development arena, including theories as well as techniques for facilitating optimum human development over the lifespan. Moreover, the book provides additional foundations for practice among all mental health professionals. And, the developmental model here is based on wellness and the positive psychology movement, a newly expanding model that appears to be changing the very foundations of counseling and clinical practice.

This book strongly supports the traditional theoretical grouping of first force psychodynamic, second force cognitive-behavioral, and third force existential-humanistic theory. All these methods, used judiciously, can make a positive difference to your clients. However, fourth force multicultural counseling and therapy (MCT) has now been added to the basic helping triad. The issues raised by MCT need to be considered in every interview, regardless of what theory is employed. Developmental counseling and therapy (DCT) is an integrative approach that allows you to use the best of each theory as appropriate for each individual client.

Developmental counseling and therapy (DCT) encourages you to build on your present theoretical and practice expertise and to give special attention to developmental issues that we all face over a lifetime. DCT asks you to start with the client and hear her or his story carefully. How does this person make sense of the world and what cognitive/emotional style do we see in the here and now of the session? What are the wellness strengths that can be used for problem resolution? Where is the client in the lifespan and what developmental transitions might be important? How might multicultural and other contextual factors affect this client?

DCT starts with a focus on wellness and positive psychology in the belief that clients grow best if we first attend to their strengths. But DCT also specifically addresses the most difficult issues that one can face in counseling and therapy, such as helping a client deal with depression and post-traumatic stress. "Handling the hard stuff" is a basic part of DCT theory and practice.

WHAT DOES THIS BOOK OFFER FOR YOUR DEVELOPMENT?

This is a highly interactive book, one that makes the counseling and therapy session clearer and will enable you to understand and work with clients at a new level of competence. However, unless you take the written word into concrete practice almost immediately, the value and potential of the ideas here will be greatly limited. Each chapter has specifics that can be used immediately in the here and now of the interview.

Table A-1 presents a listing of the 13 content chapters of this book and gives you an overview of where we are headed. Note that each chapter has a central practice objective. While based in developmental, lifespan, and wellness theory, this is a book focused on taking counseling theory directly into practice. As you review Table A-1, what goals and objectives stand out for you as most potentially valuable?

By the end of this book, you will be able to assess and treat many aspects of client thoughts, feelings, behaviors, and meanings within a developmental context. You will find a constant orientation to wellness over the lifespan. Developmental counseling and therapy (DCT) is an integrative system that is equally effective with children, adolescents, and adults. This developmental approach is also effective with those who face the typical stressors of daily life and those who are undergoing severe psychological distress. DCT will also help you to work multiculturally and with issues of spirituality.

Chapter 14 of this book returns again to Table A-1. There you will be asked to assess your mastery of the central practice competencies of this book. Thus, you may want to return to this table from time and time and reflect on your progress toward mastery of the developmental approach.

Holding in mind the practical emphasis of this book, let us turn to the issue of wellness and how it might relate to you and your work as a counselor or therapist.

THE DEVELOPMENTAL LIFELINE: AN INVENTORY OF WELLNESS

You are the central person to whom this book is addressed. As you work through the chapters, we ask you to look constantly at yourself and at your own cognitive/emotional style(s). Where are you in the lifespan? What major strengths do you bring to the interview? How do you make sense of the world? Once you have a grasp of these issues as they relate to you, you are in a good position to facilitate client development.

Developing your own lifeline is a good way to start thinking developmentally. Each client who comes to us is at some developmental stage and thus is quite likely to face issues related to that stage. But these clients also come with a developmental history that deeply affects their being and the way they interact with you in the immediacy of the interview.

Let us start the process by having you develop your own lifeline. This will help you consider your own past development and reflect on its meaning. Ideally, you will then share your lifeline with colleagues, but you need *only share those parts of your developmental past that you feel comfortable sharing.*

As you develop the lifeline, think of your life story. Where were you born? Were there any special conditions surrounding your birth? Who was/were your family/friends? What significant events do you recall from each life stage? What hardships and life challenges did you encounter? Pay special attention to the current stage at which you find yourself.

Table A-1   Central Practice Objectives of Developmental Counseling and Therapy

Chapter	Central Practice Objective
1. Our Developmental Nature	Ability to assess clients' concrete and abstract cognitive/emotional styles shown through ability to recognize and classify client statements and to distinguish them in the here and now of the interview.
2. Wellness: Optimizing Human Development Over the Lifespan	Ability to assess your wellness and that of your clients, thus providing a solid base of strengths on which to facilitate client positive movement.
3. Development Over the Lifespan: Developmental Counseling as Lifespan Therapy	Ability to conduct a lifespan review and to assess and understand clients' unique developmental history and current normative life transitions and challenges, and anticipate later developmental concerns.
4. Assessing Developmental Style	Ability to assess the four client cognitive/emotional styles through classification of transcripts and to identify client style in the here and now of the interview.
5. Developmental Interventions and Strategies: Specific Interventions to Facilitate Client Cognitive and Emotional Development	Ability to apply specific DCT questioning strategies with many types of clients and to adapt the strategies for your work utilizing many theories of counseling and therapy.
6. Assessing Client Change: Creativity, Perturbation, and Confrontation	Ability to facilitate change by perturbing and confronting client discrepancies and incongruities in a supportive fashion. Equally important, the ability to assess the impact of your confrontation on client change processes using the Confrontation Impact Scale.
7. Developing Treatment Plans: DCT and Theories of Counseling and Psychotherapy	Ability to shift your counseling style to meet the developmental needs of varying clients. You will be able to work with multiple theories of counseling and therapy and integrate DCT developmental concepts into the treatment.
8. Multicultural Counseling and Therapy	Ability to assess and to facilitate client expansion of cultural identity and multicultural consciousness. Ability to use the specific steps of psychotherapy as liberation to help clients discover, name, reflect, and act on issues related to multicultures and to oppression.
9. Reframing the *Diagnostic and Statistical Manual of Mental Disorders:* Positive Strategies From Developmental Counseling and Therapy	Ability to reframe severe distress as a logical biological and psychological response to environmental conditions. Ability to develop comprehensive treatment plans, using multiple theoretical orientations and strategies, to work with issues such as depression, personality style ("disorder"), and post-traumatic stress.
10. Early Recollections: Using DCT With Early Memories to Facilitate Second-Order Change	Ability to use the theoretical/practical Adlerian approach to early recollections as (a) a positive support base for your clients and (b) a way to help clients understand how their past relates to the present and to help them build toward the future.
11. Using Developmental Counseling and Therapy With Families	Ability to understand and work with families at various stages of the life cycle and to apply DCT questioning strategies to facilitate family development.
12. Bibliotherapy, Metaphors, and Narratives	Ability to bring more creative and artistic processes into the stories surrounding the counseling and psychotherapy process, including the use of narratives, media, and journaling.
13. Spirituality, Wellness, and Development: Applying DCT to Core Values in Clients' Lives	Ability to conceptualize and work comfortably with spiritual, religious, and meaning issues in the interview. Ability to use DCT discernment processes to help clients find direction and make meaning in their lives.
14. Epilogue: Your Future Development	You will review each of the Central Practice Objectives and assess your level of competence in and mastery of each.

Also focus on your successes in each period. What are you proud of? Keep in mind that success and accomplishment can be defined in many ways. Use the following worksheet for your notes beside the vertical lifeline.

0–5 (Birth and early childhood)

_____

_____

_____

_____

5–12 (Elementary school)

_____

_____

_____

_____

12–18 (Middle and high school)

_____

_____

_____

_____

18–22 (College or early work experience)

_____

_____

_____

_____

22–30 (Young adulthood)

_____

_____

_____

_____

31–40 (Moving on)

_____

_____

_____

_____

41–60 (Middle age)

_____

_____

_____

_____

61–80 (Late middle age to early elder status)

_____

_____

_____

_____

81– (Elder status)

_____

_____

_____

_____

Wellness inventory.   All of us face difficulty in our lives; no one gets out unscathed. Yet somehow most of us survive the difficulties and the challenges, both large and small. We endure these difficulties because we have strengths and positive assets and because we have support and encouragement from others. Some of us have had such a difficult time that it is not easy to focus on a positive wellness perspective. But in truth, it is our strengths and assets in wellness that have kept us going thus far in our lifespan journey.

The best way to review your lifespan events is with willing listeners who have also completed this lifeline. We suggest that you share your life story with others in narrative form, telling the highlights in a limited period—perhaps 10 minutes. As the others listen to your narrative, they should take notes and give you feedback on your strengths and positive assets. The strengths should be both your own and the support strengths provided by the people around you. These strengths are what carry you and others through the lifespan. Even if we have had a difficult life, each of us still has major strengths that have gotten us to this point. Listen to those strengths as others feed them back to you.

If you don't have the luxury of telling your lifeline story to others, reflect on your life and note your constructive strengths and assets here while also noting the resources and supports you have from others.

Personal wellness strengths

_____

_____

_____

_____

Self-in-relation-to-others strengths

_____

_____

_____

_____

This brief exercise in storytelling and reflection catches the essence of this book. We live in a developmental context in connection with others. If we are to continue to survive and thrive in a complex and challenging world, we can best deal with problems by starting with a positive base. This exercise can be used beneficially with your clients. It will also serve as a way to understand your clients' lives more fully.

QUESTIONING QUESTIONS:
THE IMPORTANCE OF EMPATHY AND LISTENING SKILLS

Note that the above lifespan exercise uses many questions. You will find that the developmental frame of reference of this book is also based on extensive use of questioning strategies. In some forms of counseling and therapy, such as Carl Rogers's empathic person-centered approach, questions are virtually forbidden.

Let us start with our belief and commitment that listening to clients and their stories is the most fundamental issue in counseling and therapy. Ivey and Ivey (2003) devote more than half of their book on counseling microskills to listening skills such as attending, observing, encouraging, paraphrasing, reflecting feelings, and summarizing. They include questions as one of the listening skills but point out some dangers of questions and offer critical cautions (pp. 78–79):

■ Many of your clients will have had bad experiences with questions, ranging from parents or teachers asking "Why did you do that?" to friends or supervisors who may have used questions in an intrusive manner. For some clients, "Why" questions are especially difficult.

■ Questions may appear to be grilling and can put the client on the spot.

- Many questions can be rephrased as statements. Instead of "Don't you think you and your significant other should sit down and talk frankly?" it is more straightforward to say, "It might be useful to sit down and talk."
- If trust and rapport are not there, questions can be seen as particularly intrusive. A new client in the first session needs to learn what to expect and cannot be expected to open up immediately. If you and your client come from different cultural backgrounds (e.g., gay and heterosexual, Person of Color and White, physically able and physically disabled), questions can be particularly problematic.

Why, then, do questions figure so prominently in this book? Developmental counseling and therapy is an educational approach. The word *education* comes from the Latin *educare,* to draw out. The educational approach to human change represented by DCT seeks to draw out from the client *what is already there.* Plato's *Meno* presents a dialogue in which Socrates used only questions to draw out the formulations of a complex geometric problem from a young boy. The point is that each of us contains the germ of truth if someone will help us bring out in organized form what we know. DCT speaks of co-construction between counselor and client, therapist and patient. Counseling and therapy are about the construction of new knowledge, and asking key questions in an organized way will help clients generate new ways of thinking and acting on the issues and problems they face. There is also a natural creativity in all of us that can be unleashed by appropriate questioning strategies. You will find that the systematic questions of DCT provide a framework for new learning that lasts over time. With your help, expect clients to generate their own answers to their concerns.

Nonetheless, let us close this section by returning to the importance of listening carefully to client narratives. Yes, DCT will help draw out critical information, but the listening skills of paraphrasing, reflection of feeling, and summarization remain central. The client must feel that he or she has been heard accurately. With each question you ask within DCT, balance it with careful and attentive listening.

Empathy, then, remains central. Empathy is a larger and more inclusive word than listening skills. It requires you to enter the client's world as he or she is experiencing it. Some talk about "walking in the client's shoes" as if they were your own. To have empathy,

> it is vital to listen carefully, enter the world of the client, and communicate that we understand the client's world *as the client sees and experiences it.* The client's frame of reference is central to empathic understanding. Empathy is often defined as experiencing the world as if *you* were the client, but with awareness that the client remains separate from you. (Ivey & Ivey, 2003, p. 186)

Clearly, when you use questions, it is important that your focus be on the client's perspective and worldview, not your own.

ETHICAL ISSUES AND INFORMED CONSENT

This book will be of little value if only read as an exercise. What is required for mastery is working through experiential exercises and then practicing them with role-played, volunteer, and real clients. And you need to take time with each part of the

DCT procedures. It is possible to run through an exercise quickly, but if you do, you will see superficial results. Real learning occurs only when you are willing to stay with the exercises and role-plays until you truly master them and produce specific results through your interventions.

DCT was designed to be effective with both normal and complex issues. We sometimes talk about "handling the hard stuff." You will find that addressing what DCT terms the "sensorimotor cognitive/emotional style" can result in tears and more disclosure than the client expects. In addition, discoveries about how the family or system affects the client can be equally involving. While you may be practicing with volunteer clients or other members of your class, keep in mind that ethical principles remain central.

Each practice session should be completed with a full awareness of ethical and practical issues. The websites of key human service ethical statements may be found in Box A. Keep in mind that websites change and the actual site may be different from the one in the table. We suggest that you visit www.google.com, a superior search engine. The keyword "ethics" and the name of the professional association can be used for the search.

Kaplan (2003, p. 5), addressing the issue of excellence in ethics, has said that

> 80% or more of all ethical dilemmas revolve around a single issue: informed consent. The dilemma may be disguised under the cloak of confidentiality, competence, or other issues, but it usually boils down to informed consent.
>
> What is informed consent? It simply refers to the fact that your client or student has been provided enough information about the rules so that he or she can make a knowledgeable decision about whether or not to enter into a counseling relationship with you. . . . It is important to understand that a purely

---

Box A   Internet Ethical Sites
American Association of Marriage and Family Therapy (AAMFT) www.aamft.org/resources/LRMPlan/Ethics/ethicscode2001.htm
American Counseling Association (ACA) www.counseling.org/resources/ethics.htm#ce
American Psychological Association (APA) www.apa.org/ethics/code2002.html
Canadian Association of Social Workers (CASW) – Practice Guidelines www.casw-acts.ca/swpractice.htm
Canadian Counselling Association (CCA) www.ccacc.ca/ccacc.htm
National Association of Human Service Education (NAHSE) www.nohse.com/
National Association of Social Workers (NASW) www.naswdc.org/CODE.HTM
Ethics Updates – Explores a wide variety of ethical issues http://ethics.acusd.edu/

verbal approach to informed consent is inadequate, regardless of your setting or counseling specialty.

For your practice sessions, we urge you to develop a written informed consent form and have your volunteer client sign the form for each practice session. The exact wording of the form should be worked out with your supervising professor and/or the school or agency where you may be practicing. The form needs to include information on your own preprofessional- or professional-level training that defines your level of competence. Information about confidentiality should include specific statements on audiotaping or videotaping. Information about disclosure of the interview and the nature of the supervision should be included. Dual relationships should also be noted. You may be practicing with a student in your class who may be competing with you for a grade and he or she may disclose information that needs to be handled with care. A more complete professional statement would include specifics of making and breaking appointments, charges and fees, and other relevant points according to your local and state or provincial practice.

A sample practice contract is provided in Box B.

Box B   Sample Practice Informed Consent Form

There is no standard form for informed consent. It is vital that you develop your own version of this form in consultation with your professor and supervisor(s). Consider the following a beginning framework.

I am taking an interviewing skills course and I appreciate your willingness in volunteering to meet with me in a practice session. I've had four courses in counseling, but only limited practice with skills in the interview. (Insert your own background and experience here—some suggest that you include your theoretical orientation[s].)

Real issues or role-play	You may talk about issues of real concern to you or you may prefer to role-play a problem that is quite distinct from your own experience. I do need to know as we start if you are going to role-play a real or imagined issue. I'll also inform you about the specific exercise(s) that we will go through. In several cases, I'll be able to show you the questions I'm going to ask and we can work through them together.
Emotional issues	Some of the practice exercises we will go through involve strategies that can quickly bring emotional experience to the here and now. Tears may result and that is quite common, for the roots of our issues are often emotionally based. This can happen even if you are role-playing someone else. All this is normal human reaction and we will work together should you find yourself upset. I can arrange referral to my professor, the counseling center, or elsewhere if you wish to discuss issues in more detail and depth. Again, emotions can arise in the session and becoming aware of them can be helpful.
Dual relationships	(If working with a student in your program or with someone else with whom you have a dual relationship.) The issue of dual relationships should be considered. As we both are students in the same program, we know each other and in the process of the practice session, I am also acting as your counselor. We should remain aware of this and you should disclose only what you wish in this practice session.

(continued)

Box B	*(continued)*
Confidentiality	I do not have legal confidentiality as I am a preprofessional, but rest assured that anything you say will stay with me except for important exceptions such as danger of harm to yourself or others or if you give indication of neglect or abuse of others. These types of issues I must report.
Supervision	I will be sharing this interview with my professor or supervisor for comments and suggestions on my work. The purpose of supervision is to look at my work and not to analyze you.
Audio/videotaping	I will be audio- or videotaping this session if I have your permission. This will be used for my study of my work. This tape may be shared with my professor or supervisor (insert name and phone number). At first the taping may bother you, but most people find that they soon forget it and feel comfortable. The recorder may be turned off at any time and if you wish to rescind permission to share the tape later, I will destroy the tape.
Boundaries of competence	I am a preprofessional. I appreciate your willingness to work with me and any feedback you may provide. I am being supervised by a professional counselor and he or she will be happy to meet with you should you have any questions.

Please check one:

____I give permission to record this practice session and for you to share the recording as above.

____I give permission to engage in this session, but I wish not to have it recorded.

_____   _____
Volunteer Client   Interviewer

Date_____

Not necessarily part of the ethics contract is your awareness of the key ethical issues of multicultural understanding and social justice. Throughout this book, we have made an effort to focus on multicultural competence; social justice and community action issues are an important part of DCT's dialectic/systemic style. One important therapeutic alternative for you and your clients is to move into the community and work actively toward attacking community and societal problems that have injured clients. Virtually all ethics codes now address these issues.

You will want to consult the ethical code of your professional association for more details and information. Two excellent sources of additional ethical concepts are Corey, Corey, and Callanan (2003) and Zuckerman (2003).

FROM YOUR AUTHORS AS YOU BEGIN

Allen: Feedback from those who have worked with me on DCT in the past may give you a clue as what to expect in this book. One professional commented, "I find the concepts helpful and I can use the concepts tomorrow." Another stated, "I value the emphasis on diversity." Then one said, "I couldn't decide whether the concepts were too simple or too complex." DCT is a system that works and should enable you to "handle the hard stuff."

Feel free to offer feedback and ideas for improvement at ivey@srnet.com or www.microtraining.com.

Mary: What has been valuable to me has been how well DCT works with children. Many have found that understanding the distinctions between concrete and abstract statements can be highly useful in planning intervention with younger people. At the same time, I've grown personally as I gradually have learned to be with clients, family, and friends by matching their cognitive/emotional styles. DCT is a challenging framework, but it helps me integrate multiple theories into a comprehensive treatment plan.

I would love to hear from you at maryivey@comcast.net.

Jane: I have taught DCT to both entry-level and doctoral students and supervised both in practica and internships using the DCT system for assessment, case conceptualization, and treatment planning. It is fun to watch students experience successes in counseling using this approach. They learn a lot about themselves as well as their clients, and often second-order change occurs in both. Like them, I find DCT useful in daily life as well as counseling. Integrating DCT with a wellness philosophy and wellness interventions underscores the importance of taking a lifespan, developmental approach in counseling (see Myers, 1992).

Comments are always welcome at jemyers@uncg.edu.

Tom: In 1998, many of the leaders of the counseling profession helped Chi Sigma Iota (1998) develop a national advocacy agenda. The agenda included wellness as one of six major themes to advance not only the profession of counseling as defined by CACREP, but also the public that we serve. As promoting human development over the lifespan has been a core value in counseling since its inception in the early twentieth century (Sweeney, 2002, 2003), I am delighted to help incorporate wellness into DCT. When introduced to DCT by the third author of this book, I was struck by its clinical usefulness and compatibility with my professional values and philosophy. I find the use of DCT in my teaching and practice increasingly helpful as I develop greater mastery of its various applications.

I look forward to hearing from others about the usefulness of this book as well at tjsweeney@csi-net.org.

Allen, Mary, Jane, and Tom: Thanks for joining us in this developmental venture. We wish you the very best as you contribute to the future of the counseling and psychotherapy field.

REFERENCES

American Psychiatric Association. (2000). *Diagnostic and statistical manual of mental disorders text revision (DSM-IV-TR).* Washington, DC: Author.

Chi Sigma Iota. (1998, May 27–29; December 11–12). Counselor advocacy leadership conferences, I & II. Retrieved April 28, 2003, from www.csi-net.org/displaycommon.cfm?an=5

Corey, G., Corey, M., & Callanan, P. (2003). *Issues and ethics in the helping professions* (6th ed.). Pacific Grove, CA: Brooks/Cole.

Council for Accreditation of Counseling and Related Educational Programs (CACREP). (2001). *The 2001 standards.* Alexandria, VA: Author.

Ivey, A., & Ivey, M. (2003). *Intentional interviewing and counseling: Facilitating development in a multicultural society* (5th ed.). Pacific Grove, CA: Brooks/Cole.

Kaplan, D. (2003). Excellence in ethics. *Counseling Today, 45*(10), 5.

Myers, J. E. (1992). Wellness, prevention, development: The cornerstone of the profession. *Journal of Counseling & Development, 71,* 136–139.

Sweeney, T. J. (2002). Counseling: Historical origins and philosophical roots. D. C. Locke, J. E. Myers, & E. L. Herr (Eds.), *Handbook of counseling* (pp. 3–26). Thousand Oaks, CA: Sage.

Sweeney, T. J. (2003). Milestones and history makers. In J. D. West, C. J. Osborn, & D. L. Bubenzer (Eds.), *Leaders and legacies: Contributions to the counseling profession* (pp. 23–50). New York: Brunner-Routledge.

Zuckerman, E. (2003). *The paper office: Forms, guidelines, and resources to make your practice work ethically, legally, and profitably* (3rd ed.). New York: Guilford.

SECTION I

Introduction to Developmental Counseling and Therapy

The Vitality of Lifespan Wellness

Here you will find a theoretical foundation for understanding developmental counseling and therapy (DCT), a metatheoretical perspective that will help you integrate a variety of theories in a systematic manner in order to help clients change and grow. You will learn about wellness as a positive and holistic goal of development, and will develop an understanding of lifespan development from the perspective of various theories. But, it is not just theory. This is theory that you can take directly into practice. Each chapter's Central Practice Objective focuses on specifics that you can use in the here and now of the interview.

Chapter 1. Our Developmental Nature. Counseling and therapy are presented as developmental processes underlying all methods and practices. Developmental theories and the philosophic foundations of DCT are presented. Special attention is given to the distinction between concrete and abstract personal styles and their use in the interview while the four major styles of DCT are presented in the context of philosophy, theory, and practice. Even in this first chapter, we provide specifics to help you start identifying the cognitive/emotional style of your clients.

Chapter 2. Wellness: Optimizing Human Development Over the Lifespan. We believe that clients grow in positive directions when we understand their needs from a holistic perspective. All clients have strengths in some areas, and we can use those strengths to help them address and work through problems in other areas. Wellness is a strength-based paradigm for assessing clients holistically and planning interventions to facilitate positive growth. This chapter will ask you to examine yourself and your own wellness strengths. Theory moves into practice through examples and exercises designed for the interview.

Chapter 3. Development Over the Lifespan: Developmental Counseling as Lifespan Therapy. Clients change and grow over the lifespan in both predictable and unpredictable ways. By knowing what is normative, you will be able to assess your clients more accurately and devise treatment plans to help them optimize their growth and development. Developmental blocks occur throughout the lifespan and represent an inability to cope effectively with the challenges of life. DCT provides a means to help clients remove these blocks and continue to grow in healthy ways. Applications in this chapter include drawing out a client through a life review interview and examining life transition patterns and problems.

CHAPTER 1
Our Developmental Nature

Mastery and practice of concepts in this chapter will enable you to assess clients' concrete and abstract cognitive/emotional styles, as shown through your ability to recognize and classify client statements and to distinguish them in the here and now of the interview.

Developmental counseling and therapy (DCT) is different from traditional approaches in which one starts with a theory of choice and then applies the methods and strategies of that theory to the client. The developmental approach asks you to start with the client and hear her or his story carefully. How does this person make sense of the world and what cognitive/emotional style do we see in the here and now of the session? What are the client's wellness strengths that can be used for problem resolution? Where is the client in the lifespan and what developmental transitions might be important? How might multicultural and other contextual facts affect the client?

DCT starts with a focus on wellness and positive psychology in the belief that clients grow best if we first attend to their strengths. But DCT also specifically addresses the most difficult issues that one can face in counseling and therapy, such as helping a client deal with depression and post-traumatic stress. "Handling the hard stuff" is a basic part of DCT theory and practice.

DCT is also an integrative theory in that it draws from the four major forces in counseling and therapy: psychodynamic, existential-humanistic, cognitive-behavioral, and multicultural counseling and therapy (MCT). You will find that DCT offers you specifics for organizing seemingly diverse theories and strategies into a workable treatment plan. This chapter opens the way to a developmental approach to counseling and therapy—an integrated, multitheoretical practice that is founded in wellness and theories of human development.

Knowledge of and skill in the concepts of this chapter can enable you to:

1. Explore developmental theories, with special attention to attachment theory, as foundations for culturally sensitive and effective counseling and therapy.
2. Summarize in outline form the five central developmental theories emphasized in this book.
3. Discuss the basic philosophic and practical basis of developmental counseling and therapy (DCT). Special attention will be given to the relationship of DCT to Platonic philosophy and to the Swiss epistemologist Jean Piaget.
4. Understand and work with the concepts of concretes and abstractions in counseling and therapy and receive an introduction to DCT's four information processing styles.
5. Take theory into practice through reflective and practical activities designed to help you develop a personal portfolio of competence.

INTRODUCTION: DEVELOPMENT AS A CENTRAL GOAL OF COUNSELING AND THERAPY

Our task as professional counselors and therapists is to facilitate client progression over the lifespan—to help individuals and families learn from the culture, learn how to act within that culture, and when necessary, change that culture. Becoming one with the culture and possibly changing the cultural status quo requires that we as professionals and those who seek our assistance develop maturity and mutual respect.

Our relationships with others help us navigate the passages of life. Enjoying the protection and warmth of a good parent, spending quiet time with a close friend, coming home from college, participating in weddings, having a satisfying sexual relationship, and holding a child are times of connection and attachment. It is difficult to become separate and autonomous unless we have a solid developmental foundation, which is built through our lifespan connections and attachments.

Changes and life transitions can present difficulties for individuals and their families. A small boy entering kindergarten may cry the first week of school, afraid of leaving his mother. His teenage sister may find the task of establishing her own unique personal identity too much and turn to alcohol and drugs. At the same time, the parents may be facing the challenges of middle marriage and be contemplating divorce. The grandparents may be dealing with the loss of friends and family as they cope with their own physical issues. You will find that most of the concerns your clients present relate to issues occurring over the lifespan.

Life changes represent our developmental movement over the lifespan and can also be times of celebration—a mark of achievement, of growing up. These same celebrations are also often times of separation, which bring sadness for past relationships that are changing. As each of our children matures, we mourn the loss of the child as we celebrate the birth of an adult. If attachment and trust have not solidly developed, life transitions become especially difficult.

There are also contextual multicultural issues that affect attitudes toward separation and attachment. While generalizations are incomplete and may fail to consider wide individual differences, some groups and cultures tend to be more oriented toward attachment and connection whereas others are more focused on individuation and becoming a separate individual. People from a more traditional Native American Indian, Canadian Dene, Asian, or southern Italian and Sicilian background may be expected to focus more on connection. Those of a Northern European background may emphasize autonomy and the independence of self. Women are seen as more oriented to attachment and connection whereas men are often described as more interested in separation (e.g., Gilligan, 1982, 2002). What is considered a "successful" working through of life stages and transitions may vary with your contextual multicultural background.

Twin developmental tasks of transitions—separation and attachment, autonomy and connection—guide the developmental process. Family theory is concerned with issues of enmeshment/involvement and disengagement/individuation. As helping professionals we seek to assist individuals and families to develop and find a balance between these tasks. In this effort, we need to acknowledge that each client has widely varying patterns of coping with these issues. The challenges our clients encounter as they face transitions are ably summarized by Schlossberg (2003, p. 1):

> Transitions take time, and people's reactions to them change—for better or worse—while they are under way. At first, people think of nothing but being a new graduate, a new widow, a recent retiree. Then they begin to separate from the past and move toward a new role, for a while teetering between the two. . . . For some the process happens easily and quickly, for others it might take years. There

are many people floundering for the right niche, even after years. For example it takes time to adjust to moving into any kind of retirement institution since many people define it as the last move.

Please take a moment to try the following developmental counseling and therapy sensorimotor exercise. Focus on one specific lifespan developmental transition, one that signified for you a major separation or connection in your life and the need to attach in new ways. This could be entering school, starting a new job, enduring a difficult breakup of a relationship, getting married, having or not having a child, or surviving the death of a loved one.

Take a deep breath, and gradually move your attention to a single *image* (visual, auditory, and/or bodily feeling) connected with that transition. Single images, usually visual, often provide summaries of key events in our lives. Some find that sounds, internal feelings, tastes, and key scents are helpful ways of generating images. Then allow yourself to get in touch with the thoughts and feelings surrounding your image.

What did that time of transition mean to you? How did you experience issues of separating from old attachments and patterns? How has finding new attachments and connections been for you? Who are the key people who helped you work through that time of developmental progression? How might family, contextual, and multicultural issues have affected your development?

Summarize the transition and your thoughts and feelings below as you start your journey toward integrating developmental theory into your clinical and counseling practice:

_____

_____

_____

_____

_____

_____

_____

_____

_____

_____

_____

_____

In reviewing this exercise, would you say that are you are personally more comfortable with connections or separations? How might your experience affect your work with clients facing similar developmental progressions? Does your own cultural and developmental background bias you more toward attachment and connection or more toward separation and individuation?

FIVE APPROACHES TO DEVELOPMENTAL THEORY

Developmental assessment and treatment focus on client uniqueness. What is the client's lifespan developmental history? What strengths building toward wellness can we find? What is the nature of multicultural development and social context? How can we use developmental theory itself as a way to facilitate change and growth? All of these questions guide this book.

The task of this book is to show how to apply developmental theory in the clinical and counseling interview. We explore how to use developmental approaches with developing children and adolescents. We consider adult development and examine how growth never ends. Specifics are presented for applying developmental theory to lifespan development from a wellness perspective and to complex practice issues such as working with depression and personality "disorders."

Our unique responses to transitions and change can be viewed from five theoretical approaches to development that form the basis of this book. The first four developmental theories provide essential background for understanding the lifespan. The fifth, developmental counseling and therapy (DCT), provides both theory and practice strategies. DCT will enable you to use developmental theories in your own counseling and clinical practice with all types of clients, ranging from daily concerns of living through the most complex and difficult issues. But DCT always emphasizes lifespan wellness, regardless of the challenges a client faces.

Attachment theory stresses that who we are depends first on our connections with others (Bowlby, 1969, 1973, 1990; Cassidy & Shaver, 2002). Relationship and empathy are central to the developmental approach. It is here we learn that human connectedness and attachment form the foundation for necessary separations and personal autonomy.

Wellness theory teaches us that people grow best if we focus on their developmental strengths, not just problems (Adler, 1927/1954; Myers, Sweeney, & Witmer, 2000, 2001). Chapter 2 presents detailed and specific methods to assess the strengths and wellness potential of your clients; Chapter 9 also addresses a wellness approach that reconceptualizes so-called psychopathology from a developmental and wellness perspective. Here you will learn how to apply DCT with clients who may be diagnosed within the *Diagnostic and Statistical Manual of Mental Disorders* (American Psychiatric Association, 2000).

Lifespan theory helps us understand the developmental issues we face as we make the transition through life stages (Erikson, 1963, 1994; Gilligan, 1982, 2002; Schlossberg, Waters, & Goodman, 1995; Schlossberg & Kay, 2003). Chapter 3 outlines these major theories and includes specifics for conducting lifespan interviews.

Cultural identity developmental theory enables us to think about our clients' lives contextually (Helms, 1999; Sue & Sue, 2003). As the Yakima nation proverb states,

"Education of each boy and girl is the gradual revelation of a culture." Chapter 8 speaks to these issues, but multicultural factors are also integrated throughout. *Developmental counseling and therapy* (DCT) provides us with a framework that enables us to assess client cognitive/emotional development (Ivey, 1986/2000). DCT also provides specific strategies and techniques to facilitate client attachments, to promote wellness in clients as well as ourselves, to help ourselves as well as our clients work through lifespan challenges, and to encourage all of us to think of ourselves as multicultural beings.

The attachment exercise using images at the beginning of this chapter is one of the strategies within the DCT framework to bring increased client cognitive/emotional awareness of how the here and now is affected by past history. Chapters 1, 4, and 5 focus on specifics of assessment and interview strategies using this model.

Applications of the developmental framework with a variety of clients and issues are explored in Chapters 8–13. Here you encounter developmental theory used through bibliotherapy, with children and families, and with clients in severe psychological distress; you also learn how to integrate spirituality into the interview. The remainder of this chapter introduces some basics of developmental counseling and therapy, a philosophic and theoretical framework with many specifics for action in the interview.

INTRODUCING DEVELOPMENTAL COUNSELING AND THERAPY

"There is nothing so practical as a good theory," Kurt Lewin once said. Developmental counseling and therapy (DCT) began with the observation that Piagetian theories of child development and cognition also apply to adolescent and adult development. Children go through identifiable processes of growth, and so do adolescents and adults. When we face a new developmental transition (for example, the birth of a child, a divorce, the loss of a loved one), we often "lose" our adult selves and recycle back to cognitions and feelings similar to those we had as a child. There is no definable end to development except death. DCT offers specific methods for facilitating change and developmental transitions for clients as we work with them over the lifespan (Ivey, 1986/2000).

Our first task as professional helpers is to understand how the client makes sense of the world. DCT rests on the idea that our first task is to be *with* and learn *with* clients—how do these unique people understand what is happening? How do they make meaning? Once we have joined clients' meaning-making systems, we can better comprehend their styles of being in the world.

Meaning making has two uses in this book. The first and primary use here refers to process and style—how does a person make sense of the world? DCT and meaning-making theories note that children and adults may make sense of the same event differently—for example, children may think that their behavior "caused" their parents to divorce while an adult meaning-making perspective may be very different. When working with children, we need to enter their style of making sense of the divorce; with the parents, we will need a different approach. A secondary use of meaning is closer to the traditional dictionary definitions—specifically, what is intended by what is said or done. What does the client's language mean?

By understanding the client's frame of reference and meaning-making style, we can better plan interventions to facilitate change and lifespan development within the appropriate cultural framework. *Empathy* is a word we use when we talk about understanding the world as others experience it. DCT offers techniques that can facilitate a more complete sense of empathy with clients.

DCT theory and practice are based in Platonic and neo-Platonic philosophy and the cognitive theory and studies of Jean Piaget (1923/1955, 1952/1963, 1965). Piaget is particularly important, as several meaning-making theories and systems are also derived from his thought (cf. Kegan, 1982; Kegan & Lahey, 2000; Kohlberg, 1981; Loevinger, 1998). Each of these systems uses language different from that of Piaget, but all trace their thinking to the Swiss epistemologist and focus on sequential developmental issues, heavily cognitive in orientation.

We can best join client meaning making if we understand cognitive/emotional style as shown in language and behavior. DCT's specific skills and strategies are oriented to discovering where the client "is" and how he or she constructs and makes sense of experience. Once we have a grasp of client consciousness and meaning making, we can then turn to appropriate interventions and treatment. We start with the client's organization of the world rather than from any specific theory of treatment.

By way of contrast, counselor and therapist understanding of the client's world is often shaped by our theoretical orientation (e.g., person-centered, cognitive-behavioral, psychodynamic). If you work effectively within your theoretical and meaning-making framework, you may find that your client begins thinking, speaking, and acting within your theoretical system. In a classic study, research has shown that over time in the session, clients tend to take on the language of their counselors (Meara, Pepinsky, Shannon, & Murray, 1981). Clients of person-centered therapists tend to talk about the self, cognitive clients speak of thoughts, and psychodynamic clients focus on interpretations of life history. These findings have been replicated among group leaders who also deeply impacted the meaning-making style of group members (Sherrard, cited in Ivey, Pedersen, & Ivey, 2001).

Imposing our theoretical orientation on the client may be helpful, since it can provide the client with a new or expanded frame of reference for viewing the world. The drawback is that we start with our theory rather than with that of the client. Furthermore, traditional theories have often been criticized as failing to consider multicultural issues adequately (Gilligan, 1982; Sue & Sue, 2003). We need to understand the client's way of making the world meaningful.

Piaget and Plato as Foundations for DCT

Until the turn of the century, psychology was considered part of philosophy. Perhaps it is time to bring the two together again. Developmental counseling and therapy was first derived from an alternative reading of Piaget (1952/1963). Perhaps Piaget's main contribution was his concept of the four cognitive stages or meaning-making systems that children move through as they grow: sensorimotor, preoperational, concrete, and formal (plus a stage he termed "post-formal").

Table 1-1   Platonic, Piagetian, and DCT Views of Cognitive/Emotional Development

Worldview	Plato	Piaget[1]	DCT
The concrete world of appearances	Imagining (eikasia)	Sensorimotor Preoperational	Sensorimotor/elemental
	Belief (pistis)	Concrete operations	Concrete/situational
Line between the visible concrete world and the abstract world of ideas			
The abstract world of ideas and thinking	Thinking (dianoia) Knowledge (episteme) Intelligence (noesis)	Formal operations Post-formal operations	Formal/reflective Dialectic/systemic

[1]A distinction should be made between the concepts of stage, as used by Piaget and of cognitive/emotional level, style, or orientation as used in this book. Piaget's stage concepts are related to age and cognitive competence. For example, a child must develop sufficient horizontal development (competence) in concrete cognitive tasks if he or she is to move to the next stage. Stages are considered to be sequential whereas the developmental counseling and therapy (DCT) model sees levels and styles as both sequential and holistic. DCT uses Piagetian concepts of sensorimotor, concrete, and formal operations metaphorically and we find that clients at all ages move freely from one style or orientation to another.

    In turn, Piagetian stages can be related to the four levels of consciousness and meaning making described by Plato (see Table 1-1). Plato's *Allegory of the Cave* describes what occurs as a person moves from a naïve embedded way of making sense of the world toward ever increasingly sophisticated ways of thinking. Moving through each consciousness stage can be painful and challenging. Both Plato and Piaget argue that the later stages of development are *higher* and are important developmental goals for the whole person.

    The essence of the *Allegory of the Cave* is that a slave is chained to the wall with a candle in the back providing light. The shadows on the wall become the real world for the slave as *sensorimotor* impressions form the only thing he sees. The slave develops *concrete* beliefs about the images and may tell stories about the situation. If the slave is freed and can turn to the light and see the world more fully, he can then *reflect (formal operations)* on what he had seen before as only images. As the slave becomes more accustomed to this new world, he moves to *post-formal operations* and begins to see himself in a broader systemic context. (We will be revisiting the *Allegory of the Cave* in later chapters.)

    Drawing from these roots, developmental counseling and therapy points out that our clients come to us with sometimes false sensorimotor and concrete impressions. They may reflect ineffectively on themselves and their relations to systems. Through careful listening and assessment, we can determine the cognitive/emotional style of the client and enable her or him to put aside past meaning systems and build new and more effective ways of being.

    The DCT interpretation is different in some important ways from that of Piaget and Plato. First, DCT argues that effective counseling and therapy can actually use these concepts to facilitate client growth in the here and now of the interview. Moreover, DCT is less hierarchical, arguing against Piaget and Plato's ideas of *best* or *more perfect* forms of knowledge. So-called higher forms of cognition and affect are not necessarily better. The intellectualizing client often can benefit by returning to the more direct realm of sensorimotor and concrete experience. More complete development in each consciousness style is what is sought. There is no "lower" or "higher" form of being, but the possibility of further and future development never ends.

DCT maintains that all styles of consciousness are vital for holistic development. But what of emotion? DCT focuses on cognitive/emotional development and you will see that clients present themselves and their affective world in a variety of ways. In truth, cognition cannot be separated from emotion. While emotional issues may be found in both Plato and Piaget, DCT considers emotional experience as central for understanding the client and facilitating growth.

The relationships among Plato, Piaget, and DCT are displayed in Table 1-1, which shows three critical aspects. To the right we see four levels or styles of consciousness and meaning making. These are explored in depth in Chapters 4 and 5, which will make these abstract ideas highly practical. The concrete world of appearances contains the areas of meaning that emphasize "reality" as we ordinarily think about it—what we experience through seeing, touching, hearing, or feeling. The concrete world also includes how we talk about things, often through descriptive stories with specific beginnings, middles, and endings. The second aspect of Table 1-1 is the abstract world of ideas and thinking where we reflect, deliberate, and consider the world, often from a more distant point of view.

The line between the visible concrete world and the abstract world of ideas is a critical third dimension that separates the two. Moving from Platonic images and belief or Piagetian concrete operations to formal thought involves *crossing the line* to a profoundly different way of making meaning of one's world.

The Concrete and Abstract Worlds

You will find it helpful to start your understanding of DCT theory and practice through the distinctions between concrete and abstract styles and their implications for communication in the interview. The broad concrete world includes both sensorimotor and concrete *reality* while the abstract world is that of thinking and reflection about self and self-in-system.

A client sitting in front of you is a concrete, specific person, and her or his behavior is observable and measurable. This client may describe concrete, specific events and situations, providing considerable detail about what has been seen, heard, and felt. You as a concrete person sitting before the client are something specific that the client deals with. The concrete world includes counseling words such as observables, behavior, and assertiveness, and specific verbal descriptions of problems or concerns.

At the abstract level, and equally important, are the ideas you have about this client and the ideas that the client has about her or his personal issues. Note that the word *idea* is an abstraction; an idea cannot be seen, heard, or felt. Much of counseling and therapy language concerns abstractions. Words and phrases such as *self-concept, empathy, congruence, cognition, defense mechanism,* and *personal meaning* are abstractions.

Through a complex form of reasoning, Plato points out that we could not recognize a concrete material table as a table unless we had an idea about a table. To stretch the point, the table does not exist; only an idea of the table exists. Plato argued that the abstract world of the idea is the more critical dimension for human experience. Thus he termed the concrete world of behavior and action "imaginary," as made up of mere "appearances." In a similar way, Piaget tends to talk about higher forms of knowledge as being "best."

Which is more significant: the concrete world of sensory experience and action or the abstract world of ideas, thoughts, and contemplation? Not everyone agrees with Plato on the primacy of abstractions and ideas. This question has inspired a debate that runs throughout the history of Western philosophy. Philosophers such as Locke, Bentham, and Mill argue for the primacy of the empirical, data-based, concrete, scientific world. In contrast, Kant, Fichte, and Hegel, the German idealist philosophers, and others argue for the primacy of ideas and abstractions.

Person-centered, cognitive, and psychodynamic theories tend to emphasize the world of abstract ideas whereas behavioral psychology and body-oriented therapies are more concrete in nature. All of them have a real parallel with Plato in that they seek to bring clients to new ways of thinking. By way of contrast, classical behavioral theory is concerned specifically with concrete behavioral actions. Behavioral approaches may also lead to the light and new ideas, but the focus is on doing something rather than thinking. Cognitive-behavioral theory attempts to resolve this dilemma of thinking versus action by facilitating both. The philosophical position of DCT is integrative. Cognition becomes grounded when tied to behavior. In turn, cognitive frameworks guide behavior.

However, it is useful at times to treat the concrete and the abstract as separable. With some clients, a therapist may, for a while, focus on abstract ideas about the self but may later emphasize concrete action. With other clients, it may be better to focus on concrete specifics, since subtle, abstract understanding often follows from behavioral specifics. At issue is matching one's interviewing style to the cognitive/emotional style of the client.

Examples of Concrete and Abstract Consciousness

Abstract and concrete thought and emotional patterns are revealed by client language patterns. Concrete clients will talk to you in seemingly endless detail about the facts of their life situation. For example, a teenager may say:

Yesterday, I skipped school. I went to a movie with Trey.

(Describes the movie and an important scene for five minutes.)

Anyway, after we got out, we went to get something to eat—at the diner. We had fries and a soda. It was good. I don't like school much.

This client makes meaning of skipping school by describing what happened in concrete, linear detail. You will find that clients who use the concrete style often do not respond well to a person-centered reflection of feeling or a complex Freudian interpretation. Such clients seem to understand and appreciate concrete behavioral interventions.

Many counselors and therapists are abstract, formal-operational thinkers and can become impatient with ongoing concrete description. As a consequence, it is not uncommon for professional helpers to prefer clients who observe patterns in their lives and discuss abstract ideas underlying the concretes of daily experience. For example:

> Yesterday, I skipped again. School is so boring and I generally have a great time with Trey. This time, however, it was different. Usually my pattern is to ignore that empty feeling in my stomach. But this time it got me. Even during the film, I found myself thinking about what's going on. I even felt guilty. I didn't used to do this. I think I need your help to understand myself.

This client focuses on the meaning of skipping school in an abstract way. The goal for counseling is understanding the self. Note that this client's language has few concretes, specifics, or observables. The client talks about repeating behavioral patterns and is able to examine his own behavior. Clients in this abstract mode will often respond best when an abstract theory is presented.

The point is to match the language of the therapist to the language of the client. This line of reasoning cannot be emphasized strongly enough and thus is repeated succinctly as follows:

> It is possible to identify the cognitive/emotional developmental style of a client by listening to and observing language used in the interview. Once you have observed the cognitive/emotional style of the client, match your counseling or therapeutic intervention so that the client can understand and act on what you have said.
>
> Mismatching your interventions may be equally helpful. If you have an overly abstract client, he or she may benefit from an approach that focuses on concrete specifics. Similarly, as the concrete client develops, you may help him or her toward an understanding of self and of situations by facilitating more abstract conversation.

The concrete and abstract client statements presented above could both be enlarged by examining the specific situation and what occurred during the day the person skipped school. Concrete understanding could be enriched by abstract examination of patterns of missing school and conversation oriented toward self-examination. The client who thinks abstractly may need to become aware of more concrete specifics. We are all familiar with the individual who analyzes the situation very well but does nothing to change it. Ideas and analysis are not enough. Those with the concrete style need to learn that they may be repeating the same actions again and again in a behavioral pattern. Clearly, individuals who present with a concrete style need a different type of counseling and therapy from that of clients with a more abstract orientation.

Some clients will present themselves as almost totally concrete and others as mainly abstract, but most clients are mixtures of several cognitive-developmental levels. On certain topics, they will be concrete; at other times, they may be abstract. Be flexible and ready to change your language as the client changes. Failure to be where the client is results in miscommunication, misunderstanding, and, all too often, labeling the client as resistant when it is the therapist who has failed to understand the client's way of making sense of a confusing world.

Four DCT Styles

Later chapters will clarify and explicate the essentials of the four DCT styles, but a brief summary of each may be useful at this point.

The Concrete World of Appearances, Images, and Beliefs

Sensorimotor/elemental—the immediate experiential world.   The sensorimotor world is tied to what the client receives through the senses—what is seen, heard, felt, tasted, and touched. Sensorimotor is very much a here and now immediate experience. Clients who cry and laugh and who are in touch with what is going on "right now" are representative of the sensorimotor style. Matching treatments for this type of client include meditation, body work, such as breathing and jogging, catharsis, and listening to random comments by the client.

Concrete/situational—describing reality.   Clients who give you a linear and detailed description of experience are particularly representative of this style. They can tell you what happened, but may not reflect on its meaning or implications for the self. They are also a step from here and now sensorimotor experiencing, although both dimensions will often appear at the same time. These clients may be good at acting on their world. Matching treatments for the concrete style include applied behavioral analysis, social skills and assertiveness training, and drawing out client narratives or stories in detail.

The Abstract World of Ideas and Thinking

Formal/reflective—reflecting on the self or situation.   One more step removed from direct experience, the client who presents a formal style may be quite skilled at thinking about self and reflecting on what happened. Early formal thinking often appears in the teen who starts finding that he or she has an "identity" and a "self." The ability to take multiple perspectives becomes more central with this style, but some egocentricity remains. Rogerian person-centered, psychodynamic, and much of cognitive theory may be placed in this area, although it is important to point out that all these theories also operate at multiple levels.

Dialectic/systemic—integration and/or seeing self-in-system.   These clients tend to think contextually and use multiple perspectives. They are good at meta-cognition—thinking about thinking. Family therapy, feminist theory, multicultural counseling and therapy (MCT), and DCT are all oriented toward helping clients see self-in-system. The family and community genograms are examples of useful strategies with this type of client. Direct work to change social systems with a social justice orientation may be highly useful activities for some clients.

Both clients and the cognitive/emotional styles are multilevel. While clients may present their issue at one level (and it is important to match that level in your therapy), expect them to shift style, often within a minute or so. Your ability to shift your counseling and therapeutic style and treatment is critical if you are to be empathic with clients and help them grow. Style-matching could be termed *precision empathy,* being with clients more completely as they share themselves in their own style. Expect recycling and movement among styles. Clients move through varying cognitive/emotional levels and tasks again and again as they learn and develop.

A CASE EXAMPLE

A client, Derryl, works as a manager of a computer firm. He is clearly formal-operational and abstract when he deals with complex problems at work. Yet, as is true for some, he is highly concrete and sometimes insensitive in his relationships. The following words are central to DCT and we repeat them here again for emphasis. *Most therapy and counseling clients will talk about their lives and issues from more than one cognitive/emotional style.* Although most clients have a primary style, expect most to change the levels or style as they present varying issues. You should not expect "single-style" clients, nor should you use a single style of interacting with them. Meet them where they are on the issue, help them explore their concerns in more depth, and, perhaps, mismatch your style to help them move to new levels and ways of thinking and being.

Derryl comes to us for marriage counseling. He is facing the developmental task of generating a sense of intimacy and caring with Shera, his wife of two years. He may be very concrete and nonreflective as he describes his problems with her ("We argued last night and she refused to have sex"). But Derryl has other developmental tasks on which he may be further along than he is with this relationship. He may be effective at abstract tasks such as listening to his staff and helping them perform at a higher level. He may be able to plan a complex budget having a variety of economic contingencies.

The counseling or therapeutic goal may be both concrete (obtain more specific details of the relationship and help him find new behaviors) and abstract (help him think about himself and the relationship in new ways). His racial/ethnic background, his spiritual orientation, and many other factors inform his meaning making. Intimacy for an orthodox Christian, Jew, or Muslim may have a very different meaning from liberal traditions in each religious orientation. Multicultural factors will help determine what is an effective form of intimacy. And we should be aware that his wife, Shera, might very well be in a "different place" from the one he is in for making sense of what intimacy really means.

Recall that as a manager, Derryl operates using a primarily abstract formal-operational style, but in his relationships he is mainly concrete in orientation. Differences in cognitive/emotional processes appear repeatedly in daily conversation and also in the helping interview. Failure to understand these differences often results when one person views the world from a concrete standpoint and the other takes an abstract point of view.

Following is an ineffective first interview in which Derryl works with an abstractly oriented therapist who does not match his concrete meaning-making style. The importance of matching your interviewing style to the world of the client should be apparent.

Client and Counselor Conversation	Process Comments
1. *Derryl:* Last night I had a fight with Shera. I wanted to have sex, but she said "no" again.	Concrete description.
2. *Counselor:* That seems to be a pattern. You talk about your needs and desires but fail to take her frame of reference and how she feels into account.	The counselor does not match Derryl's language system in his abstract reframing of the problem. The reframe may be correct, but does not match Derryl's present concrete orientation.
3. *Derryl:* But, it's me that isn't satisfied. Like last night we went to a sexy movie. (He describes the movie plot in some detail.)	The counselor listens, silently wishing that Derryl understood his abstract and important observation. Don't expect people who present concretely to reflect and think about themselves and the situation easily.
4. *Derryl:* Well, anyway, when we got home, I kissed her and she actually kissed me back. Then I reached for her breast, and she pulled away. "If you're going to be that way," I said, and I started rubbing her. She really got mad. Damn woman is frigid.	In the concrete style, expect linear description and the failure to see points of view other than one's own.
5. *Counselor:* Derryl, that's a pattern with you. You want sex very much. Last night is another situation where you didn't think of her feelings. How do you feel about yourself when you think of it from her point of view?	The counselor again tries to help Derryl sees Shera's point of view. Until the concrete story is explored fully and in detail, it will be difficult for Derryl to reflect on the situation more adequately.
6. *Derryl:* Really ticked! I don't see why she is that way. We used to get along fine. All she needs to do is relax and go along.	The abstract counselor remains out of touch with the concrete style of the client.

The following example illustrates a counseling approach that matches the client's concrete cognitive/emotional style. Using DCT's concepts of matching and mismatching cognitive/emotional style, it is possible to facilitate reflection among clients who are primarily concrete in orientation. Note especially that the counselor is willing to listen to Derryl's concrete comments and through this is able to begin to move Derryl to a more reflective and abstract style.

Counselor and Client Conversation	Process Comments
1. *Derryl:* Last night I had a fight with Shera after we went to a good film. I wanted to have sex, but she said "no" again.	The client starts with a brief concrete summary of what happened last night.
2. *Counselor:* Could you tell me more specifically what happened? I'd like to hear what happened at the movie and afterward.	The counselor is searching for concretes and specific sequences of action and thought. With most clients, concrete or abstract, we need to know the linear story.

(continued)

Counselor and Client Conversation	Process Comments
3. *Derryl:* We went to a sexy movie. It was great and let me tell you about it. . . . (Derryl describes the movie plot in some detail and talks about Shera holding his hand and even leaning close to him.)	The counselor listens intently and paraphrases and reflects feelings, accepting that it is necessary to listen to details as part of work with concrete clients.
4. *Counselor:* So, Derryl, it was a great film and it really turned you on and perhaps Shera as well. I hear that the two of you were feeling good about each other—Shera held your hand in the movie and put her head on your shoulder. The two of you felt close at the movie.	The counselor stays concrete in his summary, but focuses on positive relationship strengths. He uses the client's main words.
5. *Derryl:* (Nods his head) Well, anyway, when we got home, I kissed her and she actually kissed me back. Then I reached for her breast, and she pulled away. "If you're going to be that way," I said, and I started rubbing her. She really got mad. We had a bad argument. Damn woman is frigid.	Continued concrete description, but Derryl is willing to get into useful specific detail so that the counselor can better understand what is really going on. You will find that the concretes of your client's situation are invaluable, regardless of the person's cognitive/emotional style.
6. *Counselor:* Derryl, you really feel angry because she turned you away last night.	The reflection of feeling is concrete and focuses on a single situation, "you feel angry because . . ." While this may be a pattern, it is more appropriate to focus on the single event before the pattern itself. Pattern and abstract thought can come later, especially after emotions have cooled.
7. *Derryl:* Right; it hurt.	Having been heard, Derryl's nonverbal behavior becomes a bit calm and he adds a new word, "hurt."
8. *Counselor:* And when you got home she even responded to a kiss for the first time in almost a month. Right?	This concrete paraphrase of a key issue may be useful in helping Derryl look at his situation more comprehensively.
9. *Derryl:* Yeah.	A questioning look appears on Derryl's face and he seems to be more open.
10. *Counselor:* Now let's see, after just one kiss you reached for her breast, she pulled away, and then you got angry and reached for her again, and then the two of you had a terrible argument again and certainly sex wasn't going to work.	The concrete paraphrase continues.
11. *Derryl:* Yeah.	He calms down a bit more.
12. *Counselor:* Derryl, let me repeat again what happened between you and Shera. You start off feeling good about your wife and she seems to respond. You move faster than she wants, *and then* an argument starts.	The counselor's lead here is intended to help Derryl move toward more complex concrete thinking. He so far has been *describing* what happened. The counselor is now looking for "if . . . , then . . ." statements. Once this is accomplished we are better prepared for the reflective thought in abstract thinking.

Client and Counselor Conversation	Process Comments
13. *Derryl:* Yeah, she calls me "fast Eddie" and says I never wait for her to catch up.	Derryl is able to show the beginning of patterned abstract thought.
14. *Counselor:* So, *if* you move fast and don't wait for her, *then* the two of you have an argument, and certainly there isn't any sex.	This summary catches the essence of both the situation last night and the general pattern between Derryl and Shera.
15. *Derryl:* I guess so. She says she wants me to keep paying attention to her rather than just think of myself.	Note that Derryl is finally starting to talk about how Shera might be thinking and not just about himself. He remains basically concrete in thought but clearly is moving toward thinking of the sexual difficulty in new perspectives and abstract thought. Taking the perspective of the other can be challenging for clients who work primarily with a concrete style. As interviewer, you need patience and skill to help them think in new ways.

In this second example, the counselor has chosen to work in a more deliberate fashion and talk about the problem at a more concrete level. Interviews with concretely oriented clients can be agonizingly slow for the formal-operational, abstract counselor or therapist unless he or she becomes aware of necessary cognitive/emotional progressions in development.

DCT maintains that with clients such as Derryl, it may be necessary to listen to several concrete examples of repeating behavior while paraphrasing and summarizing what has been said. It does little good at this point to ask Derryl, "Is that a pattern?" Once the client has been listened to thoroughly, the therapist can help the client understand the situation by using late concrete, causal (if/then) reasoning. *If* Derryl moves too fast, failing to note where Shera is, *then* she will reject him. Derryl must first understand the ineffectiveness of his present behavior before he can look at his self-defeating, repeating patterns.

Seeing the world as someone else sees it (empathy) requires Derryl to engage in formal-operational, abstract thinking. At this point, Derryl is simply is not able to make this cognitive/emotional leap. DCT provides a framework for systematic progressions that will help you first identify the cognitive/emotional style of the client. You can join the client's level of meaning making and once that is fully explored, you can help the client move to other frames of reference and new cognitive/emotional levels.

SUMMARY

The purpose of counseling, therapy, and all helping interventions is the facilitation of human development over the lifespan. When we integrate counseling with development, we find ourselves focusing on the clients' unique way of knowing the world and making meaning of their experience. Our task is to help individuals, families, groups, and organizations reach their developmental potential. We hope that they will expand their cognitive/emotional and behavioral repertoires and develop new alternatives for thought and action, since flexibility and resilience are required for living in a changing world.

Developmental counseling and therapy (DCT) offers an integrative approach for working with typical lifespan issues and also difficult therapeutic challenges. The developmental approach asks you to start with the client and hear her or his story carefully. Then, you can assess the client's style of meaning making and provide interventions designed to meet the client where he or she is. DCT draws from all theories and provides an integrative rationale for choosing one intervention over another.

We need to balance independence and dependence, connectedness and separation. Becoming attached to others and becoming separate from others are twin developmental tasks that face us throughout our lives. Differing balances of separation and attachment are required for varying life tasks. Empathic understanding of our clients also requires a delicate balance of appropriate attachment and connectedness plus equally appropriate separation and boundaries.

Five approaches to developmental theory are emphasized in this book as being vital to successful clinical and counseling work.

- Bowlby's attachment theory reminds us that we are selves-in-relation, persons-in-community.
- Wellness theory helps us maintain awareness that a focus solely on problems is not only incomplete but also allows us to miss important strengths for resolving our issues and building for the future in a positive way.
- Lifespan theory enables us to think of the person's history and where he or she is going. Many client issues relate to lifespan developmental tasks and transitions.
- Cultural identity theory and multicultural theory remind us that context and social history are vital to who we are.
- Developmental counseling and therapy provides us with specific assessment and treatment tools to facilitate life process and movement.

Parallels among Platonic thought, Piagetian theory, and DCT theory and strategies have been presented. Western thought and philosophy have consistently argued over the primacy of ideas as contrasted with concrete reality. Four levels of meaning making have been presented, but for this chapter the emphasis has been on the concrete and abstract worlds. The four levels are explored in Chapters 4 and 5.

DCT's approach to concrete and abstract meaning-making systems have been presented with specific examples of what to look for in your clients, whether children or adults. Both modes of being are considered vital, but being fixed in one style is usually limiting. An important task of counseling and therapy is to open client consciousness to new ways of viewing the world. Your first task is to be able to identify abstract and concrete consciousness; later you can learn how to facilitate development with clients who may present using either mode of meaning making. DCT's four cognitive/emotional styles have been summarized within the context of concrete and abstract meaning-making systems—sensorimotor/elemental, concrete/situational, formal/reflective, and dialectic/systemic.

THEORY INTO PRACTICE: DEVELOPING YOUR PORTFOLIO OF COMPETENCE

This book is about learning intentional and purposeful assessment tools and interventions that facilitate client development. You will learn how to recognize developmental and cognitive/emotional style variations in clients, and how to change your interviewing style to match their needs. You will find that meeting your clients where they are enables them to see the world in new ways and to act more effectively.

Each chapter concludes by asking you to reflect on what you have read and experienced. Generally, the reflective exercises are oriented to the broad abstract notions as described by DCT whereas the practice exercises seek to take abstract notions into concrete practice.

We suggest that you take notes on your early thoughts here and then expand them in a more complete fashion in a formal portfolio of competence on your computer disk.

Self-Assessment Exercises

Exercise 1. Are you oriented to concreteness or abstractions?

Do you see yourself more as a concrete or an abstract person? Will you be able to be patient with the client who needs concrete specifics and behavioral action? Will you be able to challenge and work with the abstractly oriented, intellectualizing client? In terms of therapy theory, do you tend to favor more concrete, behaviorally oriented approaches or more abstract, self-reflective approaches? Will you be able to shift your helping style as client needs vary?

_____

_____

_____

_____

Exercise 2. Wellness and lifespan reflections

What is healthy about you and what are your strengths? How might good things that have occurred in your lifespan history affect the counseling relationship? Let us start work with our clients from a wellness perspective. We can explore developmental challenges and problems best after we have identified strengths both in ourselves and in our clients.

_____

_____

_____

_____

Identifying and Classifying Concrete and Abstract Statements

Exercise 3. Classifying concrete and abstract statements

Classify each client statement as primarily concrete or primarily abstract. (Answers to the exercise may be found at the conclusion of this chapter.) Circle C (concrete) or A (abstract) below:

C A   1. I cry a lot. I couldn't sleep last night. I can't eat.

C A   2. I feel really depressed lately. I'm thinking about myself all the time.

C A   3. I feel guilty because I'm late so often for our counseling sessions.

C A   4. Sorry I'm late for the session. Traffic was very heavy.

C A   5. I feel really awkward on dates. I'm a social dud.

C A   6. Last night I went on a date. I didn't know what to say, so I just started talking and then we had dinner. We had steak and . . . (continues). Then we (continues).

C A   7. The police stopped me yesterday. I wasn't even speeding. They got me out of the car and pushed me over the hood.

C A   8. The police are always after People of Color and treat them unfairly.

C A   9. My family is very loving. We have a pattern of sharing and always try to do something for each other.

C A   10. My mom just sent me a box of cookies.

Interviewing Practice Exercise

Exercise 4. Separation and attachment interviewing practice

Ask a friend or family member to share a time of life transition and change with you. Listen to the story carefully and note whether the person describes that transition in concrete or abstract language. Some potentially useful ideas and questions that you may consider as an outline include the following:

- Before you start, obtain permission from the volunteer client and, as appropriate, ask him or her to sign a release allowing you to record or take notes on the session. Work within the ethical framework in your classroom, school, or agency.
- You could start the session by asking "Could you tell me about an important life event that involved a transition from one stage of your life to another? For example, this could be entering school at any age, starting a new job, getting married, having a child, or losing a loved one through death."
- Listen to the client's story and note concrete and abstract styles.
- You can facilitate concrete conversation by asking questions such as the following: "Could you give me an example?" "What specifically happened?" "What occurred next?" "What was the result?"
- You can facilitate abstract conversation through variations of the following examples: "What did you think about that?" "What was going on inside your

head?" "Is that a pattern in your life?" "What does this mean when you think about yourself?"

■ You may wish to add wellness dimensions to your practice exercise by asking questions such as these: "What strengths helped you deal with this situation?" "What personal strengths or important new learnings came from this experience?"

Use the following space for your planning and/or summary of your experience.

_____

_____

_____

_____

Toward Multicultural Competence

Exercise 5. Development as a cultural expression

The theologian Paul Tillich points out that we are literally thrown into the world. By the act of being born, we become part of a cultural script that directs many of our actions. Individual and family development does not occur in a vacuum. A middle-class White person develops certain frames of reference from his or her culture. Men are expected to be more individualistic; women are often seen as more relational. In the United States, this can represent a highly individualistic frame of reference. African American, Asian American, Native American, and Latina/o cultures often stress relationship and communal development. What is appropriate development in one culture may be inappropriate in another. At the same time, we must avoid stereotyping as you will find wide individual variations in the individualistic and re-lational developmental frames.

The following are some key multicultural areas over which we have little control when we are born or "thrown into the world." Yet these cultural dimensions have immense impact on our personal development. First, fill in the left column, which itemizes the givens of your life experience. Second, imagine and note how your life might have been different if your path of development had occurred with different givens in a different cultural or societal setting.

Societal/cultural	*How would your life be changed if your social context and cultural conditions were different?*
Gender _____	_____
Race/ethnicity _____	_____
Religion _____	_____
Socioeconomic status _____	_____
Nationality _____	_____

How would your life be changed if your social context and cultural conditions were different?

Societal/cultural

Disability/ability————————————   ————————————————

Sexual orientation————————————   ————————————————

Age ————————————————   ————————————————

You may notice that these societal and cultural variables at times may affect human development as much as or more than individual or family interactions. How might these multicultural issues affect your counseling and therapy practice?

——

——

——

Generalization: Taking Abstract and Concrete Ideas Home

Exercise 6. Observation skills of DCT

The only real way to learn and master a theoretical system such as DCT is to take the concepts home and make sure they are clear to you. Most basic are observation and the ability to recognize cognitive/emotional style. During this coming week, spend time each day noting the conversational style of those whom you meet. Who is concrete, likes to tell stories, and provides linear, detailed information? Who is reflective, thinking about self and situation and perhaps analyzing as well?

Portfolio Reflections

Exercise 7. Your reflections on a developmental approach to counseling and therapy

So, what do you think? What stood out for you from this chapter? What sense do you make of what you have just read? What are your key points? Write your ideas here and consider establishing a Portfolio Folder in your computer that you will gradually develop as you work through this text.

——

——

——

——

——

——

REFERENCES

Adler, A. (1954). *Understanding human nature* (W. B. Wolf, Trans.). New York: Fawcett. (Original work published 1927)

American Psychiatric Association. (2000). *Diagnostic and statistical manual of mental disorders: Text revision (DSM-IV-TR).* Washington, DC: Author.

Bowlby, J. (1969). *Attachment.* New York: Basic Books.

Bowlby, J. (1973). *Separation.* New York: Basic Books.

Bowlby, J. (1990). *A secure base.* New York: Basic Books.

Cassidy, J., & Shaver, P. (2002). *Handbook of attachment.* New York: Guilford.

Erikson, E. (1963). *Childhood and society* (2nd ed.). New York: Norton.

Erikson, E. (1994). *Identity and the life cycle.* New York: Norton.

Gilligan, C. (1982). *In a different voice.* Cambridge, MA: Harvard University Press.

Gilligan, C. (2002). *The birth of pleasure.* New York: Knopf.

Helms, J. (1999). *Using race and culture in counseling and psychotherapy.* Needham Heights, MA: Allyn & Bacon.

Ivey, A. (2000). *Developmental therapy: Theory into practice.* North Amherst, MA: Microtraining. (Original work published 1986)

Ivey, A., Pedersen, P., & Ivey, M. (2001). *Intentional group counseling.* Pacific Grove, CA: Microtraining.

Kegan, R. (1982). *The evolving self.* Cambridge, MA: Harvard University Press.

Kegan, R., & Lahey, L. (2000). *How the way we talk can change the way we work.* San Francisco: Jossey-Bass.

Kohlberg, L. (1981). *The philosophy of moral development.* San Francisco: Harper & Row.

Loevinger, J. (Ed.) (1998). Technical foundations for measuring ego development. Mahwah, NJ: Erlbaum.

Meara, N., Pepinsky, H., Shannon, J., & Murray, W. (1981). Comparisons of stylistic complexity of the language of counselor and client across three theoretical orientations. *Journal of Counseling Psychology, 26,* 181–189.

Myers, J. E., Sweeney, T. J., & Witmer, J. M. (2000). Counseling for wellness: A holistic model for treatment planning. *Journal of Counseling and Development, 78,* 251–266.

Myers, J. E., Sweeney, T. J., & Witmer, J. M. (2001). Optimization of behavior/promotion of wellness. In D. Locke, J. E. Myers, & E. H. Herr (Eds.), *The handbook of counseling* (pp. 641–652). Thousand Oaks, CA: Sage.

Piaget, J. (1955). *The language and thought of the child.* New York: New American Library. (Original work published 1923)

Piaget, J. (1963). *The origins of intelligence in children.* New York: Norton. (Original work published 1952)

Piaget, J. (1965). *The moral judgment of the child.* New York: Norton.

Schlossberg, N. K. (2003). *Transition works.* Unpublished manuscript. Washington: DC: Transition Works, www.transitionguide.com

Schlossberg, N. K., & Kay, S. (2003). *The transition guide: A new way to think about change.* Washington, DC: Transition Works, www.transitionguide.com

Schlossberg, N. K., Waters, E., & Goodman, J. (1995). *Counseling adults in transition: Linking practice with theory.* New York: Springer.

Sue, D. W., & Sue, D. (2003). *Counseling the culturally different* (4th ed.). New York: Wiley.

Answers to Concrete/Abstract Classification Exercise

1. C	4. C	7. C	9. A
2. A	5. A	8. A	10. C
3. A	6. C		

CHAPTER 2
Wellness

Optimizing Human Development Over the Lifespan

Thomas Sweeney and Jane Myers

CENTRAL PRACTICE OBJECTIVE | Mastery and practice of concepts in this chapter will enable you to assess your wellness and that of your clients, thus providing a solid base of strengths on which to facilitate client positive movement.

C lients change and grow best from a base of strength and wellness. We can work with their most difficult issues more effectively if their capabilities and resources are clearly identified. More than a decade ago the need for a paradigm shift to wellness rather than pathology was recognized (Larson, 1999), and lifespan wellness theory and practice is increasingly seen as the wave of the future in counseling and mental health services (Locke, Myers, & Herr, 2001; Myers, Sweeney, & Witmer, 2001; Palmo, Shosh, & Weikel, 2001). However, bringing about a change that focuses on wellness rather than on problems and psychopathology will require a renewed understanding of development as a personal journey that involves the whole person in all aspects of life.

This chapter presents a wellness paradigm, illustrated by two models. Both models seek to promote development beyond what is "normal" or "dysfunctional." If your counseling and therapy sessions first center on wellness and positive psychology, you will find that your clients will respond more readily to your interventions. With a positive wellness base, you'll find that they respond more readily to you and that positive change will be more likely.

Knowledge of and skill in the concepts of this chapter can enable you to:

1. Discuss two conceptual models for the wellness paradigm—the theoretical Wheel of Wellness model and the empirically based Indivisible Self model.
2. Conceptualize human development and wellness holistically, thus avoiding reductionist strategies common in the physical and medical sciences influencing contemporary theory.
3. Utilize wellness theory as a model for theory, research, and practice. The wellness paradigm is based on traditional Adlerian theory and practice; research across disciplines; and contemporary theory, research, and practice using developmental counseling and therapy.
4. Apply the concepts of this chapter in real life through practice, exercises, personal reflection, and development of a portfolio of competence.

INTRODUCTION: FROM ILLNESS AND REPAIR TO THE PROMOTION AND ENHANCEMENT OF WELLNESS

There is a common axiom that if you do not know where you are going, you can end up someplace else! In the fields of education, psychology, and counseling, there is a common goal for our efforts to help others with their human journey. The goal is to facilitate their human development through understanding of self, others, and life. We use various methods, techniques, and mechanisms to explain, identify, and illuminate topics related to each of these areas. Traditionally, counselors and therapists solve problems, remediate difficulties, and seek to alleviate pathology. A wellness approach attacks the same issues, but seeks to work with human health rather than human illness. Such an approach builds on client strengths and resources.

During the last decades of the 20th century in the United States, the changing and complex nature of society, increases in violence and person abuse, and competition in the mental health marketplace for adequate funding for health needs led to an increasing adoption of a medical, illness-based model among health care professionals. Until suffering and dysfunction are present, no intervention is available. When pain is moderated and a modicum of "normalcy" is attained, no further assistance is required. Frustration, needless human suffering, and high costs have all shown the illness-based model to be incomplete. New advocates for change are being found among business, industry, insurance, and government agency personnel who see rising costs as a compelling reason to seek relief. As a consequence, there is an opportunity for helping professionals to redefine the purposes for their interventions from repair and crisis intervention to prevention and optimization of human development (Myers, Sweeney, & Witmer, 2000).

In 1989 the governing council of the American Association for Counseling and Development (AACD), now the American Counseling Association (ACA), adopted a resolution affirming the counseling profession as advocates for optimum health and wellness (ACA Governing Council, July 13, 1991). While historically consistent with the underlying philosophy of counseling as a discipline, this resolution rededicated counseling's position among the helping professions as proactive, positive, and developmentally based (Myers, 1992; Sweeney, 2001). As a result, the American Counseling Association (ACA) adopted as its 1990–91 theme an emphasis entirely focused on promoting wellness throughout life. In addition, an entire special issue of the *Journal of Counseling and Development* was devoted to methods of promoting wellness throughout the lifespan (Myers, Emmerling, & Leafgren, 1992).

The positive psychology movement is yet another illustration of professional movement toward wellness. Martin Seligman, a past president of the American Psychological Association, summarized the essence of positive psychology (2002b, p. 1): "Modern psychology has been co-opted by the disease model. We've become too preoccupied with repairing damage when our focus should be on building strength and resilience, especially in children." Seligman (1998a) points out that we have overemphasized self-esteem and individualism with a resulting loss of awareness of others. He speaks of the "I-We" balance and the importance of individuals' being fully conscious of their connection to and responsibility for others. Positive psychology is oriented toward connection to others and the world and helps clients find personal strengths to cope with self and others (Seligman 1998b, 2002a). An extensive body of literature, research, and instrumentation has developed around positive psychology (Snyder & Lopez, 2001) and wellness (Myers, Sweeney, & Witmer, 2000).

This chapter provides an overview of a wellness model that draws on the work of Alfred Adler (1927/1954) and advocates for his theory of personality, including the writings of Rudolph Dreikurs (1971) and Thomas Sweeney (1998). A new model of wellness (Myers & Sweeney, 2002, 2004) is used to integrate Adler's Individual Psychology (IP) and wellness with developmental counseling and therapy. Individual Psychology and DCT have been cited as the most culturally appropriate of all the various approaches to counseling (Arciniega & Newlon, 1999; Sweeney, 1998). Not surprisingly, they blend well together in practice as well as theory.

Adler proposed a theory of holism, or indivisibility of the individual, in which work, love, friendship, spirit, and self are central to understanding human growth and development. An exploration of Adler's theory provides an essential foundation for understanding wellness—philosophically, as well as in your own daily life and in your clinical work. These philosophical and practical approaches provide skills in strength-based assessment and intervention for promoting and enhancing positive development across the lifespan.

Myers, Sweeney, and Witmer (2000) define wellness "as a way of life oriented toward optimal health and well-being, in which body, mind, and spirit are integrated by the individual to live life more fully within the human and natural community" (p. 252). Ideally, it is the optimum state of health and well-being that each individual is capable of achieving. Through the development of a theoretical model, assessment instrument, research, and practice, these authors have defined and promoted a practical approach to helping people optimize their behavior and achieve wellness across the lifespan. Two models of wellness associated with Individual Psychology have been published (Myers et al., 2000; Sweeney & Witmer, 1991; Witmer & Sweeney, 1992) and a number of studies using instruments based on these models have been conducted (Myers & Sweeney, 2004).

A new model evolving from these earlier efforts is also outlined and illustrated in this chapter as it relates to both Individual Psychology and developmental counseling and therapy. This is the first time DCT has been identified with a model of wellness but the practitioner should find it a logical extension of the theory into practice.

THREE KEY ADLERIAN DEVELOPMENTAL CONSTRUCTS: SOCIO-TELEO-ANALYTIC

Adlerian theory espouses three major developmental constructs. They help us understand how we can empower individuals toward self-discovery, their connections with others, and a sense of personal power. These three dimensions are briefly defined and then described in greater detail.

Socio. Humans have a social need for connectedness and belonging.

Teleo. Humans are goal oriented in their thoughts, feelings, and behavior. There is always a reason and a purpose for what we do.

Analytic. Human behavior is predicated upon much that is not understood or conscious. This biases individual perceptions and actions.

Socio. Adler believed that human beings have a basic inclination toward *Gemeinschaftsgefuhl*—that is, a striving to feel belongingness, a willingness to serve the greater good for the betterment of humankind. The closest interpretation of this German word in English is "social interest." An expression of this inclination is observed in each person's striving to make a place for himself or herself and to feel a sense of belonging. Understanding individuals' striving is significant in helping them to overcome their own self-defeating behaviors or the actions of society that thwart their development. Individuals successful in making a place for themselves socially tend to live long and well. Likewise, individuals who struggle with developing successful social relationships tend not to live as long or as well as other persons.

Alienation, prejudice, and isolation have negative consequences for positive health and diminish hope for optimizing one's development. Regardless of circumstances, however, everyone has a desire to belong, to be someone of significance to others, to experience respect and worth. Behavior, then, can be understood as a part of one's striving to be in community with others. From infancy in the family throughout later life, each person seeks a place to fulfill this motivation.

Adler was a phenomenologist who believed that this social motivation to belong was understood best through the eyes of the beholder. He referred to the basic notions that guide us through life as our style of life or, as more commonly referred to now, *lifestyle*. He characterized lifestyle as "unity in each individual in his thinking, feeling, acting; in his so-called conscious and unconscious, in every expression of his personality. This (self-consistent) unity we call the style of life of the individual" (Ansbacher & Ansbacher, 1956, p. 175).

Lifestyle is not determined by heredity or environment, but both are important antecedents. Individuals decide how they think, value, and feel about their gender, family position, or ethnicity. Each lifestyle is unique. An individual develops a lifestyle in accordance to its usefulness in helping the person cope with other people and the world. Through an understanding of their unique perceptions, individuals also come to understand the consistency in their behavior. We strive to understand the *private logic* of the individual, including what is commonly referred to as one's "self-talk."

DCT theory and practice have proven particularly effective in helping individuals to participate in this process of self-discovery through examination of assumptions, practices, and results of their behavior that otherwise escape their understanding. It is useful in conjunction with Individual Psychology in helping us understand the language (i.e., self-talk) and cognitive/emotional processes of the client. Through such understanding, the counselor can be intentional and effective in matching the self-talk of clients to establish rapport, and he or she can use mismatching as needed to help them learn to overcome blocks in their processing of information, feelings, and experiences.

Teleo.   Human beings have a goal-striving nature. Behavior is purposive even though the "why" and "what" we are striving for may be obscure to both the individual and the observer. Individuals choose to act or not act because it is useful to them. As Ansbacher (1969, p. 1) writes:

> The science of Individual Psychology developed out of the effort to understand that mysterious creative power of life—that power which expresses itself in the desire to develop, to strive and to achieve—and even to compensate for defeats in one direction by striving for success in another. This power is teleological—it expresses itself in the striving after a goal.

This teleological orientation has an optimistic and encouraging nature. As Rudolf Dreikurs (personal communication, June 1970) once said, "Tell a person what they are, schizophrenic, so what? Tell a person how they feel, sad or bad, so what? But, tell a person what they intend! Now that is something they can change!"

Because goals of behavior can be understood and anticipated, they can be changed. Individuals may choose to change the valuing of their goals or the behavior they use in their striving. Individuals, therefore, are not victims of circumstances beyond their control in any absolute way. Through the DCT assessment process, clients—regardless of age, gender, or culture—can learn the motivation guiding their behaviors and decide whether it is always in their best interest to pursue these behaviors as they have in the past. This is an empowering process that affirms the individuals' right and capacity to choose new goals and practice new behaviors at any time in life that doing so serves their purposes for living life more fully.

Analytic.   Individuals frequently report that they do not understand their behavior or motives. Closer inspection reveals that they often understand more than they willingly admit. The analytic aspect of Individual Psychology is derived from the observation that most behavior is based on what is unconscious or not understood (Mosak & Dreikurs, 1973). In a helping relationship, however, individuals more readily accept direct challenges about the purposes of their behavior, including purposes of which they were not consciously aware. One of the positive attributes of a DCT intervention is that the helper guides clients in challenging their own mistaken ideas rather than attempting to do this for them. The helper works "with" rather than "on" the client.

With this as a background, let us turn to two models of wellness, one theoretical and one empirical. Both have validity in explaining human behavior and lifespan development.

THE WHEEL OF WELLNESS: A HOLISTIC MODEL OF HUMAN DEVELOPMENT

The history of science is full of discoveries and contributions for improving the quality of human life. One of its legacies, however, has been the tendency to objectify and dichotomize the human condition. Individuals are seen as a combination of parts that work in concert. When a part is diseased or damaged, it is removed or repaired. Hence, the person is once again "whole" or healthy. In reality, nothing could be further from the truth.

The tendency to conceptualize human nature as divisible and even at odds with its parts might be illustrated best by Freud's conceptualization of personality development. Certainly no personality theory has had more influence or notoriety than Freud's psychoanalysis. His contemporary, Alfred Adler (1927/1954), took exception to Freud's theory and its portrayal of human beings as parts at odds with one another (id, ego, and superego). Instead, Adler taught that individuals are mind, body, and spirit, indivisible, unique, creative, and purposeful. *Equally important, whether for good or bad, one aspect of self affects the other aspects of self within this holistic interaction.*

With the exception of Carl Jung, Adlerian acknowledgment of the soul or spirit side of human existence seemed to run counter to the efforts of other 20th-century theorists to present human growth and development as measurable, malleable, and linear. The spirit side of human nature defies measurement. In spite of racism, oppression, or physical destruction, it cannot be "molded." Likewise, it eludes linear thinking as experienced in the human condition. Spirituality (not religiosity, per se) is as vital to wellness as any attribute of mind and body. Research findings suggest

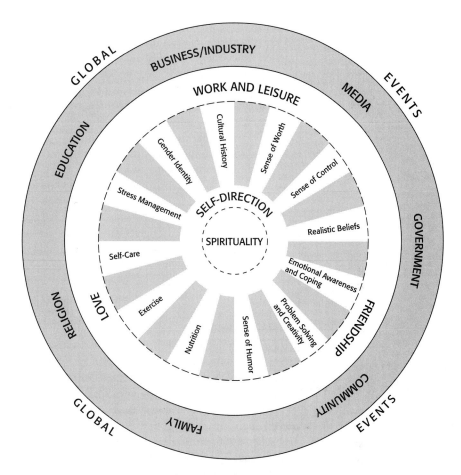

Figure 2-1   The Wheel of Wellness (Copyright © J. M. Witmer, T. J. Sweeney, & J. E. Myers, 1998. Reprinted with permission.)

that spirituality is an essential component for healthy development for all individuals (see Myers et al., 2000; Myers & Willard, 2003).

The original Witmer and Sweeney (1992) Wheel of Wellness model was hypothesized based on the theoretical life tasks identified by Adler (1927/1954) and Dreikurs (1967; Mosak & Dreikurs, 1967) that everyone must address (i.e., work, friendship, love, self, and spirit). The model incorporated research results; theoretical perspectives from personality, social, clinical, health, and developmental psychology; and stress management, behavioral medicine, psychoneuroimmunology, ecology, and contextualism. This model was later modified to further define subtasks in the major life task of self-direction (see Myers et al., 2000), as shown in Figure 2-1.

The Wheel of Wellness depicted in Figure 2-1 is hypothetical and assumes that life tasks located in the center of the model (i.e., spirituality) are more central and important to human functioning than are tasks located around the rims of the

Wheel. In other words, the model assumes a circumplex structure in which a hierarchy exists in the salience of life tasks. In this model, the 12 subtasks of self-direction function much like the spokes in a wheel to provide stability and support for the entire structure. Moreover, these tasks are the essential means through which we manage our lives and address Adler's three main life tasks of work, friendship, and love. The model is contextual in that life forces, such as family and community as well as global events, affect individual functioning and in turn are affected by each individual. This contextual description is similar to that provided in Bronfenbrenner's (1999) well-known model of human growth and development.

This holistic circumplex model has found considerable practical support because it is useful in conceptualizing the client's world (Sweeney, 1995). Practitioners and many clients have found the core emphasis on spirituality to be profoundly useful in building relationships and in examining life goals. Again, think of spirituality in the broadest sense—what gives meaning to one's life is obviously central. Viktor Frankl's *Man's Search for Meaning* (1959) and his logotherapy focus on the *will to meaning*, which is often considered a spiritual quest. More recent writings in spirituality clearly indicate that this is an important adjunct to counseling and therapy (cf. Richards & Bergin, 2000; this book, Chapter 13). As you work with the wheel model, please constantly think about your own personal definitions of spirituality and meaning and use this as a guide to understanding this section in your own way.

Each person has both the power and means to create ways of coping, managing, and transcending circumstances. As we know, however, not all do (Frankl, 1959; Prochaska, DiClemente, & Norcross, 1992). Our goal in helping, then, is to facilitate the optimization of each individual's capacity to grow and develop. This includes helping to moderate personal and systemic obstacles that inevitably enter everyone's journey through life. Adler speaks eloquently about the *will to power* (Ansbacher & Ansbacher, 1956, pp. 111–119). In some sense, this is like a spiritual journey or search for meaning. The person with a strong self-concept and awareness of others will use that will in positive ways whereas those with a sense of inferiority may be destructive to themselves and others—thus the need for a positive wellness approach.

Personal obstacles can be conceived as phenomenological—self-created thoughts about life, self, and others. Adler posits the idea that people create their own realities but with a purpose—that is, for reasons meaningful to the individual if not to others who live or work with them. Understanding that purpose allows one to discover the *private logic* of the individual. In DCT, we likewise attempt to understand the unique self of the individual as expressed through her or his efforts to make meaning, belong, participate, and share in social interactions with others. These conceptualizations are manifest in "rules" about life similar to those discovered in the private logic of individuals through Adlerian lifestyle assessment (Sweeney, 1998).

Meaning is the way we make sense of the world. By "making meaning" we organize reality and our reactions to it. Meaning could be described as a spiritual force in that each of us has a "will to meaning" (Frankl, 1959). Equally important, individuals are more than a "responding" mechanism. Human beings create changes in their behavior whenever change is perceived as being in their best interests (Ansbacher & Ansbacher, 1956; Ivey, 1986/2000).

Systemic obstacles are the result of both deliberate and unintentional inequities and oppression within society (Dreikurs, 1971; Ivey & Ivey, 2003). As helpers, we are obligated to do all that we can to make it possible for those we help to overcome inequities that thwart personal development. Social "rules" that emanate from prejudice of whatever persuasion become a part of the private logic that limits human development. These may be stereotypic depictions of race, gender roles, age appropriate behaviors, or physical characteristics that carry the connotation that superiority, not social equity, is an underlying value. The helper using a wellness approach will be able to root out such prejudice and challenge the logic, appropriateness, and validity of such faulty notions. Through such examination, individuals are not only freed of the limitations of prejudice but are invited to develop new meanings in which they think more equitably and compassionately about others who are different from them.

Although early research on the circumplex Wheel of Wellness model was promising, more recent data analyses do not fully support the hierarchical model (Hattie, Myers, & Sweeney, in press; Myers, Luecht, & Sweeney, 2003; Myers & Sweeney, 2003). We suggest that you use the diagram in Figure 2-1 as a useful way to think about the many systems that affect the way your clients make meaning and sense of the world. An updated wellness model, presented later in this chapter (Figure 2-2), is supported by empirical research based on the Wheel of Wellness model.

Nonetheless, the circumplex wheel model based on Adlerian theory and its wellness orientation lead us to think in an "I/We" contextual framework rather than a naïve focus solely on an autonomous individual. In particular, we suggest that an I/We meaning-making system may be an important foundation for an individually and culturally relevant view of holistic lifespan development.

THE INDIVISIBLE SELF MODEL FOR WELLNESS (IS-WEL)

The Indivisible Self model is portrayed in Figure 2-2. Based on research, this model provides a comprehensive wellness framework for counseling and therapy practice. You'll find assessment tools with which to examine yourself and a practical system that you can use immediately in the session to help clients sort out their strengths and wellness assets. At the same time, you'll identify areas of need for further development. You'll find that starting your sessions with a positive, goal-oriented frame will make therapy and counseling with even the most difficult clients more productive.

While the earlier Wheel of Wellness model (Figure 2-1) hypothesized a hierarchical, circumplex construct (Witmer & Sweeney, 1998), subsequent data analyses have revealed essentially one overarching factor (wellness) with five components and each of their elements contributing to this factor (Hattie, Myers, & Sweeney, in press; Myers & Sweeney, 2002; Myers & Sweeney, 2003). In short, all items and all components are related to wellness. None could be considered statistically more (or less) important than the other components of the model. Contrary to traditional linear thinking, this outcome is entirely consistent with DCT as well as Adlerian theory, both of which emphasize the indivisibility of the individual. As a consequence, the new model is appropriately named the Indivisible Self (see Figure 2-2).

CONTEXTS:

Local (safety)
   Family
   Neighborhood
   Community

Institutional (policies & laws)
   Education
   Religion
   Government
   Business/Industry

Global (world events)
   Politics
   Culture
   Global Events
   Environment
   Media
   Community

Chronometrical (time-focused)
   Perpetual
   Positive
   Purposeful

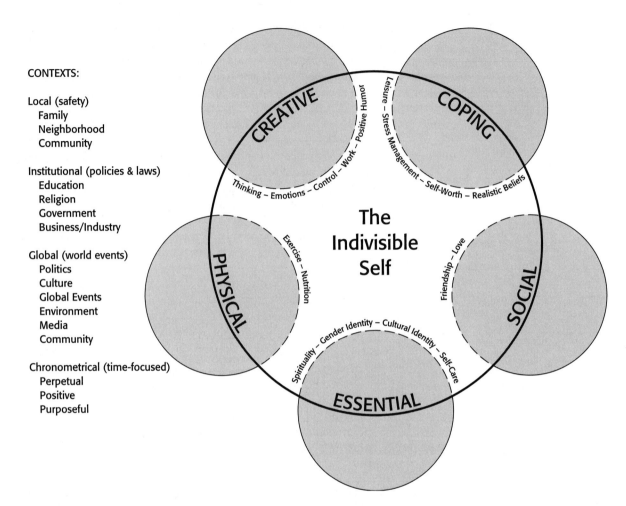

Figure 2-2   The Indivisible Self: An Evidence-Based Model of Wellness (From *The Indivisible Self: An Evidence-Based Model of Wellness.* Copyright © T. J. Sweeney & J. E. Myers, 2003. Reprinted with permission.)

Central to the idea of the Indivisible Self is the conviction that positive change in one area of one's being can have positive benefits in other areas as well. Change, then, can be incremental, cumulative, and self-paced in one or more areas of life but all areas may benefit. What we have learned is that we may focus on five factors essential to personal wellness. These activities central to well-being are conceptualized within the construct of *Self*: Essential Self; Coping Self; Social Self; Creative Self; and Physical Self. Within the five factors are 17 components; research findings across disciplines suggest that each of the 17 contributes to both longevity and quality of life (Myers et al., 2000).

In other words, people who live longest and best have mastered some specific attributes, habits, and competencies in each of these 17 components. Mastery of these attributes, habits, and competencies helps buffer them from the harm that inevitably comes in life. Again, we suggest that focusing on the positive throughout the lifespan will enable us to cope more effectively with the negative. Both spirituality and meaning making remain important constructs in our wellness research. Note that the *Essential Self* is based on three meaning issues: spirituality, gender issues, and cultural identity. The *Coping Self* includes self-worth and realistic beliefs. Aspects of the *Social Self,* the *Creative Self,* and even the *Physical Self* rely on issues of meaning.

Someone may ask how many of the 17 components one needs to enhance to be considered "well." We are reminded of a sign in our dentist's office, "You don't need to floss all of your teeth, only the ones that you wish to keep!" On other occasions, individuals want to know how they compare with others: how "well" am I compared to others like me? An answer to that question suggests that there is a "norm" for well-being, and there is not! Even one individual's norms change with time, circumstances, and conditions. You may be limited by illness, injury, organic difficulties, or environmental conditions that work against your optimal well-being. These may be temporary or moderated by lifestyle choices and changes. This realization alone can be terrifically empowering. It can liberate one from an otherwise somber outlook on life and its gifts.

The Four Contextual Dimensions of Wellness

As you examine Figure 2-2, notice that four contexts are identified that act individually and collectively to affect the indivisible self and all aspects of wellness within the self. These contexts include local, institutional, global, and chronometrical (time-focused) components. Local contexts are forces close to one's home and family. While the Indivisible Self Model for Wellness (IS-Wel) includes friendship and love as essential aspects of wellness, the context of friends, family, and neighbors refers to how these elements external to the self influence one's well-being on a daily basis. This influence can be for better or worse. When we assess the effects of contextual variables, feelings of personal safety, as defined by Maslow (1954/1970), reflect personal reactions to the local context.

The institutional context includes agencies and institutions in areas as diverse as religion, education, government, and business/industry. Laws, policies, rules, and regulations within these contexts may empower or limit individuals in their daily lives. For example, the effect of fundamental religious institutions is particularly strong in the southeastern and midwestern United States. Persons moving from other areas of the country to some parts of these geographic regions may find that stores do not open on Sundays, alcohol cannot be purchased within a city or county, and employees prefer not to work on Wednesday nights as this is a common time for church activities. In other areas, a local government may decide that employees cannot take paid leave for personal religious or cultural holidays.

Global contexts reflect our understanding that we are part of a global community and that worldwide events affect us in ways we sometimes do not even understand. Armed conflict and war that occur halfway around the world and far away from our homes and communities can have a significant affect on our daily lives. Recent wars in the Middle East are felt in the United States in rising oil and gasoline prices and the separation of families due to the requirements of military service. The media allow us to experience wars as if we were there, with embedded journalists providing coverage of conflict the moment it occurs. Post-trauma reactions as a consequence of television viewing are increasingly common, both in terms of news coverage of events such as the terrorist attacks of September 11, 2001, on the World Trade Center and the Pentagon, and in terms of violence in movies and even cartoons.

The fourth context, chronometrical, refers to the element of time. We grow and change over a lifetime, and like it or not, change is inevitable. Those who experience the greatest wellness view change as positive and approach change in an intentional or purposeful manner. With these contextual dimensions in mind, let us turn to how you might use wellness concepts in your own interviewing practice.

Assessing Personal Wellness: Practical Applications

We use both informal (e.g., clinical interviews, behavioral observations) and formal assessment tools (e.g., Indivisible Self Wellness Inventory, or IS-Wel; Myers & Sweeney, 2002) to help bring focus to the various components of well-being, but they are at best only approximations of the many thoughts, behaviors, and practices that can be conceptualized within each component. Equally important, genetics, age, gender, culture, and other circumstances moderate what may be said about one individual versus another.

Contrary to some people's outlook on life, even those with a severe disability or terminal illness can enhance the quality and longevity of life by focusing, for example, on what they can do (control) and how they can contribute to others (work, friendship, love); they can practice self-care and spirituality, and seek to be fully functioning in their thinking and emotions. This leads to the need for further illumination of the components that comprise wellness and how they can be addressed to enhance their positive effect on human development over the lifespan.

One of the best ways to become acquainted with the components of wellness is through a personal assessment. Once you understand how the IS-Wel model applies to you personally, you are better equipped to apply wellness ideas in your own practice. In the following pages, each component of the Indivisible Self is defined. As you read each definition, think about how it applies to you in your daily functioning and interactions with others. Below each description are two rating scales. As you reflect on your personal wellness in relation to each component, you are asked to make two self-report assessments:

> First, rate your perception of your overall wellness on a scale from 1 (very low) to 10 (very high). Although your feelings about your wellness may change from day to day or week to week depending on your activities, in this assessment you are asked to evaluate your wellness in general, perhaps over the past three months.
>
> Second, think about your level of satisfaction with your wellness in that area. Then, using the second rating scale, circle your level of satisfaction with your wellness.

We have found that some individuals report mid to low levels of wellness in an area, and also report that they are quite content with their score at a particular point in time and have no desire for change. On the other hand, you might rate yourself as being high in a wellness area such as gender or cultural identity, but because of difficult personal experiences of oppression, your satisfaction may be lower. Discrepancies may or may not be areas where you could seek intervention through counseling and therapy sessions.

Essential Self

There are four components to this factor: *spirituality, gender identity, cultural identity*, and *self-care*. Spirituality, not religiosity, has positive benefits for longevity and quality of life. Conceived as a core component of the factor by virtue of its existential meaning, purpose, and hopefulness toward life, one's identity as male or female affects one's sense of worth and place within all life. Likewise, cultural identity is conceptualized as both a filter through which life experiences are seen and an influence on how others are experienced in response to our identity. Self-care relates to the Essential Self as attention to proactive efforts to live long and live well. Conversely, carelessness, avoidance of health-promoting habits, and general disregard of one's well-being are potentially signs of despair, hopelessness, and alienation from life's opportunities.

Spirituality.   This is defined as an awareness of a being or force that transcends the material aspects of life and gives a deep sense of wholeness or connectedness to the universe. For many, this is equated with meaning. Spirituality is associated with hope, optimism, seeking meaning and purpose in life, and practices that express these through prayer, meditation, and worship. A distinction is made between spirituality, a broad concept representing personal beliefs and values, and religiosity, a more specific concept that refers to institutional beliefs and behaviors. Religious affiliation is a public matter, often expressed through group religious participation; spirituality is a more private issue that may or may not be expressed publicly. Most people will agree on a definition of religion, but you will find wide variation in the way the word *spirituality* is characterized.

Recent studies suggest that there is a significant, positive relationship between spirituality, of which religion is only one part, mental health, physical health, life satisfaction, and wellness. Consistent with these studies, recent meta-analyses by the Fetzer Institute–National Institute on Aging Workgroup (1999) resulted in the following "key domains of religiousness/spirituality as essential . . . because of the strength of their conceptualization and theoretical or empirical connection to health outcomes: daily spiritual experiences, meaning, values, beliefs, forgiveness, private religious practices, religious/spiritual coping, religious support, religious/spiritual history, commitment, organizational religiousness, and religious preference" (p. 4).

Spirituality

Overall Wellness	1	2	3	4	5	6	7	8	9	10
Satisfaction	1	2	3	4	5	6	7	8	9	10

Gender Identity.   Gender identity refers to subjective feelings of maleness or femaleness and is culturally constructed or defined. Gender role socialization, a process that begins at birth and continues throughout the lifespan, results in culturally appropriate gender role behaviors' being rewarded for both males and females. These differences have been linked to wellness as well as illness in adulthood. Feelings of satisfaction with one's gender, feeling supported and valued in relationships with persons of both genders, and being competent to respond appropriately to gender-related stressors in life are characteristics of those who have a positive gender identity.

Gender Identity
Overall Wellness   1   2   3   4   5   6   7   8   9   10

Satisfaction   1   2   3   4   5   6   7   8   9   10

Cultural Identity.   Culture may be broadly defined as "a multidimensional concept that encompasses the collective reality of a group of people" (Lee & Richardson, 1997, p. 11). Cultural identity, a concept that incorporates racial identity, acculturation, and an appreciation for the unique aspects of one's culture, is positively related to well-being. Cultural identity affects self-perceived health and wellness since concepts of health differ according to culture. Feelings of satisfaction with one's cultural heritage, feeling supported and valued in relationships with persons of one's own and other cultures, and being competent to respond appropriately to culture-related stressors in life are characteristics of those who have a positive cultural identity. This closely relates to the ideas of cultural identity development, discussed in depth in Chapter 8 on multicultural counseling and therapy (MCT).

Cultural Identity
Overall Wellness   1   2   3   4   5   6   7   8   9   10

Satisfaction   1   2   3   4   5   6   7   8   9   10

Self-Care.   Self-care relates to concern and attention to one's well-being in all of its dimensions. Choosing to develop safety habits, including practicing preventive medical and dental care, wearing seat belts, and avoiding harmful substances including those in the environment, improves quality of life and extends longevity; failure to engage in these preventive health habits leads to declines in physical functioning and increased mortality. More than a sign of concern for one's physical well-being, however, the practice of safety habits may be interpreted as behavioral evidence of an existential desire for living. Conversely, the absence of self-care to whatever extent circumstances permit may be considered a sign of essential discouragement with life.

Self-Care
Overall Wellness   1   2   3   4   5   6   7   8   9   10

Satisfaction   1   2   3   4   5   6   7   8   9   10

Coping Self

There are four components to the Coping Self: *realistic beliefs, stress management, self-worth,* and *leisure.* Irrational beliefs are the source of frustrations and disappointments with life for many individuals. Even those who hold to such beliefs as "I need to please others" can cope successfully with life's requirements if they learn to manage the inevitable stress that they will experience. Likewise, self-worth can be enhanced through effective coping with life's challenges (Branden, 1994). As self-efficacy is experienced through success experiences, self-worth increases as well.

Finally, leisure is essential to this concept of wellness and continual development. Learning to become totally absorbed in an activity that makes time stand still helps one not only cope with but transcend the more difficult requirements of life. Leisure opens pathways to growth in both creative and spiritual dimensions. The Coping Self, then, encompasses elements that regulate the responses to life events and provides a means for transcending their negative effects.

Realistic Beliefs.   Healthy people are able to process information accurately and perceive reality as it is rather than as they wish it to be. They actively entertain thoughts that help them avoid conflict with others, find solutions to life's inevitable vexations, protect them from harm, achieve worthwhile personal goals, and maintain a positive emotional balance. People who have realistic beliefs are able to accept themselves as imperfect and to challenge irrational thoughts about "always, never, or should" in relation to themselves, others, and life circumstances. They can view others and life events from more than one perspective. From the DCT perspective, they cultivate and utilize their capacity to be dialectic, and they recognize that strivings for perfection will inevitably result in frustration as humans will always be less than perfect in most ways.

Realistic Beliefs

Overall Wellness	1	2	3	4	5	6	7	8	9	10
Satisfaction	1	2	3	4	5	6	7	8	9	10

Stress Management.   Stress affects both psychological and physiological functioning, and has a specific depressant effect on immune system functioning. People who are stress resistant experience more positive and beneficial immune system responses, greater resistance to psychosocial stressors, a more internal locus of control, more positive mental health, and greater physical health. Effective managers of stress include the capacity to experience change as positive, regulate one's time and energy to maintain balance, set realistic limits, self-monitor effectively, and be proactive in responding to life events.

Stress Management

Overall Wellness	1	2	3	4	5	6	7	8	9	10
Satisfaction	1	2	3	4	5	6	7	8	9	10

Self-Worth.   Self-worth is variously referred to in the literature as self-concept, self-esteem, and self-worth. Its essence, however, may be summed up simply as acceptance of oneself both in gifts and imperfections. Neither inflated nor discounted in value, one is unique, worthwhile, and deserving of all of life's benefits and confident in dealing with its disappointments. Faulty self-evaluation may be seen in behaviors that reveal a private logic devoted to excuses, blaming, complaining, fears, and "disabilities" designed to avoid meeting life's most basic tasks.

Self-Worth

Overall Wellness	1	2	3	4	5	6	7	8	9	10
Satisfaction	1	2	3	4	5	6	7	8	9	10

Leisure.   Leisure activities, including physical, social, intellectual, volunteer, and creative, have a positive effect on self-worth and overall wellness. Life satisfaction also is influenced by leisure congruence, defined as the selection of leisure activities consistent with one's personality type. This may be best represented by activities through which one loses track of time, feeling totally immersed in an activity that brings out one's innate creativity, talents, and personal passions for beauty, life, and creation.

Leisure

Overall Wellness	1	2	3	4	5	6	7	8	9	10
Satisfaction	1	2	3	4	5	6	7	8	9	10

Social Self

There are two components to this factor: *friendship* and *love*. Friendship and love can be conceived of as existing on a continuum and, as a consequence, not clearly distinguishable in practice. Sexual intimacy is sometimes thought to be a distinction between love and friendship but no such distinction seems appropriate as physical attraction and true love can sometimes (or often) have little in common. What is clear, however, is that friendships and intimate relationships do enhance the quality and length of one's life. Isolation, alienation, and separation from others generally are associated with all manner of poor health conditions and greater susceptibility to premature death, whereas social support remains in multiple studies as the strongest identified predictor of positive mental health over the lifespan. The mainstay of this support is family, with healthier families providing the most positive sources of individual wellness (Berg & Seeman, 1994). Importantly, healthy families can be either biological or families of choice.

Friendship.   This motivation is reflected in the need for frequent, positive interactions with the same persons, and the search for a long-term, stable, and caring support network. There is a strong positive connection between friendship quality and sense of well-being, including physical as well as mental health. This includes connectedness with others in nonsexual relationships, having a social support system in times of need or celebration, being able to give support to others, feeling comfortable with others, and possibly most important, not feeling lonely, alienated, or neglected.

Friendship

Overall Wellness	1	2	3	4	5	6	7	8	9	10
Satisfaction	1	2	3	4	5	6	7	8	9	10

Love.   Characteristics of healthy love relationships include the ability to be intimate, trusting, and self-disclosing with another person and the ability to receive as well as express affection with significant others. The life task of love also necessitates having a family or family-like support system that has the following nine characteristics: shared coping and problem-solving skills, commitment to the family, good and frequent communication, encouragement of individuals, regular expression of appreciation, shared religious/spiritual values, social connectedness, clear roles, and shared interests, values, and significant time together.

Love

Overall Wellness	1	2	3	4	5	6	7	8	9	10
Satisfaction	1	2	3	4	5	6	7	8	9	10

Creative Self

Adler spoke of the creative self as the combination of attributes that each of us forms to make a unique place among others in our social interactions (Adler, 1927/1954; Ansbacher & Ansbacher, 1956). We believe that the concept of a creative self is also appropriate to how each of us uniquely addresses being alive and sustaining life (Myers & Sweeney, 2004). From a DCT perspective, cognition, affect, and one's interpreting of life experiences has everything to do with one's capacity to develop and grow across the lifespan. Therefore, the Creative Self is in a constant state of processing, capable of changing cognitions, affective responses, and behaviors. However, as an outcome of being purposive (goal oriented), individuals seek to make a unique place among others that can either facilitate or thwart development, growth, and well-being.

There are five components to this factor: *thinking, emotions, control, positive humor,* and *work*. As research and clinical experience suggest, what one thinks affects the emotions as well as the body. Likewise, one's emotional experiences tend to influence one's cognitive responses to similar experiences. Control is a matter of perceived capacity to influence events in one's life. Positive expectations influence emotions, behavior, and anticipated outcomes. Enriching one's ability to think clearly, perceive accurately, and respond appropriately can decrease stress and enhance the humor response that medical research has shown affects the immune system positively. Likewise, work is an essential element in human experience that can enhance or undermine one's capacity to live life fully.

Work from an Adlerian perspective is a major life task of all persons. The term *work* is more inclusive than paid employment, however. Children "work" at play to master their environment. Older persons contribute to the well-being of others through a variety of volunteer and personal services that require working for them— that is, effort in service to others without remuneration or expectation of gain. Work, however, can and often does involve compensation for services and in everyday commerce some compensation is expected. The following describes the five components of the Creative Self in more detail.

Thinking.   Active thinking including analytical and creative activity is necessary for healthy brain functioning and hence quality of life across the lifespan (i.e., use it or lose it). Effective problem solving has been correlated with lower anxiety and depression, and greater overall psychological adjustment. Creativity has been identified as a universal characteristic of self-actualizing people, all of whom demonstrate originality, a special kind of creativeness, inventiveness, and problem-solving ability.

Thinking

Overall Wellness	1	2	3	4	5	6	7	8	9	10
Satisfaction	1	2	3	4	5	6	7	8	9	10

Emotions.   Individuals who are spontaneous in their behavior and emotions are able to experience a range of both positive and negative affect: anger, anxiety (fear), sadness, guilt, shame, disgust, interest/excitement, love/compassion, happiness/joy in a way that is conducive to positive human relations. With the freedom of children in expressing themselves, they reflect the wisdom of life when expressing emotions—such as anger or intimacy—appropriately.

Emotions

Overall Wellness	1	2	3	4	5	6	7	8	9	10
Satisfaction	1	2	3	4	5	6	7	8	9	10

Control.   The results of numerous studies indicate that people experience positive outcomes when they perceive themselves as having an impact on what happens to them and negative outcomes (e.g., depression) when they perceive a lack of personal control. Perceived control is associated with emotional well-being, successful coping with stress, better physical health, and better mental health over the lifespan.

Control

Overall Wellness	1	2	3	4	5	6	7	8	9	10
Satisfaction	1	2	3	4	5	6	7	8	9	10

Positive Humor.   Positive humor, a cognitive and emotional process, includes both recognition and appreciation of humorous events and creation of humorous situations. Positive humor neither hurts nor deprecates self or others. Quite the opposite, positive humor releases tension so that new insights may be gained, intimacy can be enhanced, and cohesiveness and trust can be established. Especially when accompanied by laughter, humor causes the skeletal muscles to relax, boosts the immune system, increases heart rate, stimulates circulation, oxygenates the blood, massages the vital organs, aids digestion, and releases chemicals (endorphins) into the brain that enhance a sense of well-being. This includes laughing at oneself, laughing with others (not at others), seeing the contradictions, oddities, and predicaments of life in an objective yet "funny" way, and learning new ways of coping as a result of life's surprises.

Positive Humor

Overall Wellness	1	2	3	4	5	6	7	8	9	10
Satisfaction	1	2	3	4	5	6	7	8	9	10

Work.   Work satisfaction, comprised of challenge, financial reward, coworker relations, and working conditions, is one of the best predictors of longevity as well as perceived quality of life. This involves feeling that one's skills are used appropriately, experiencing satisfaction and some degree of influence with both the process and product, feeling that time and resources are available to achieve what is expected, feeling valued by others in the effort, feeling secure with one's place as a contributing participant, and benefiting (by receiving pay or recognition) when appropriate to an extent at least equal to the task assigned or attempted.

Work
Overall Wellness   1   2   3   4   5   6   7   8   9   10

Satisfaction   1   2   3   4   5   6   7   8   9   10

Physical Self

The two components within this factor, Physical Self, are *nutrition* and *exercise*. These are widely promoted and, unfortunately, often overemphasized to the exclusion of other components of holistic well-being reported here that also are important. The research evidence is compelling with regard to the importance of exercise and nutrition, especially with changes over the lifespan. Not surprisingly, preliminary data suggest that "survivors," individuals who live longest, attend to both exercise and diet/nutrition. Counseling and psychotherapy theory and practice give insufficient attention to this area. Because of this, we suggest that you give it special attention in your own practice so that you can provide your clients with a more holistic and comprehensive view of successful progress through the lifespan.

Nutrition.   There is a clear relationship between what we eat and our health, moods, performance, and longevity. The eating and drinking habits of Americans have been implicated in 6 of the 10 leading causes of death, including the fact that more than one in every two Americans is considered to be overweight. Eating breakfast regularly, eating a variety of the food groups recommended, maintaining one's ideal weight, and drinking water in sufficient quantity each day are basic rules of thumb corroborated by research findings on healthy diets.

Nutrition
Overall Wellness   1   2   3   4   5   6   7   8   9   10

Satisfaction   1   2   3   4   5   6   7   8   9   10

Exercise.   Regular physical activity is essential in the prevention of disease and enhancement of health as well as for healthy aging. Exercise increases strength as well as self-confidence and self-esteem. Stretching, exercising for 20–30 minutes a day, and generally leading a physically active life are beneficial beyond what the effort seems to require.

Exercise
Overall Wellness   1   2   3   4   5   6   7   8   9   10

Satisfaction   1   2   3   4   5   6   7   8   9   10

Examining Your Self-Ratings

How do your wellness scores "feel" to you? What sense do you get out of this exercise thus far? What occurs for you as you reflect on your self-ratings? Allow thoughts and feelings to enter your mind freely.. In addition, confirm that these ratings are accur in terms of how you see your wellness at this point in time. Determine how representative the scores are of your total wellness.

_____

_____

_____

_____

What patterns do you note? Once you have completed your self-ratings, reflect on the scores to determine themes and patterns. Next, reflect on the pattern of your high and low scores. Select one or more of your lower scores as areas in which you would like to change in the direction of greater wellness. Alternately, you may wish to choose an area in which you received a high score yet would like to enhance your personal wellness further. Deliberately consider high score areas as assets that will be a source of strength when coping with those found less satisfactory (e.g., a good sense of humor can go a long way toward ameliorating discouragement when you find change in another area is difficult for you).

_____

_____

_____

_____

Developing an Intentional Personal Wellness Plan. Once wellness in each dimension has been assessed, either informally or formally, choose one or more areas of wellness that you would like to change and improve. We do not recommend trying to effect change in all areas simultaneously for two reasons. First, choosing to change in more than two or three areas will likely be overwhelming for anyone. Second, awareness of wellness needs combined with change in any one area is likely to increase overall wellness and wellness in specific additional areas of the model. Once you have identified the dimensions you would like to change in the direction of greater wellness, you can develop a personal wellness plan in each targeted area.

_____

_____

_____

_____

Both short- and long-range plans to improve your wellness are necessary: Patience is a virtue! We have found that many people are able to develop and implement their own wellness plans after a short while given only a blank worksheet whereas others prefer a more focused, step-by-step process involving discussion with a professional. Some areas of wellness are popular in the media today, such as the Physical Self wellness areas of nutrition and exercise, and little outside intervention may be required to help you experience positive change in these dimensions. Other areas, such as those within the Creative Self and the Coping Self, may benefit from traditional counseling interventions to facilitate change.

PROMOTING WELLNESS: A CASE ILLUSTRATION

The client, Victoria, is a 34-year-old Hispanic female. She is the oldest of six children, raised in a predominantly Hispanic neighborhood in a large metropolitan city in the Southwest. Religion has been very important in her early development. She attended Catholic schools and her family has strong traditional Catholic beliefs. She is a single parent raising two children, an 8-year-old son and a 10-year-old daughter. She is bilingual, graduated from college with honors, has a teaching degree, and has taught middle school math and science for six years. She and her husband of six years divorced three years ago after a separation of two years. She receives no financial assistance from her former husband and the only knowledge the children have of their father is through communication with their paternal grandparents.

Victoria arrived for her appointment accompanied by her son and daughter. She was eager to begin talking and did so easily but she appeared very intense and her voice was strained. She had been referred to the mental health agency by her physician because of insomnia and frequent unexplained crying spells. During the intake process, she stated that she was depressed, unable to sleep because of recurring nightmares, not eating, losing control of her two children, and having difficulty dealing with family members. She said that she has thought about suicide but stops due to the guilt she feels about abandoning her children. She has difficulty concentrating and this is impacting her teaching. She has been absent frequently from work and her principal is recommending that she take a leave of absence. This decision is causing her great distress as she needs the income to support her children.

If she leaves her teaching position, she will be forced to move back with her family. She is unable to maintain meaningful relationships with various males she has been dating and views her future as very negative.

Based on information gathered during the intake process, Victoria describes her family of origin as very close-knit, held together by both cultural and religious values. She was raised to be proud of her Hispanic heritage, her language, and her cultural traditions. She has three younger brothers and two younger sisters all of whom look to her for advice and support. Education was stressed in her home and her academic success was the source of much family pride. She was held up as a model to her siblings and was expected to perform in an exemplary way not only in school but also in other aspects of her life.

Her family, with the exception of one sister, was very opposed to Victoria's marriage and made their opposition known not only to Victoria, but also to Mark, her former husband. Victoria and Mark also experienced opposition from his parents. To avoid further confrontations, Victoria and Mark eloped and were married by a justice of the peace in a nearby state. Now, after her divorce, even her sister who had supported her decision to marry is unhappy with Victoria.

After even a brief opportunity to listen and observe Victoria, we perceive th for her to be at peace, she would be functioning as a caring, competent person a professional meeting her responsibilities with satisfaction to herself and others. She has the intelligence, education, and basic values needed to be successful. However, she has embedded within her basic life convictions the sources of her discouragement. An oldest child with high expectations for herself reinforced by "success" at home and school in meeting these expectations throughout her early years, she finds that she is cut off from everything that helped her to be what she is today.

Worse yet, she feels no peace within her spiritual self from which to draw strength and even unworthy of seeking it. It is not possible here to fully develop a treatment plan and illustrate specific techniques in the process. However, we will use some of the wellness model components to illustrate that regardless of a person's current level of functioning developmentally, through deliberate encouragement, we can enhance that person's capacity to meet her or his life tasks and increase enjoyment in doing so.

Reorientation to Wellness

After appropriate rapport, reflection, and empathy with Victoria's predicament, we would invite her to consider reframing the help she needs from crisis control to wellness. As we will learn in later chapters, a variety of both Adlerian and DCT methods can be employed to facilitate readiness for such a reframing of her purpose for counseling. When presented with the question, "Tell me, Victoria, what is more important to you after we address your immediate issues today: to learn how to cope with crises or instead how to become more able to live life fully with less stress and more joy?" This simple question offers hope, not for simple solutions but more desirable outcomes. With higher level purpose, greater sustained effort can be attained.

After addressing the emotional need for support and understanding, clients are invited to respond to a brief self-assessment on each of the components of the IS-Wel. Each component is explained and they select one on which to work immediately. In this case, Victoria gave herself low ratings for self-worth (Coping Self), control, and emotions (Creative Self). She was invited to learn the "push button" technique for relaxation by relaxing and imagining herself in control, safe, and at peace in whatever environment she chose. Likewise, she was invited to experience the challenge of pushing the button metaphorically and seeing, for example, her children "talking back" to their mother (or another image if we judge that one image is too emotionally stressful). The objective is to have her practice taking charge of her own images and, consequently, her emotions. We also worked with her to introduce a pleasant thought or scene just before fully falling asleep, giving her subconscious a directive to implement a new outcome to her sleep.

On other components of wellness, we would attend to the needs of Victoria with respect to exercise, nutrition (Physical Self), and self-care (Essential Self). In addition to any needed medical care, Victoria will benefit from stress relief, enjoy better sleep, experience less depression, and have more energy through attention to her own physical needs. She apparently needs permission to do so and instruction on where and how to begin.

Regarding work issues (Creative Self), we would ask Victoria if, after some rest, she thought she could imagine herself going back to teaching for perhaps a one-week trial. If this seemed too much, we would negotiate down to what she found comfortable. Naturally, her principal would need to understand that she was getting assistance and that this was a part of the plan. Our expectation would be for her cooperation with this modest goal and through it the beginnings of recovery and empowerment. We would teach Victoria to think about doing things "as if" she had all the confidence and support that she required. She would be asked to practice thinking this way outside the counseling sessions and reporting how she felt about it. As an aside, we note that as a responsible, oldest child in the family (Sweeney, 1998), she will be a willing learner. In fact, one of our admonitions will be to moderate her tendency to please and to do what is asked "perfectly"!

With respect to the friendship life task (Social Self), Victoria has friends but she has been so dispirited that she has been unavailable to them. We would invite her to rediscover the joy and satisfaction she feels in being with others who respect and care for her, especially those who help her laugh. We would make a short list of individuals whose company she enjoys. She would be asked to pick one or two to invite to dinner, a movie, or a similar activity for a specific time. We may talk about what she wishes to share with those she trusts the most and what she might reasonably expect from them in the way of support as caring friends.

We would help her identify colleagues at school with whom she could spend time at school during lunch, recess, and after school to help recreate a professional network of friends from whom she can get support. We would rehearse when and how she would act on some specific behavioral goals to achieve these contacts.

We would address male companionship, dating, and courting in due course. Victoria's "tool box" for relationship skills is based on what she observed between her parents and, possibly in this case, more of what she did not observe—what went on between her parents that she did not see or could not understand as a child. Helping her to assess her assets and needs realistically for further development will be a part of the process. We always build on assets, however, and as a consequence it is an encouraging process.

Victoria's most intimate relationships have been with her family. We would expect the children to be counseled with a purpose to winning their cooperation in reestablishing a happy home environment for all of them. We would invite Victoria to observe an Adlerian family counseling session and eventually to participate in a parent study group. Through these experiences, she will learn how her challenges with her children are shared by other families as well. Equally important, the children will be given support for the fact that they are not "bad" children and encouraged to feel loved and empowered as positive contributors to the household.

Naturally, the extended family is an important if not crucial component of Victoria's present crisis. We would hope to invite the entire family to join us for family counseling once we determine that Victoria is sufficiently strong to participate without undue risk. Because a full explanation of the family process goes beyond the scope of this chapter, the major point we wish to convey is the appreciation for a systemic approach to understanding and intervening with such a situation. Both the intrapsychic and interpersonal perspectives have validity when engaged in such a case. We wish to understand and empower Victoria while acknowledging the powerful influence and potential of the family system to either facilitate or thwart her progress toward maturity and good health. Our goal would be to help all the family members heal from the estrangement; affirm Victoria in her differentiation of self within the family; and encourage all to share their love, support, and common values once again, including celebration of grandchildren, spiritual practices and holidays, and open hearts.

Finally, Victoria has such a deep faith on which to draw for strength and comfort that we would encourage her to focus on it early in the counseling process (Essential Self: spirituality). As a Catholic, she learned in her formative years that a contrite confession would absolve all "sins" and even the worst sinner would be worthy of communion with her Lord once again. As a youngster, she was much admired by all who knew her as a responsible, even pious, young woman. Her parish priest would be one resource for her to reestablish her spiritual bonds and spiritual practices. In addition, there will be a divorced Catholics support and social group to which she can belong. Her pastor also may help the family appreciate that what the church teaches is an ideal, but it is also aware of the human condition and ministers to all as God's children as did Jesus. Victoria is her parents' child still and needs their support, love, and understanding.

Case Caveat

Adler had an expression that "everything can be something else!" or words to that effect. By touching on only a few illustrations within these paragraphs, we run the risk of omitting someone's preferred method or not illustrating adequately those that are mentioned. Therefore, attempting to provide a brief overview related principally to wellness alone does an injustice to the depth and breadth of these approaches in theory as well as practice.

In addition, we have deliberately touched on components of the wellness model as we have integrated them into the Adlerian constructs of life tasks. As presented in the case of Victoria, we see the use of the wellness model to help Victoria move from a deficit mode of functioning to what is considered more "normal." In point of fact, we would continue to work with Victoria using both Adlerian and DCT methods to take her to new levels of functioning in as many areas as she found desirable, including those mentioned and more. Her sense of humor, for example, could be enhanced to her great benefit. In short, Victoria is a terrific candidate not only to "get better," but to live life more fully, joyfully, and with greater satisfaction and peace of mind and spirit.

SUMMARY

In this chapter, a new holistic human development paradigm for helping is presented. The whole is greater than the sum of the parts and that "whole" is the sum of each individual. In lieu of the more traditional concept of facilitating development to a goal of "normalcy," given that what is "normal" is defined based on what is most common, and what is most common is not always optimum (e.g., more than half of the population is overweight, which does not make being overweight desirable), wellness was presented as a new paradigm for optimizing development.

Wellness is the most desirable outcome goal of helping interventions. This is an encouraging, positive position that helps client grow throughout the lifespan. Wellness is neither normative nor finite but rather is idiographic and ongoing for each person. Wellness choices made at any point in the lifespan will affect subsequent development in positive and holistic ways. Development, then, is truly an individual journey without end.

Three key aspects of Adlerian theory are stressed in this chapter—socio (connectedness), teleo (goal-oriented), and analytic (the unconscious). The healthy individual develops in relation to others, with specific goals, but often in a fashion and direction of which he or she is not fully conscious.

The Wheel of Wellness model of human development places spirituality and wellness at the center in how we manage our lives. This model may be particularly useful for you as you work with clients who are struggling with meaning or spirituality as a central issue.

The Indivisible Self Model for Wellness (IS-Wel), based on research, stresses the connectedness of all dimensions of wellness. A special feature of this model is its emphasis on contextual dimensions and its immediate applicability to the interview.

Self-assessment of wellness patterns is a vital part of a healthy and holistic lifespan plan. You were asked to engage in a self-assessment and we encourage you to work through this same self-assessment with your clients.

Challenges: Counseling, psychology, social work, and other human service professions often take an illness or deficit approach to human problems. Wellness and developmental counseling and therapy take an alternative approach in the firm belief that clients grow from strengths. One of your professional challenges will be to maintain the wellness approach in the face of those who seek to maintain the primary focus on human weakness rather than strength.

Research issues: How might wellness, and the meaning of wellness, differ among people of different ages? How does the meaning of concepts such as spirituality differ over the lifespan? To answer these and related questions, interview people of different ages to determine their perceptions of wellness. You might consider using available formal assessment instruments (e.g., the IS-Wel) to collect data and pursue statistical comparisons across groups.

THEORY INTO PRACTICE: DEVELOPING YOUR PORTFOLIO OF COMPETENCE

Self-Assessment Exercises

Exercise 1. Reflections on theory

Take a moment to review the three key Adlerian constructs of socio-teleo-analytic. What are examples from your own life that validate these three concepts? Think about your own behaviors, thoughts, feelings, and personal history as you consider these areas.

Socio: _____

_____

_____

_____

Teleo: _____

_____

_____

_____

Analytic: _____

_____

_____

Exercise 2. Wellness assessment

Review the self-assessment of wellness completed earlier in this chapter. Recall that you were asked to do two ratings, each on a scale of 1 to 10. First, you rated *your perception of your overall wellness in an area*, then you rated *your level of satisfaction with your wellness in that area*. For which two or three areas of wellness did you report the *highest* perceptions of your own wellness?

_____

_____

How did your level of satisfaction with your wellness compare to your rated levels of wellness in these areas?

_____

_____

For which two or three areas of wellness did you report the *lowest* perceptions of your own wellness?

_____

_____

How did your level of satisfaction with your wellness compare to your rated levels of wellness in these areas?

_____

_____

For which two or three areas did you report the most satisfaction with your own wellness?

_____

_____

Are there any areas of wellness you would like to change or improve? What are those areas?

_____

_____

Exercise 3. Developing a wellness plan

Develop a plan for change for the area(s) of wellness identified in Exercise 2 above.

What is your baseline of behavior, thought, and feeling in this area (i.e., what are the specific behaviors, thoughts, and/or feelings you have now that you would like to change)?

_____

_____

What is your goal for change? What will life be like when you have made this change toward greater wellness?

_____

_____

What are some self-help strategies and resources you can use to help you change (e.g., books, behavioral charts/records, special food, clothing, exercise equipment)?

_____

_____

What people can serve as resources to help you change (i.e., family, friends, professionals, counselors)?

_____

_____

When and how will you evaluate the change process?

_____

_____

Toward Multicultural Competence

Exercise 4. Understanding life experiences of persons from other cultures and backgrounds

Interview persons of varying age, gender, spiritual/religious beliefs, and ethnic background to determine their perceptions of the meaning of "wellness." How do their descriptions inform your understanding of personal and cultural influences in the meaning-making processes of individuals and groups? How do their responses affect your understanding of wellness across the lifespan?

Exercise 5. Group practice

Divide into small groups. Assign each group one or more of the five factors in the Indivisible Self wellness model. Interview persons of varying age, gender, spiritual/religious beliefs, and ethnic background to determine their perceptions of the meaning of each factor and its subcomponents. Develop a list of observed healthy and unhealthy behaviors related to cultural issues. Discuss how wellness differs across cultures, and how those differences could affect your counseling interventions.

Interviewing Practice Exercises

Exercise 6

With a partner, discuss the meaning of wellness. Examine the two models of wellness presented earlier and discuss your reactions to each one and in particular to the hypothesized and empirical relationships among the various wellness constructs. Which model is most useful in explaining your personal view of wellness?

Exercise 7

Divide into small groups. Assign each group one or more of the five factors in the Indivisible Self wellness model. For each component of the factor, develop a list of observed healthy and unhealthy behaviors in others. Discuss how you can help people become aware of unhealthy behaviors. What strategies could you use to promote healthier development in regard to the 5 factors and 17 components of wellness?

Generalization: Taking Adlerian and Wellness Concepts Home

Exercise 8. Practice and observation with life choices

During the next week, pay close attention to your daily choices and decisions relative to the areas of wellness in the Indivisible Self model. It may be easy to notice what you choose to eat and when and how you choose to exercise. Though more difficult, it is also important to be aware of when you laugh and what makes you laugh, when you feel a need to be perfect and when you allow yourself the courage to be imperfect. Be aware of when you feel satisfaction with your work and leisure activities, and what brings you satisfaction. Also, pay attention to your relationships with others. What are the components of wellness in those relationships that help you live your life more fully?

Portfolio Reflections

Exercise 9. Reflections on your wellness

What stood out for you from this chapter? What sense do you make of the exercises on your wellness? What are the key points you want to remember from this chapter? Record your thoughts below and in your Portfolio Folder.

_____

_____

_____

_____

_____

_____

_____

_____

_____

REFERENCES

Adler, A. (1954). *Understanding human nature* (W. B. Wolf, Trans.). New York: Fawcett. (Original work published 1927)

American Counseling Association. (1991, July 13). *Minutes of governing council meeting.* Alexandria, VA: Author.

Ansbacher, H. L. (Ed.). (1969). *The science of living: Alfred Adler.* Garden City, NY: Doubleday.

Ansbacher, H. L., & Ansbacher, R. R. (Eds.). (1967). *The individual psychology of Alfred Adler.* New York: Harper & Row.

Arciniega, G. M. & Newlon, B. J. (1999). In D. Capuzzi & D. R. Gross (Eds.), *Counseling and psychotherapy* (pp. 435–455). Upper Saddle River, NJ: Merrill.

Berg, M. M., & Seeman, T. E. (1994). Families and health: The negative side of social ties. *Annals of Behavioral Medicine, 16,* 109–115.

Branden, N. (1994). *Six pillars of self-esteem.* New York: Bantam.

Bronfenbrenner, U. (1999). Environments in developmental perspective: Theoretical and operational models. In S. L. Friedman & T. D. Wachs (Eds.), *Measuring environment across the life span: Emerging methods and concepts* (pp. 3–28). Washington, DC: American Psychological Association.

Dreikurs, R. (1967). *Psychodynamics, psychotherapy, and counseling.* Chicago: Alfred Adler Institute.

Dreikurs, R. (1971). *Social equality: The challenge of today.* Chicago: Regnery.

Fetzer Institute–National Institute on Aging Workgroup. (1999). *Multidimensional measure of religiousness/spirituality for use in health research: A report of the Fetzer Institute–National Institute on Aging Workgroup.* Kalamazoo, MI: Fetzer Institute.

Frankl, V. E. (1959). *Man's search for meaning.* New York: Beacon.

Hattie, J. A., Myers, J. E., & Sweeney, T. J. (in press). A multidisciplinary model of wellness: The development of the wellness evaluation of lifestyle. *Journal of Counseling & Development.*

Ivey, A. (2000). *Developmental therapy: Theory into practice.* North Amherst, MA: Microtraining. (Original work published 1986)

Ivey, A., & Ivey, M. (2003). *Intentional interviewing and counseling: Facilitating client development in a multicultural world* (5th ed.). Pacific Grove, CA: Brooks/Cole.

Larson, D. D. (1999). The conceptualization of health. *Medical Care Research and Review, 56,* 123–136.

Lee, C. C., & Richardson, B. (1997). *Multicultural issues in counseling: New approaches to diversity.* Alexandria, VA: American Counseling Association.

Locke, D. C., Myers, J. E., & Herr, E. L. (Eds.). (2001). *The handbook of counseling.* Thousand Oaks, CA: Sage.

Maslow, A. (1970). *Motivation and personality* (2nd ed.). New York: Harper & Row. (Original work published 1954)

Mosak, H. H., & Dreikurs, R. (1967). The life tasks III, the fifth life task. *Individual Psychologist, 5*(1), 16, 22.

Mosak, H. H., & Dreikurs, R. (1973). Adlerian psychotherapy. In R. Corsini (Ed.), *Current psychotherapies.* Itasca, IL: Peacock.

Myers, J. E. (1992). Wellness, prevention, development: The cornerstone of the profession. *Journal of Counseling and Development, 71*(2), 136–139.

Myers, J. E., Emmerling, D., & Leafgren, F. (Eds.). (1992). Wellness throughout the lifespan. *Journal of Counseling and Development* (special issue), *71.*

Myers, J. E., Luecht, R. M., & Sweeney, T. J. (2003). *Reexamining the Wellness Evaluation of Lifestyle: Defining new constructs for assessing wellness.* Manuscript submitted for review.

Myers, J. E., & Sweeney, T. J. (2002). IS-Wel: Indivisible Self-Wellness Inventory. Lexington, NC: Authors.

Myers, J. E., & Sweeney, T. J. (2004). *Counseling for wellness: Theory, research, and practice.* Alexandria, VA: American Counseling Association.

Myers, J. E., & Sweeney, T. J. (In press). The indivisible self: An evidence-based model of wellness. *Journal of Individual Psychology.*

Myers, J. E., Sweeney, T. J., & Witmer, J. M. (1998). *Workbook for the Wellness Evaluation of Lifestyle.* Greensboro, NC: Authors.

Myers, J. E., Sweeney, T. J., & Witmer, J. M. (2000). The Wheel of Wellness counseling for wellness: A holistic model for treatment planning. *Journal of Counseling and Development, 78*(3), 251–266.

Myers, J. E., Sweeney, T. J., & Witmer, J. M. (2001). Optimization of behavior: Promotion of wellness. In D. C. Locke, J. E. Myers, & E. H. Herr (Eds.), *The handbook of counseling.* Thousand Oaks, CA: Sage.

Myers, J. E., & Williard, K. (2003). Integrating spirituality into counseling and counselor training: A developmental, wellness approach. *Counseling & Values, 47,* 142–155.

Palmo, A. J., Shosh, M. J., & Weikel, W. J. (2001) In D. C. Locke, J. E. Myers, & E. H. Herr (Eds.), *The handbook of counseling* (pp. 653–668). Thousand Oaks, CA: Sage.

Prochaska, J. O., DiClemente, C. C., & Norcross, J. C. (1992). In search of how people change: Applications to addictive behaviors. *American Psychologist, 47*(9), 1102–1114.

Richards, P., & Bergin, A. (2000). *Handbook of psychotherapy and religious diversity.* Washington, DC: American Psychological Association.

Seligman, M. (1998a). Depression and violence. Comments to the National Press Club, Morning Newsmaker series, September 3, 9:00 AM, Washington, DC.

Seligman, M. (1998b). *Learned optimism.* New York: Pocket Books.

Seligman, M. (2002a). *Authentic happiness.* New York: Free Press.

Seligman, M. (2002b). *Positive psychology.* Washington, DC: American Psychological Association. Available online: http://www.apa.org/releases/positivepsy.html

Snyder, C., & Lopez, S. (2001). *Handbook of positive psychology.* Oxford: Oxford University Press.

Sweeney, T. (1995). Adlerian theory. In D. Cappuzi & D. Gross (Eds.), *Counseling and psychotherapy.* Columbus, OH: Merrill.

Sweeney, T. J. (1998). *Adlerian counseling: A practitioner's approach* (4th ed.). Muncie, IN: Accelerated Development.

Sweeney, T. J. (2001). Counseling: Historical origins and philosophical roots. In D. C. Locke, J. E. Myers, & E. H. Herr (Eds.), *The handbook of counseling* (pp. 3–27). Thousand Oaks, CA: Sage.

Sweeney, T. J., & Myers, J. E. (2001). A new model of wellness: The IS-Wel. Lexington, NC: Authors.

Sweeney, T. J., & Witmer, J. M. (1991). Beyond social interest: Striving toward optimum health and wellness. *Individual Psychology, 47*(4), 527–540.

Witmer, J. M., & Sweeney, T. J. (1992). A holistic model for wellness and prevention over the lifespan. *Journal of Counseling and Development, 71,* 140–148.

Witmer, J. M., & Sweeney, T. J. (1998). Toward wellness: The goal of counseling. In T. J. Sweeney, *Adlerian counseling: A practitioner's approach* (4th ed.). Muncie, IN: Accelerated Development.

CHAPTER 3
Development Over the Lifespan
Developmental Counseling as Lifespan Therapy

CENTRAL PRACTICE OBJECTIVE | Mastery and practice of concepts in this chapter will enable you to conduct a lifespan review with clients, to assess and understand their unique developmental history and current normative life transitions and challenges, and to anticipate their later developmental concerns.

This chapter focuses on theories of development and concludes with methods for taking developmental theory into concrete practice. Lifespan development is more than linear growth over time. We do not just move through a series of events in our lives. Our early individual and family experiences shape us and may empower us to face the future. The manner in which we have connected with others in the past provides us with resources as we move toward autonomy and individuation. But autonomy and individuation are not enough. We need to reattach with others throughout our lives—with friends and lovers, children, and coworkers. Balancing the twin needs of separation and attachment, connection and autonomy, is core to all the lifespan developmental tasks we all face.

Knowledge of and skill in the concepts of this chapter can enable you to:

1. Develop a context for understanding comprehensive lifespan developmental patterns by examining some key ideas from Bowlby's attachment theory.
2. Expand the concept of self and how each of us relates to our developmental history through ideas such as self-in-relation, Ogbonnya's person-as-community, and the Wellesley Stone Center concept of being-in-relation.
3. Utilize a foundation for understanding the complexities of human development and change, starting with a brief review of Erikson's lifespan theory.
4. Examine the theoretical foundations of cognitive developmental theories proposed by Kohlberg, Loevinger, and Kegan.
5. Consider the impact of gender on developmental processes, as introduced by Gilligan.
6. Utilize Schlossberg's transition theory as an organizing framework for understanding human reactions to changes that occur over the lifespan.
7. Move theory into practice using Tamase's introspective developmental counseling.
8. Integrate wellness as the goal of optimum lifespan development.

INTRODUCTION: ATTACHMENT AND SEPARATION—DEVELOPMENTAL CHALLENGES ACROSS THE LIFESPAN

John Bowlby's attachment theory (1969, 1973, 1990) provides a strong foundation for developmental theory, and this chapter starts with basics from this theory that are important for practice. Our past relationships with others become organized into patterns that tend to repeat again and again. Both positive and problematic aspects of the self can often be traced back to critical events in a person's life that later manifest as repeating behaviors, thoughts, and feelings. A developmental approach to counseling and therapy requires an awareness of these patterns manifested as the person-in-context or being-in-relation (Baker Miller, Stiver, & Hooks, 1998). This chapter presents several approaches to enriching our understanding of lifespan development, but all are based on the way we relate to and attach to one another.

Bowlby (1990) described attachment as a close emotional bond between an infant and a caregiver (usually the mother). He suggested that infants are active in creating attachment behaviors, using biological behaviors such as smiling and crying to elicit nurturing behaviors from the caregiver. How caregivers respond to infant needs has a lifespan impact on the development and maintenance of all relationships. The self does not develop by itself spontaneously. Rather, the relationships we have with others are the critical elements in nurturing and developing us as unique biological human beings. The self exists in context.

Attachment develops during infancy through repeated interactions between caregivers and the child and is most important during the first year of life. Schaffer (1996) described the development of attachment through four phases. During the first two months of life, attachment is instinctive, and most humans are likely to elicit smiling and crying behaviors from the newborn child. Between the ages of 2 and 7 months, the baby learns to distinguish among caregivers, and attachment focuses on the primary caregiver. Between 7 months and 2 years of age, the child develops more specific attachments to additional figures, such as the father. He or she now desires regular contact with the primary caregiver(s). From 2 years of age on, children become increasingly aware of themselves as separate from others and start taking the concerns, ideas, and/or feelings of others into account in their own choices and actions.

Mary Ainsworth (1978) studied attachment theory and was the first to place it on a secure research footing. She noted that some infants are more positively and securely attached to caregivers than other infants. Her research and that of others based on her hypotheses conclusively demonstrated that the actions of caregivers have a significant and lasting impact on the development of infants. For example, infants who are securely attached during the first year of life experience more positive emotionality, particularly in relation to others, and are more able to explore their world without fear of abandonment by their caregiver than are infants with less secure attachments. Infants who are insecurely attached may avoid their mothers, engage in excessive clinging (i.e., dependent) behavior, or develop patterns of avoidance and fearfulness. Research reveals that attachment pattern styles continue into adulthood. See Cassidy, Shaver, and Main (1999) to review the extensive research supporting attachment theory.

For some children, there is consistency between early caregiver behaviors and later development; for others, the link is not so clear. This may be because attachment develops during a preverbal stage; thus the sensorimotor period that Piaget describes, when the child relates to the world through senses and motor behavior, offers another avenue to understanding this early critical developmental period. Feelings at this point (as well as later in development and throughout life) are clearly physically embedded. Whereas most counseling and therapy approaches reflect an inability to access these early body experiences, developmental counseling and therapy (DCT) provides an avenue for helping individuals understand the impact of preverbal learning on their adult development and functioning. Of course, this is especially significant in helping people develop healthy relationships, which emerges as a central goal of the counseling and therapy process.

SELF AND/OR SELF-IN-RELATION

When you conduct counseling and therapy from a developmental point of view, the very nature of the word *self* changes. Traditionally, the field has viewed the self from an individualistic frame of reference with a focus on building client self-esteem, self-actualization, and self-efficacy. All these constructions of the self are important within a developmental context, but we are more than an individual and autonomous self.

Developmentally, the idea of an autonomous, separate self is ultimately incomplete. All the strands of developmental theory presented in this book emphasize the connected, related self. Attachment theory and its extensive research reveal clearly that the healthy individual develops in connection with others. Object relations theories, of course, make the same point. The infant and child develop a sense of self in relationships with their mother and other key caregivers (cf. Greenberg & Mitchell, 1983; Mahler, 2000; Winnicott, 1987).

Lifespan and wellness theory also reminds us that we can find mental health only in relation to others. Developmental counseling and therapy stresses the dialectic between interviewer and client, and you will find many of your clients reenacting the developmental history of attachment and separation theory with you in the interview. DCT argues that the development of the self continues as a central dimension of the here and now of the interview, recognizing that the self is not fixed, but rather is constantly changing as context and relationships shift.

The multicultural view, often termed multicultural counseling and therapy (MCT), could be described as an overarching and expanded framework for everything discussed so far in this chapter. We develop as selves-in-relation in a cultural/environmental context. Thus, attachment, lifespan, and other developmental theories all exist in connection to our multicultural world (Sue, Ivey, & Pedersen, 1996).

If we are to help individuals become autonomous and self-actualized, an important part of that process is helping them become aware of their connections with others. Consciousness of self in social context is central and essential. The individualistic word *self* is replaced by *self-in-context, self-in-relation, person-as-community* (Ogbonnya, 1994), or *being-in-relation* as described by the Wellesley Stone Center (Baker Miller, Stiver, & Hooks, 1998) and reflected in the Indivisible Self Model of Wellness discussed in Chapter 2.

Other-esteem, or esteem for others, has been introduced as a solution for a society that is too focused on self and self-esteem (Hwang, 2000). Other-esteem focuses on respecting, caring for, and valuing all human beings. It is obviously a key dimension of empathy—learning and accepting what the other person feels and thinks. Self-esteem and self-actualization remain important, but only if they are balanced by awareness of the self-in-relation.

Developmental counseling and therapy (DCT) points out that internal emotional distress is often related to external stressors. So-called disorder is often a reaction to disordered environmental or social conditions such as trauma, racism, and oppression. If we are to work successfully and positively with our clients, we need to become more fully aware of their lifespan experience. It does little good to treat an individual for depression or post-traumatic stress without consideration of her or his external stressors and developmental history.

From the DCT frame of reference, counseling and psychotherapy give insufficient attention to Oneness—the wholeness of the individual, the interconnectedness of the family, and the contextual aspects of the group. As we develop and work our way through life, there are multiple ways of viewing the journey. Some perspectives and ways of thinking and being are more useful than others, but the ability to flex intentionally and move with a constantly changing world is invaluable. We need to think both of the individual and of the multiple contexts within which that person lives—family, group, culture, and the impact of life experiences.

The Buddhist view of development also supplies additional insights into the nature of the connected self:

> Western psychology studies the development of the ego (as a structure) horizontally, in terms of stages spanning a number of years in childhood. Buddhist psychology looks at the egoic self in a more vertical, immediate way—as the activity of recreating and reinforcing our concept of self over and over again at every moment. (Welwood, 2002, p. 42)

Those of us in the helping professions can have an important part in helping our clients develop both a sense of connection with others and a sense of appropriate boundaries and separateness. The self is always under construction.

LIFESPAN THEORY: THE DEVELOPMENTAL TASKS OF INDIVIDUALS

Erikson (1963, 1994) lists eight key stages of development, with accompanying developmental tasks at each age. Each stage has a corresponding critical developmental issue. If these developmental tasks are not completed and the critical issue not resolved (adequate horizontal development), achieving maturity at the next stage (vertical development) will be difficult, perhaps impossible.

Erikson's life stages and developmental tasks are presented below. As you review these stages, think about what stage you are in currently and identify some of your own key developmental tasks.

Infancy (ages 0 through 2)—the developmental issue is generating a sense of trust versus mistrust. If the child does not develop a sense of trust at this stage, this failure will impact the forming of attachments with others throughout life.

Early childhood (ages 2 through 4)—the developmental issue is autonomy versus shame and doubt, or in Eriksonian terms, "letting go" versus "holding on." In this critical separation task, can the child find a unique personal space among many demands made by family and culture?

Preschool/kindergarten (ages 4 through 7)—the issue is initiative versus guilt. Can the child start to direct her or his own life or will others make these determinations on how the child lives?

Elementary school (ages 7 through 12) the issue is industry versus inferiority. Can the child develop a sense of competence and capability?

Adolescence (ages 12 through 19)—the issue is identity versus role confusion. Can the adolescent define a separate and distinct role identity as an individual? If earlier developmental tasks are incomplete, accomplishing this task may be impossible.

Young adulthood (ages 19 through 30)—the issue is intimacy versus isolation. Building on the past foundation, can the young adult find a sense of closeness with others?

Middle adulthood (ages 30 through 60)—the issue is generativity versus stagnation. The midlife adult experiences a need to give back to others, family members (children) as well as society; thus Adler's concept of social interest discussed in Chapter 2 aids in understanding the central challenge of the middle years.

Later adulthood (ages 60 +)—the issue is ego integrity versus despair. The fully mature adult accepts both failures and successes and is able to integrate them into a meaningful life pattern.

Erikson's lifespan theory maintains that the major developmental tasks of early childhood are to develop a sense of trust, autonomy, and initiative. To master these tasks requires a supportive family and cultural environment. If early life stages are not negotiated successfully, difficulties will develop later for the child, adolescent, or adult and may preclude the development of a sense of autonomy, an individual identity, or generativity. Each life stage requires a varying balance of separation and attachment.

Erikson also theorizes that all developmental conflicts are present throughout the lifespan. Each life stage has certain developmental tasks that are most critical at that time, but uncompleted developmental tasks may manifest themselves as problems later in life. At each life stage, the conflicts that come with other life stages are still factors. That is, although the infant's major life issue may be trust versus mistrust, other developmental tasks also exist. An infant begins developing a sense of autonomy and capability as it matures physically, emotionally, and cognitively. All infants gain more impact on the world and thus achieve a sense of initiative. If parents squash this initiative, a sense of guilt and inferiority may begin to emerge. The development of trust or mistrust between a child and caregiver can affect later developmental tasks, but if a child generates a sense of trust, later generation of a satisfactory personal identity and intimacy with others is more easily accomplished.

Upon deeper examination, Erikson's model shows that all life issues are present all the time. At first glance, the model seems linear, but in truth it is holistic. The developmental tasks of life repeat themselves again and again as patterns that eventually become what we call "personality." The adult struggling with the central issue of generativity versus stagnation still deals with issues of intimacy versus isolation, identity versus role confusion, and trust versus mistrust. The young child, in very different ways, deals with intimacy (being close with parents), role (sex role, family role), and even generativity (children are always creating as they learn and develop).

Different cultures resolve developmental conflicts in different ways. The predominantly White North American culture, for example, emphasizes individual autonomy. Autonomy is often less important for Hispanic and African American people. In many cultures, autonomy is more relational and family centered. In Japanese culture, dependence on the group is the traditional goal, and totally autonomous individualism is discouraged.

Using Erikson's lifespan framework with no consideration of cultural differences can result in serious error. The definition of healthy trust, autonomy, initiative, and other life-stage issues varies among cultural groups. Also, men and women may differ significantly in their developmental issues at Eriksonian stages. For example, you will find in the following section that some serious criticisms are made of the Eriksonian model as it relates to women in the adolescent and later years. Even in infancy females

Table 3-1   Comparisons of Cognitive Developmental Theories

Developmental Theory/Theorist	Concrete		Abstract	
	Stage or Style 1	Stage or Style 2	Stage or Style 3	Stage or Style 4
DCT	Sensorimotor	Concrete	Formal	Dialectic/systemic
Piaget	Sensorimotor/ preoperational	Concrete	Formal	Post-formal
Maslow's hierarchy	Survival and safety	Belonging	Self-esteem	Self-actualization
Erikson's lifespan	Trust vs. mistrust	Initiative vs. guilt, industry vs. inferiority	Identity vs. role diffusion	Intimacy vs. isolation, integrity vs. despair
Kohlberg's moral development		Punishment and obedience, instrumental orientation	Interpersonal and concordance	Societal and principled orientation
Kegan's evolving self	Incorporative, impulsive	Imperial	Interpersonal	Interindividual
Loevinger's ego development	Impulsive	Self-protective, conformist	Self-aware, conscientious, individualistic, autonomous	Integrated

and males are treated differently, by family members as well as strangers. Even well-meaning individuals can counteract parental desires to raise children outside of gender stereotypes by bringing presents such as blue items for males and pink items for females, and by encouraging gender-stereotyped play activities.

As a helping professional, you will need to address the specific life tasks of your clients. Many adult clients have never developed an adequate foundation of trust, autonomy, industry, and identity. Your therapeutic task is to help them complete and build an adequate developmental foundation. A foundation of trust is essential for full generativity in life.

Table 3-1 compares Erikson's life stages with those of Piaget, showing the individual's cognitive and affective development as he or she works through Eriksonian developmental tasks. The first row of the table relates the two models to the action dimensions of developmental counseling and therapy. Trust is generated primarily in the sensorimotor stage. At this stage, the child is particularly vulnerable to the environment. The generation of initiative and control occurs when the child is particularly likely to engage in magical thinking (late sensorimotor). A sense of industry and competence is generated during the concrete operational period.

The relationship between Erikson's and Piaget's frameworks becomes particularly clear in adolescence, the period of identity development. To develop a clear identity, one must step outside oneself and think about oneself from a new perspective; this is an abstract, formal-operational task. If adolescents do not feel good about themselves, owing to previous life experience (for example, the failure to develop trust or a sense of industry earlier), generating a positive identity will be difficult. As this lack of positive self-identity continues over the lifespan, individuals will experience problems in adulthood and maturity.

Clients come to psychotherapy stuck in old, unworkable life patterns, patterns they have learned throughout their lives. One of the important tasks of the therapist is to find the relationship between present styles of behaving and past developmental history. Armed with this understanding, the therapist can encourage behavioral and cognitive action that will help the client overcome past developmental blocks.

Developmental and counseling therapy focuses on the basic concrete and formal life tasks of sensorimotor, concrete operational, and formal-operational development; DCT practitioners generally prefer the word *style* to the more linear *level* or *stage*. The therapy is oriented toward a holistic view, reflecting the idea that all styles have value, rather than one style being "better than" another. The systematic learning sequence of DCT provides an opportunity for the therapist and client to return to the beginning of development and learn about the nature of trust and mistrust (sensorimotor), industry and inferiority (concrete), and identity versus role confusion (abstract/formal). The abstract dialectic/systemic style focuses on issues of ego integrity and the organization and meaning of experience. Failure to integrate successfully can result in despair.

The dialectic style represents post-formal thinking. Such thinking is complex and reflective. Interestingly, considering Piaget's observation that only three-fourths of people achieve fully abstract formal-operational thought, it is likely that an even smaller percentage is able to engage in truly dialectic thinking. DCT interventions and questioning style can help people learn to think more abstractly and to use both formal and dialectic/systemic concepts.

Finally, formal and dialectic/systemic thought are closely related to perspective taking—seeing the situation from another person's point of view. You will find that even concretely oriented children can still see other perspectives if you use concrete questions. For example, "How would you feel if you had been hit or teased?" often enables the child to imagine how another child might feel and think. Children and adolescents who experience prejudice as a result of systemic racism often are able to discuss these issues in a dialectic/systemic fashion, perhaps prompted by those in their home environment.

COGNITIVE DEVELOPMENTAL THEORIES

Three major cognitive theories are presented in this section. Like developmental counseling and therapy (DCT), all of them are derived from Piagetian thought. The idea that cognitive style changes over time appears to be well grounded in the three theoretical perspectives discussed in this section and in research on Piagetian constructs. Together, they strengthen the idea that it is appropriate for therapists to match therapeutic style with the cognitive/emotional style of the client. The three theories presented here, however, tend to be descriptive rather than suggesting specific modes of treatment that may be useful in meeting client needs. Chapters 4 and 5 focus on how to take cognitive/emotional developmental theory into concrete and specific action in the interview.

Perry (1970) studied the transition from adolescence to young adulthood, noting the tendency of adolescents to engage in absolute, dualistic thinking. As they enter adulthood, most people become aware of diverse points of view among others and the multiple perspectives of others. Thus, there is movement from either/or thinking to the reflective or relativistic thinking of adults. This new way of thinking has been defined as post-formal thought, a new, fifth stage of cognitive development. It may be best understood through the work of theorists such as Kohlberg, Loevinger, and Kegan. These perspectives are summarized in Table 3-1, along with the work of Piaget (discussed in Chapter 1), Erikson, and the DCT perspective. Maslow's (1954/1993) work is also summarized in the table as the levels in his hierarchy correspond closely with the DCT paradigm.

Kohlberg's Theory of Moral Development

Kohlberg (1981) extended Piaget's theory of cognitive development to explain what he termed a universal sequence of stages in the development of moral reasoning. Similar to Piaget, Kohlberg's stages are hierarchical, linear, and invariant. His theory is based on the rules that people use to make moral decisions and to cope with moral and ethical dilemmas.

Kohlberg identified three levels of moral reasoning, each of which is further divided into two sublevels or stages. The first level, preconventional, corresponds to Piaget's stage of preoperational thought. Children in this stage reason based on external sanctions. They begin with an obedience orientation, believing that those in authority "know" what is right and wrong. As they move into an instrumental orientation, consistent with concrete thought processes, they begin to be concerned with their own needs and justify their actions based on those needs.

At the second level, termed conventional morality, moral reasoning is based on societal or interpersonal norms. This is consistent with early formal thinking. The later stage in this level, termed social system morality, is also known as a "law and order" orientation. People choose to follow laws and rules because they believe that laws exist to promote the common good.

Moral reasoning based on a personal moral code marks the postconventional level. Rather than look for external guidance, in the fifth stage people make moral decisions based on a social contract. This type of reasoning is consistent with fully formal-operational thinking. It is only in Kohlberg's final stage, that of universal ethical principles, that dialectic thinking is achieved. In this stage, abstract principles such as justice create the foundation for a personal code of ethical conduct. Kohlberg suggested that few people reach this final stage of reasoning. Again, not everyone reasons in a dialectic manner.

Loevinger's Theory of Ego Development

Loevinger (1976, 1998) proposed and tested a theory of ego development over the lifespan that includes several discrete stages of cognitive change. The early stages in this theory reflect simple and undifferentiated modes of construing events; the later stages represent complex and differentiated cognitive functioning and decision making.

Presocial Stage—At this stage the child lacks a full awareness of self as differentiated from others. Ego development begins with the end of this stage.

Impulsive Stage—Children in this stage act on their impulses and control of their behavior is largely external. Reward and punishment are the primary means used for control.

Self-Protective Stage—During this stage, children learn that they can get what they want by manipulating others in their environment. Need gratification occupies the child's attention, and others are viewed as persons who can satisfy needs.

Conformist Stage— The conformist stage reflects the development of socialization and an awareness that one's well-being is intertwined with that of a social group. Rules are obeyed because they arise from the group.

Self-Aware Stage—Along with an increase in self-awareness, individuals develop an ability to consider multiple perspectives in moral decision making. Limited exceptions to the rule of group conformity may occur.

Conscientious Stage—The fully adult conscience emerges in this stage. The individual is able to formulate rules based on personal values regardless of whether they conform to social rules.

Autonomous Stage—Autonomous individuals can take multiple perspectives and are not bound by absolutist thinking. They are able to tolerate ambiguity and also are able to set and work toward long-range goals.

Integrated Stage—In the integrated stage, people are able to recognize and resolve multiple and competing as well as contradictory realities. Few people ever reach this stage, which may in fact be an ideal.

Kegan's Theory of the Evolution of the Self

Kegan (1982; also see Kegan & Lahey, 2000) described the evolution of an independent and unique self as a process of development in which qualitative changes occur in one's meaning-making system. Truly a constructivist thinker, Kegan (1982) defined five assumptions underlying constructivist thought:

> (1) Human being is *meaning making*. (2) *These meaning systems shape our experience.* (3) *These meaning systems to a great extent give rise to our behavior.* (4) Except during periods of transition and evolution from one system to another, to a considerable extent *a given system of meaning organizes our thinking, feeling, and acting over a wide range of human functioning.* (5) Although everyone makes meaning in richly idiosyncratic and unique ways, *there are striking regularities to the underlying structure of meaning-making systems* and to the sequence of meaning-making systems that people grow through. . . . Development is always a process of outgrowing one system of meaning by integrating it (as a subsystem) into a whole new system of meaning. What was "the whole" becomes "part of a new whole." (pp. 202–203)

Based on a constructivist paradigm, Kegan proposed five stages through which individuals develop. A dynamic interplay between inclusion and independence, integration and differentiation, constitutes a driving developmental force within and across the stages. As shown in Table 3-1, Kegan's stages may be described as follows:

Stage 0, Incorporative—In this sensorimotor developmental stage, the self senses and moves through reflexes. The child and his or her environment seem to be extensions of each other rather than independent.

Stage 1, Impulsive—In the impulsive stage, which ends by the age of 7, the self is defined in terms of impulses and perceptions; these coordinate one's reflexes. Consistent with preoperational thought, objects are understood as presently perceived.

Stage 2, Imperial—The imperial stage lasts through adolescence and is characterized by an emerging awareness that one is unique and that others do not know what one is thinking. There is a private life that is not shared with others. Empathy is absent, as the individual is unable to imagine the internal responses of others (i.e., dialectic thinking is absent).

Stage 3, Interpersonal—In this stage, the self is viewed as interpersonal, and existing in mutual relations with others. These relations are not necessarily intimate in nature.

Stage 4, Institutional—In the institutional stage, individuals are self-reflective and aware of the self as a regulator of relationships. Consistent with fully formal-operational thought, the self is viewed as the author of one's identity.

Stage 5, Interindividual—In Kegan's final stage, there is an awareness of the roles one plays in relation to others and systems, and of the genesis of these roles. Dialectic thought is the hallmark of this stage.

This brief discussion of cognitive theory reveals the importance of understanding how cognitions and emotions grow, change, and develop over the lifespan. Individuals can be in any of a number of different cognitive/emotional developmental stages regardless of their age or life circumstances. Thus they may present a variety of explanations for their behaviors that are unique to their level of cognitive/emotional development. In counseling, cognitive/emotional developmental style may be the key to understanding clients and to helping them change. Strategies for determining cognitive developmental level and for encouraging cognitive/emotional growth clearly are needed. DCT is one such strategy that is useful across the lifespan, regardless of a client's gender or culture. However, inclusion of both gender and cultural issues is critical to understanding individuals and their development.

GENDER ISSUES IN DEVELOPMENT

Women follow a developmental path different from that of men. This statement rapidly became an axiom of the helping professions when Carol Gilligan wrote her groundbreaking book, *In a Different Voice* (1982). Gilligan points out that Erikson's conception of development focuses on separateness, and Erikson's emphasis on such words as *autonomy, initiative,* and *industry* tend to focus on individuals doing or accomplishing things by themselves. Interestingly, Gilligan worked as Erikson's teaching assistant and came to believe that his concepts, while helpful in viewing the lifespan, did not recognize gender differences and that Erikson had unwisely failed to differentiate developmental paths of men and women.

Women's developmental orientation, Gilligan maintains, is more relational in nature. She believes that women in adolescence are actually working simultaneously on issues of identity and intimacy. She talks about women as being more relational, or more attached, to use the language of Bowlby. In effect, the cultural developmental task of men is to become relatively more autonomous and separate while the task of women is to become relatively more attached and relational. Extensive research has been completed on the complexity of women's development, which seems to bear out Gilligan's thesis (see, for example, Gilligan, Ward, & Taylor, 1988).

Gilligan et al. (1988) propose two separate models of the self. The first is the *separate/objective self,* which is autonomous in relation to others. This model tends to be characteristic of male development in North American culture with an emphasis on relationships between highly separated individuals, a morality based on rules and fairness, and roles based on duty or obligation.

The *connected self* is interdependent and responds to others with a sense of concern. This response is mediated through a morality of caring and connection in relationships. Gilligan et al. (1988) note that women's development in North American culture is more difficult than men's because the relational connected self requires more complex thought patterns.

It seems clear that developmental theory must be constantly informed by an awareness of differences between men's and women's roles in North America. Even the most cursory review reveals that values of differing cultural groups in terms of the connected self and the interdependent self must be considered in the future. For example, many Native American, Black, Hispanic, and Asian families call more attention to the connected self than does the "mainstream" White male culture.

Some see women's development over the lifespan as interconnected rather than linear. Differences in male and female development exist throughout the lifespan. It is clear that boys and girls are treated differently from infancy and experience different types of relationships and expectations from caregivers and culture; however, gender-oriented theory is critical of Erikson's development framework as it applies to adolescence and adult life. Neugarten (1979), for example, points out that women's development could be considered as a fan in which you can see all the pieces moving out from a central core with all the parts related to the rest. An adolescent woman, for example, may indeed be working on issues of identity, but intimacy may be a higher priority. A woman in the working world may deal with issues of generativity during her 20s, intimacy in her 30s, and perhaps rework issues around identity when she reaches 40.

Women's development may touch on some parts of Erikson's framework and in more or less detail than he suggests. Needless to say, the same variations in developmental transitions can occur with men; life is not a straight line and taking the Erikson framework too literally can cause problems.

TRANSITIONS: WHAT HAPPENS BETWEEN LIFESPAN STAGES?

Developmental transition is an important term in the Eriksonian framework and refers to our growth over the lifespan. This concept is considered too simplistic by Nancy Schlossberg, who outlined six types of developmental transitions showing that change occurs in many ways besides aging (Schlossberg, 1984; Schlossberg & Kay, 2002; Schlossberg, Waters, & Goodman, 1995). All of the following transitions regularly appear in counseling and therapy sessions. These are issues you will face constantly in the daily practice of counseling and psychotherapy. Working through these and other issues is critical if a person is to move through the lifespan with some degree of mental health.

Each of the following transitions (and nontransitions) presents your client with major challenges. As you read the following list, think about the many clients you will face who will consult with you about these issues:

Elected transitions: graduating from school, changing jobs, having a baby, retiring, moving, divorcing.

Surprise transitions: car accident, death of a child, plant closing, an unexpected raise or significant promotion, a reduction by the state in welfare benefits for poor mothers.

Nonevents (when the expected doesn't happen): a couple experiences infertility, a promotion or raise doesn't come through, child does not leave home.

Life on hold (transition "waiting to happen"): long engagement, waiting to die in a hospice, waiting for the "right person" to come along, waiting for an important other person to make a key decision.

Sleeper transition (occurs almost without your awareness): becoming fat or thin, falling in love, getting bored at a job you once loved, gradually tiring of a relationship; for a neighborhood, deteriorating or becoming overrun with drugs.

Double whammies: retiring and losing a spouse by death; having a baby and reverting to one income; caring for ill parents at home at the same time that one of your children divorces and moves back home; suffering through a house fire in the winter at the same time the welfare office has lost your file. (Schlossberg notes that daily life "hassles" such as a difficult commute, a sick child, a bounced check, or a difficult boss can produce considerable stress in themselves.)

The combined implications of Gilligan, Neugarten, and Schlossberg cannot be ignored. Certainly women do move through the lifespan, but we need to broaden our constructs of development with special attention to issues of gender and culture.

You will work with many people, both men and women, who seek help from you because of difficult and problematic transitions and nontransitions. We all face constant change throughout life. *The Transition Guide* (Schlossberg & Kay, 2002) is a useful tool to help you and your clients think about change. The authors have developed a four-step process to facilitate moving more successfully through difficult life transitions. *The Transition Guide* focuses on the following dimensions:

Situation: Here you need to listen to clients' stories and help them organize their thinking on the transition—facts, feelings, and meanings. The concrete narratives of DCT, of course, are important in helping them examine their situations. Once the story is told, Schlossberg and Kay recommend reflecting on such topics as the difficulty and challenges in the situation, ways clients have worked successfully with other transitions, goals for a successful transition, other problems and stresses they currently face, and how their cultural background might lead to varying views on what an appropriate resolution might be. In some cultures an active, problem-solving style might be considered appropriate; in others, acceptance and just living with the problem as it is may be more suitable. Not all issues around a transition or nontransition can be resolved. At times a healthy solution is to help the client accept "what is."

Self: What does the client bring to the situation? What are the person's skills, degree of resiliency, and self-knowledge? The wellness assessment of Chapter 2 is an example of a positive, strength-based approach to effective management of transitions. In addition, how optimistic is the client? What sense of control does this person feel? How realistic are her or his expectations?

Supports: All too often clients think they face transitions alone. Transition theory and methods encourage exploration for support from spouse/partner, family, friends, and groups. These systems can be very problematic or quite supportive when a person is working through some transitions. Given the presence or absence of support systems, how does this client accept affections, assistance, and feedback? Does the client have special interests, recreational and physical activities, and spiritual supports as he or she faces difficult situations?

Strategies: There are many counseling and therapeutic strategies to help manage life transitions and nontransitions. Among many others, consider the following: negotiating skills, assertiveness, ability to take advice and feedback, and goal setting. Understanding the nature of the transition and naming it for what it is can be extremely helpful to many clients. For example, a person who has just lost a job through cutbacks can benefit from knowing that this is a transition and, in this way, partially distance himself or herself from the situation and think of it in a new light. Therapeutic techniques drawn from many theoretical orientations are, of course, highly useful. See Chapters 7, 8, and 9 for many specific suggestions.

Once these four aspects of transition work are understood, you and the client can work together toward an action plan for the future.

INTROSPECTIVE DEVELOPMENTAL COUNSELING: MOVING LIFESPAN THEORY TO DAILY PRACTICE

Introspective developmental counseling (IDC) provides a systematic framework for examining the foundations of development in the interview. This approach, elaborated by Tamase (1989, 1998), draws on Japanese Naikan therapy, the work of Erikson, and DCT theory and practice. Tamase argues that client personality trends and behavioral dispositions depend on life history. The goal of introspective developmental counseling is to discover how past history repeats itself in present-day life, then to use this information to help the client move intentionally toward greater wellness.

Our basic attachments to others and our sense of self and other esteem are based in the earliest stages of life, for it is here that we become *selves-in-relation*. Our esteem for ourselves and for others is founded in our early life experiences. Introspective developmental counseling involves four highly structured sessions, each focusing on four foundation phases of life development: birth through preschool, elementary school, high school, and the recent past and future. These periods correspond to Eriksonian life stages and describe developmental experiences common to Western and Asian culture.

The series of structured interviews is presented to the client as a developmental learning opportunity. The goal is to facilitate the client's understanding of personal life history in the hope that this will bring about a better understanding of current life patterns. As the client works through the four-interview series, he or she reviews life issues, such as family and peer relationships, life accomplishments, and problems experienced.

As clients think about their life histories, they gradually see patterns from the past that continue in their present-day lives. Clients often find that many of the issues they currently face can be better understood in the context of past life events. To put it another way, introspective developmental counseling is oriented toward cognitive/emotional understanding of the past and the past's repetition in the present. In IDC, the questioning process itself is a critical therapeutic intervention.

Introspective developmental counseling can be contrasted with historical approaches to therapy such as Freudian analysis and other psychodynamic theories. Traditional approaches to therapy typically begin with an exploration of current life problems and then return to the past to search for the developmental roots of these difficulties. Tamase argues that we can review our cognitive/emotional developmental history as a natural progression of random and concrete life events that we organize into patterns of thought and action. Through the process of introspective developmental counseling, clients can gain new knowledge of themselves and their relations with others from a more positive, developmentally oriented frame of reference.

Introspective developmental counseling began as a counselor training program in which beginning counselors worked through four one-hour sessions. In pairs, these counselors interviewed each other for half an hour, asking seven specific questions designed to elicit information about the individual's experiences from birth through the present. The IDC process proved to be a helpful growth experience for the counselor trainees, and it was found that the model could be expanded and used in counseling and therapy with clients seeking to understand themselves more fully.

You can use the questioning strategies of IDC with your clients as a route toward understanding their background. Out of this can come awareness of how their developmental past affects the present. The first session focuses on the birth through preschool period. The following list, based on Tamase's research in Japan and the United States, presents a revised and expanded version of his original seven IDC questions for this period. Please read these questions slowly and thoughtfully, as you will later be asked to reflect on them yourself.

Introspective Developmental Counseling Questions (birth to preschool)

1. Could you tell me about your family members, the people closest to you, during your life from the time you were born to just before you entered elementary school? What particular important life events were they experiencing during your earliest years? What key events were happening for them on a personal level? What was going on in the broader society such as economic change, war, or social trends? (These questions are particularly important as they provide the context for the client's developmental history.)
2. Is there anything about your birth that you have heard from your mother or other family member?
3. Could you tell me about your life from the earliest age you can remember?
4. What is the most impressive thing that happened prior to kindergarten?

5. What kind of behavior bothered your mother when you were a preschool child? What positive behaviors do you recall her talking about?
6. How did you feel about your parents when you were a preschool child?
7. Did you struggle with your brothers or sisters at this age?
8. Is there any particular event that made you feel either very happy or afraid at this age?
9. What single event do you recall most positively from this period of your life?
10. What patterns from this early period continue in your present life?

The last question is designed to facilitate client reflection on how the past relates to present behavior, thoughts, and feelings. If you have a good relationship with your client and your interviewing skills are effective, you'll find that clients start to think about the implications of their early life experience before they reach question 10. Tamase puts special emphasis on listening skills such as paraphrasing, reflection of feeling, and summarization. Introspective developmental counseling does not make interpretations of the client's life history but rather helps the client make sense of his or her own life. Tamase's emphasis on listening and natural development is in marked contrast with psychodynamic orientations, which are highly interpretive and may encourage the client to adopt a particular way of viewing the world.

The questions in the list are about preschool sensorimotor issues and as such relate to Erikson's stages of trust versus mistrust and autonomy versus shame and doubt. The first question is designed to identify the family context at this particular stage. These questions elicit random information without any particular organization. However, as the client hears data fed back and summarized by the counselor, concrete events descriptive of the period become apparent. As the session continues, clients are able to see patterns in the preschool period that subsequently affected their development in elementary school and in later life stages.

Appendix 1 of this book contains IDC questions for all four developmental stages. Questions for the elementary school period focus on issues of competence (industry versus inferiority). Questions for the high school period emphasize relationships with friends and family as well as academic achievement. The final session focuses on the recent past and the future. Questions are about current vocation and personal adjustment, relationships with friends and family, and current problem issues. Theoretical concepts from Erikson, Perry, Kegan, Schlossberg, and other theorists discussed in this chapter are reflected in the IDC model. As you consider the goal of facilitating optimum development and wellness in clients, you will discover the inherent value of Tamase's approach in helping clients develop more fully as they participate in the life review process.

It is particularly important in such a systematic life review to maintain a positive orientation. There is a danger that the focus can remain solely on problems. The next to last question in each period, "What single event do you recall most positively from this period of your life?" is particularly important. A developmental review should not focus just on problems; it should also emphasize strengths and positives. Clients can draw on these positive events as they cope with real difficulties from the past or present. Introspective developmental counseling can be a beneficial growth experience if the counselor is careful to pay attention to positive assets of the client throughout the lifespan.

The first clinical evaluation of IDC reviewed audiotapes of counselor trainee interviews (Tamase, 1988). The researcher found that all his counselor trainees were at the formal stage—that is, they were able to identify continuing patterns in their lives. The fact that all clients reported seeing new patterns and continuities in their lives raises an interesting question: Did Tamase's systematic step-by-step framework enable clients to see the patterns, or is this method effective only with abstract clients who are already formal-operational? Experience has shown that the sequential, developmentally oriented questions described in Chapter 5 help clients with a concrete style find abstract patterns in their lives. What seems to be most critical is for the therapist to make systematic interventions and follow logical cognitive/emotional progressions. With clients who use the concrete style, the counselor should move more slowly through the life review process and should elicit more examples from the client before attempting to help the client recognize these patterns.

Tamase also observed in this first study that strong feelings and images often surface during the initial session (the birth through preschool period). As might be anticipated, clients tended to talk about elementary school experiences in a more concrete way, saving their formal, patterned thinking primarily for the discussion about the high school period. Finally, in the fourth session, which allows for more reflection and integration of the past, clients demonstrated more dialectical/systemic thinking—that is, they were able to examine more complex patterns of their past life and see how these related to the present.

The comments of two of Tamase's clients reflect the usefulness of the process (Tamase, 1988, pp. 14–15).

> The process was very valuable to me, even though I had three previous years of therapy. It was especially useful to concentrate on one period of life at a time. This helped me to see the overall progression of my development from beginning to the present.
>
> One of the most predominant feelings from doing these exercises is amazement at the differences in emotions that each session brings back. The first and third seemed especially good, while the second seemed bad. Prior to introspective developmental counseling, I was aware of a generally good childhood and past life history. I was not aware, however, of how strongly different my emotions were in regard to the different periods.

IDC has helped student clients develop increased self-consciousness and feelings of self-efficacy (Tamase, 1993). Two investigations found that the specific questioning framework enabled clients to discuss their issues from multiple perspectives and expand their worldviews (Tamase & Rigazio-DiGilio, 1997). This finding is particularly important as it reveals that careful sequencing in the interview can lead most clients to at least some form of dialectic/systemic complex thought. Even children, with careful guidance, can learn a type of reflective formal thinking—something that Piaget did not adequately anticipate. Tamase and Fukuda (1999) discovered that college students did less irrational thinking if they used a formal-operational style as they viewed their lives.

We suggest that you now reread each birth through preschool question silently and think about your own responses. Then write down a few key words to remind you of your responses to each of the first nine questions.

1. _____

2. _____

3. _____

4. _____

5. _____

6. _____

7. _____

8. _____

9. _____

You have now listed several seemingly unrelated events, perhaps using sensorimotor and concrete examples. If you have not included concrete examples in your responses to the questions, do so now, indicating specific experiences and events for each question on the above list.

Review your list and reflect on what you wrote. Write down the patterns you see that you have carried over to later periods of your life. How does your past affect the present? Are there specific events from your past that affect your overall wellness?

10. _____

   _____

   _____

   _____

Now consider what you have written from a broader family perspective. How were your traits and patterns related to your own family history? Were there important crises and events that affected the family and you? Were the individual tasks your family members struggled with important in your own development?

   _____

   _____

   _____

   _____

Introspective developmental counseling clearly shows that a lifespan review can be organized systematically. Tamase does not see his work as therapy, although it may be therapeutic. Instead, he considers it a method for reviewing life patterns and opening the way for more extended analysis and problem examination, if desired. Many clients find that answering the questions in brief individual or group sessions is helpful in making sense of their lives.

The series of four sessions outlined by Tamase could serve as part of a larger program of treatment. For example, for a client who has discovered a pattern of nonassertiveness going back to earlier periods of life, cognitive understanding may not be enough. The counselor may utilize concrete assertiveness training so that the formal or reflective knowledge can become specific, concrete action. Later, rational disputation and cognitive-behavioral methods may be useful in challenging and changing the formal thought patterns.

Each of Tamase's questions can be explored in more depth using the systematic questioning sequence of DCT. The four-session program can be expanded into a major program of systematic therapy if developmental crises and family events are explored further. Many people who go through the IDC process will identify key developmental events that are still affecting their day-to-day lives. They may need to work through their discoveries at a more emotional level. For example, a client who reveals a traumatic event at the preschool period may be helped by carefully going through the systematic questions of DCT. The client can be asked to think of a sensorimotor image connected with the experience and the resulting emotions may then be explored in depth. The event can then be explored within the concrete, formal, and dialectic/systemic styles.

Finally, you may want to emphasize family background and family systems thinking when employing the introspective developmental approach to counseling. The awareness of how one's life has been affected by one's family may create the desire to work through old remaining issues in family therapy. At the same time, awareness of these issues can be an important means of identifying strengths. Strength-based assessment can be important in helping clients successfully negotiate many of the transitions and changes of life while maintaining a positive, wellness orientation.

SUMMARY

Attachment theory provides a new way for us to think about counseling and therapy. Most research and work with John Bowlby's concepts have focused on child development; yet this same research shows that attachment patterns in childhood manifest themselves throughout the lifespan. The way a client relates to you in the session provides you with a mini-picture of how he or she relates to others.

A broader definition of "self" focuses on self-in-context, self-in-relation, being-in-relation, or person as community. The contextualized self is related to family, community, and multiple cultural groups. We suggest that your interviewing style will change with this one central awareness. Your client does not have a fixed self but one that can and will change in response to environmental events, including the counseling and therapy session.

Erikson's lifespan theory is foundational. Our developmental tasks change as we move through the lifespan. The developmental needs and problems vary with how well each person has mastered earlier central life tasks. Age-related issues are central and tend to be given insufficient attention in most counseling and therapy theory. What is needed, of course, is to take this theory into concrete practice. Erikson was one of the first to emphasize cultural factors in human development, but his theory still needs reinforcement through more emphasis on multicultural factors that deeply affect human development. Nonetheless, we should remain aware that lifespan events do not always follow Erikson's linear patterns.

The cognitive/emotional developmental theories proposed by Kohlberg, Loevinger, and Kegan are, like DCT, all derived from Piaget. Together, these theories provided additional support for the idea of matching our work with the client's individual cognitive/emotional style.

The works of Gilligan and Neugarten remind us that as we work with lifespan developmental theory, we need to be constantly aware of issues of gender. Erikson's framework remains valuable but clearly must be adapted to stand the test of viability for work with women and people of varying cultural backgrounds.

Transition theory reminds us that the most challenging lifespan tasks, particularly prominent in counseling, are times of change. Schlossberg and Kay suggest that we need to analyze and understand the situation, examine the nature of the self, consider support systems, and select from many strategies to develop a plan that works to help clients move through transitions. Naming the transition as a "transition" itself can be helpful.

Tamase's introspective developmental counseling helps us move lifespan theory into counseling and clinical practice. Tamase focuses on the foundation life stages of birth through preschool, elementary school, and high school and provides a highly specific, systematic program for developmental counseling over a four-interview series. Our basic attachments to others and our sense of self- and other-esteem are based here; it is in the early stages that we become *selves-in-relation.*

Remember that the goal of lifespan development is optimum wellness. Through understanding the various lifespan theories we are better able to assess our clients' needs and help them work through a variety of developmental challenges. At any point in life a variety of developmental processes may be affecting one's daily life. Assessing strengths as well as challenges provides a foundation for selecting interventions to help clients continue to grow in healthy ways and successfully negotiate developmental tasks.

Challenges: The major issue at this point is being willing to *practice* and master the applications of developmental theory in the clinical interview. Understanding the concepts is at best a beginning. A developmental approach to counseling and therapy makes sense, but will be only as relevant as your clinical and counseling skills in actually using the concepts in the session. Understanding is not competence. Can you make it happen?

Research issues: Do your clients change their cognitive/emotional style when you speak about issues during childhood? Do they tend to be more concrete? When speaking about adolescent experiences, are your clients more abstract? Are you able to help concrete clients speak more abstractly—or abstract clients more concretely?

THEORY INTO PRACTICE: DEVELOPING YOUR PORTFOLIO OF COMPETENCE

Self-Assessment Exercises

Exercise 1. Erikson's eight stages

Listed below are Erikson's eight life stages and the associated key developmental tasks. Identify an issue in your own life or that of a client that is associated with each stage. For example, how trusting are you? Where does that trust or lack of trust come from?

0–2 years: Trust versus mistrust

Example of a life issue and experiences that relate to your present lifestyle:

_____

_____

_____

On a separate sheet of paper, list examples of concrete and abstract life issues for each stage below. For each stage, include past life experiences that relate to your present behavior on these issues. If you have not reached that stage, think of someone you know who is at that stage and reflect on that individual's style and how he or she might have developed present feelings and thoughts (e.g., identify an elder and reflect on this person's balance of integrity versus despair. What life experiences might have resulted in her or his present status?)

2–4 years: Autonomy versus shame and doubt
4–7 years: Initiative versus guilt
7–12 years: Industry versus inferiority
12–19 years: Identity versus role confusion
19–30 years: Intimacy versus isolation
30–60 years: Generativity versus stagnation
60+ years: Ego integrity versus despair

Exercise 2. Your experience of transitions

Erikson's framework will almost always be useful, but it is clear that the linear step-by-step framework is not appropriate for all. You may find that transition theory and practice is more useful at times. Give an example of transitions that occurred for you that may have changed the way you went through a developmental stage. For each transition you select, briefly indicate the situation, your self-assessment as you examine yourself in that situation, your support system, and the strategies that worked and didn't work.

- *Elected transitions*: graduating from school, changing jobs, having a baby, retiring, moving, divorcing
- *Surprise transitions*: car accident, the death of a child, plant closing, an unexpected raise or large promotion, reduction by the state in welfare benefits for poor mothers
- *Nonevents (when the expected doesn't happen):* a couple experiences infertility, a promotion or raise doesn't come through, a child does not leave home
- *Life on hold (the transition "waiting to happen"):* the long engagement, waiting to die in a hospice, waiting for the "right person" to come along, waiting for an important other person to make a key decision
- *Sleeper transition (this occurs almost without your awareness)*: becoming fat or thin, falling in love, getting bored at a job you once loved, gradually tiring of a relationship; for a neighborhood, deteriorating or becoming overrun with drugs

- ■ *Double whammies*: retiring and losing a spouse by death; having a baby and re-verting to one income; caring for ill parents at home at the same time that one of your children divorces and moves back home; suffering through a house fire in the winter at the same time the welfare office has lost your file

Describe the transition situation:

_____

_____

_____

_____

Self-assessment:

_____

_____

_____

_____

Nature of support systems:

_____

_____

_____

_____

Strategies for dealing with the transition:

_____

_____

_____

_____

Identification and Classification Exercise

Exercise 3. Self-in-relation, self-esteem, person-in-community, and esteem for others

Note that these items reflect the Adlerian lifestyle beliefs relating to self, life, and others discussed in Chapter 2.

Identify the following items as related to a client who is talking about her or his experience in different ways. Answers may be found at the end of the chapter. Circle SIR (self-in-relation), SE (self-esteem), or OE (other-esteem).

SIR SE OE   1. I'm very proud of what I've accomplished in my life.

SIR SE OE   2. My parents have made me what I am and I've been able to build on their example.

SIR SE OE   3. I'm so proud of my parents.

SIR SE OE   4. We build ourselves on the shoulders of others.

SIR SE OE   5. I've done it all by myself.

SIR SE OE   6. Others have done so much for the world.

SIR SE OE   7. I've grown and developed through adversity.

SIR SE OE   8. People of cultures different from my own offer me a chance to grow.

SIR SE OE   9. Other cultures than my own offer a lot.

Classify the following for lack of self-esteem (LSE) or lack of other-esteem (LOE).

LSE LOE   10. I'm feeling bad about myself.

LSE LOE   11. I don't like men (women).

LSE LOE   12. Sometimes I just don't think as well as other people do.

LSE LOE   13. In truth, I think I'm better than most people around me.

LSE LOE   14. People whose color is different from mine are less able than I am.

LSE LOE   15. My racial/ethnic background makes it almost impossible for me to succeed.

Toward Multicultural Competence

Exercise 4. Gender and culturally related issues of development and transition

You may wish to repeat the exercise on developmental transitions above while giving special attention to possible differences among men and women. In addition, consider how one's multicultural background affects lifespan development and the way transitions are negotiated.

Exercise 5. Variations in transitions

List examples of life issues that might affect men and women and those of varying cultural backgrounds differently when they appear for counseling or therapy.

Elected transitions _____

Surprise transitions _____

Nonevents (when the expected doesn't happen) _____

Life on hold (the transition "waiting to happen") _____

Sleeper transition (without your awareness) _____

Double whammies _____

Interviewing Practice Exercises

Exercise 6. Group practice with introspective developmental counseling

In this practice session, be sure to follow the ethical guidelines and confidentiality practices of your class or workshop.

Step 1: Divide into Practice Groups

Get acquainted with each other informally.

Step 2: Select a Group Leader

The leader's task is to ensure that the group follows the specific steps of the practice session. It often proves helpful if the least-experienced group member serves as leader first.

Step 3: Assign Roles for the Practice Session

- Role-played client: The role-played client will talk freely about one of the four life periods outlined by Tamase.
- Interviewer: The interviewer will ask the specific questions suggested by Tamase. Have the questions available on a sheet of paper on your lap to look at from time to time. The interviewer's task is to encourage reflection. Remember to use listening skills frequently and help the client organize information through reflection of feeling and summarization.
- Observers 1 and 2: The observers will write down key words of each client response and classify the response as concrete or abstract. At the conclusion of the interview, each will note life-stage patterns that seem to recur.

Step 4: Plan the Session

The interviewer and client must first agree on the specific stage of Tamase's introspective developmental counseling model to be reviewed. The two observers can examine the feedback form (Box 3-1). The interview need not just follow Tamase's questioning sequence. Each individual is different, and the skilled interviewer will naturally use follow-up questions and interventions to help the client talk about his or her issues using appropriate developmental styles.

Step 5: Conduct a 30-Minute Interviewing Session

It is helpful to videotape and/or audiotape practice sessions.

Step 6: Provide Immediate Feedback and Complete Notes (5 Minutes)

Allow the client and interviewer time to provide immediate personal reactions to the practice session. At this point, the observers should turn the session over and let the participants take control. Use this time to complete your classification and notes.

Step 7: Review Practice Session and Provide Feedback (15 to 30 Minutes)

The interviewer should be the person to ask for feedback rather than getting it without being asked. The observers can share their observations from the feedback form on the next page and from their observations as the session progressed. Avoid judgmental feedback.

Exercise 7. Group practice using Erikson's stages in a role-played session

Use the seven steps above to review one or more of Erikson's lifespan stages.

Exercise 8. Group practice interviewing around transitions issues

Once again, use the same seven steps, but change the topic to key developmental transitions and their impact on one's movement through traditional life stages. Consider situation, self, supports, and strategies.

Box 3-1 Introspective Developmental Counseling Interview

Mapping Developmental Styles in the Session

Feedback Sheet

Developmental Stage Presented by Client (check one)

___ Birth through preschool

___ Elementary school

___ Junior through senior high school

___ Recent past and current life situation

IDC's stage questions range from 10 to 12. For each question associated with that stage, summarize the main points made by the client. Circle the cognitive/emotional style or styles used by the client in response to the interviewer's questions. Encourage the interviewer to aim for complete discussion of each question.

IDC Question 1. Central thoughts/feelings expressed by client:

_____

_____

Concrete/Abstract

IDC 2. Question 2. Central thoughts/feelings expressed by client:

_____

_____

Concrete/Abstract

(Use a separate piece of paper to continue the record.)

What cognitive/emotional style(s) did the client use to discuss this life stage? Often clients discuss the birth–preschool period using an early concrete style (sensorimotor), the elementary period in a concrete style, and junior through senior high school with a late concrete or early formal style. Current life patterns are often discussed in a formal style and occasionally at the post-formal (dialectic/systemic) level.

Pattern analysis: What continuing patterns from early life appear to be continuing in this client's present-day experience?

_____

_____

What did the interviewer do right?

_____

_____

What might the interviewer add to her or his work in the future?

_____

_____

Generalization: Taking Lifespan Development Home

Exercise 9. Practice and observation with individuals in daily life

As you go through the coming week, use one or more of the following ideas to help reinforce the concepts of this chapter.

- Observe individuals at different stages of the lifespan. Can you identify specific examples of children (or adolescents or adults) working through issues of trust versus mistrust, autonomy versus shame and doubt, and so on?
- Note transitions issues that people around you are dealing with. You'll likely find that virtually everyone is dealing with transitions issues constantly.
- Talk with professional therapists and counselors. Is their practice developmental? Do they use developmental concepts daily in their practice? Most use the concepts for case conceptualization but not for direct intervention in the interview. How do these therapists respond to the idea of developmental counseling and therapy?
- Note how people talk about themselves in relation to life challenges. Do you hear a focus on strengths or difficulties??

Exercise 10. The interview

Apply your knowledge of lifespan developmental theory in the here and now of the interview.

- Take a client through Tamase's four interviews as a supplement to your regular practice. Inform the client of your purpose and discuss the effectiveness of each session after completing the 30- to 50-minute interview.
- Try out your own questions, using Erikson's framework, on appropriate clients. What do you observe and what do they learn? Are the clients able to identify patterns that relate to their current life style?

Help clients focus on developmental transitions. What do you learn and what do your clients discover? How many of your clients are working through transitions in developmental stages or the many surprises that can occur over a lifespan? What strengths are evident in their self-talk?

Portfolio Reflections

Exercise 11. Your reflections on lifespan development

What stood out for you from this chapter? What sense do you make of what you have just read? What are your key points? How would you integrate lifespan theory, into your own practice? Record your thoughts here and in a Portfolio Folder.

_____

_____

_____

_____

_____

_____

REFERENCES

Ainsworth, M. (1978). *Patterns of attachment.* Mahwah, NJ: Erlbaum.

Baker Miller, J., Stiver, I., & Hooks, T. (Eds.). (1998). *The healing connection: Women in relationships in therapy and life.* Boston: Beacon.

Bowlby, J. (1969). *Attachment.* New York: Basic Books.

Bowlby, J. (1973). *Separation.* New York: Basic Books.

Bowlby, J. (1990). *A secure base.* New York: Basic Books.

Cassidy, J., Shaver, P., & Main, M. (1999). *Handbook of attachment.* New York: Guilford.

Erikson, E. (1963). *Childhood and society* (2nd ed.). New York: Norton.

Erikson, E. (1994). *Identity and the life cycle.* New York: Norton.

Gilligan, C. (1982). *In a different voice.* Cambridge, MA: Harvard University Press.

Gilligan, C. (2002). *The birth of pleasure.* New York: Knopf.

Gilligan, C., Ward, J., & Taylor, J. (1988). *Mapping the moral domain.* Cambridge, MA: Harvard University Press.

Greenberg, J., & Mitchell, S. (1983). *Object relations in psychoanalytic therapy.* Cambridge, MA: Harvard University Press.

Hwang, P. (2000). *Other esteem: Meaningful life in a multicultural society.* Philadelphia: Accelerated Press.

Kegan, R. (1982). *The evolving self.* Cambridge, MA: Harvard University Press.

Kegan, R., & Lahey, L. (2000). *How the way we talk can change the way we work.* San Francisco: Jossey-Bass.

Kohlberg, L. (1981). *The philosophy of moral development.* San Francisco: Harper & Row.

Loevinger, J. (1976). *Ego development: Conceptions and theories.* San Francisco: Jossey-Bass.

Loevinger, J. (Ed.). (1998). *Technical foundations for measuring ego development.* Mahwah, NJ: Erlbaum.

Mahler, M. (2000). *The psychological birth of the human infant.* New York: Basic Books.

Maslow, A. (1993). *The farther reaches of human nature.* New York: Viking. (Original work published 1954) (Currently available through Arkana Publishers, New York)

Neugarten, B. (1979). Time, age, and the life cycle. *American Journal of Psychiatry, 136,* 887–894.

Ogbonnya, O. (1994). Person as community: An African understanding of the person as an intrapsychic community. *Journal of Black Psychology, 20,* 75–87.

Perry, W. (1970). *Forms of intellectual and ethical development in the college years.* New York: Holt, Rinehart, and Winston.

Piaget, J. (1955). *The language and thought of the child.* New York: New American Library. (Original work published 1923)

Piaget, J. (1963). *The origins of intelligence in children.* New York: Norton. (Original work published 1952)

Piaget, J. (1965). *The moral judgment of the child.* New York: Norton.

Schaffer, H. R. (1996). *Social development.* Oxford, UK : Blackwell.

Schlossberg, N. (1984). *Counseling adults in transition.* New York: Pantheon.

Schlossberg, N., & Kay, S. (2002). *The transition guide: A new way to think about change.* Washington, DC: Transitions. Available online: www.transitionguide.com

Schlossberg, N., Waters, E., & Goodman, J. (1995). *Counseling adults in transition: Linking practice with theory.* New York: Springer.

Sue, D. W., Ivey, A., & Pedersen, P. (Eds.). (1996). *A theory of multicultural counseling and therapy.* Pacific Grove: CA: Brooks/Cole.

Tamase, K. (1988). *Introspective-developmental counseling.* Unpublished manuscript.

Tamase, K. (1989). Introspective developmental counseling. *Bulletin of Nara University of Education, 38,* 166–177.

Tamase, K. (1993, October). *The effect of the introspective-developmental interview on career consciousness.* Presentation to the 35th Annual Conference of the Japanese Association of Educational Psychology, Nagoya.

Tamase, K. (1998). Introspective developmental counseling. *L'esprit d'aujourd'hui, 12,* 78–86.

Tamase, K., & Fukuda, I. (1999). The relationship between cognitive-developmental orientation and irrational beliefs of college students. *Bulletin of Nara University of Education, 48,* 161–172.

Tamase, K., & Rigazio-DiGilio, S. (1997). Expanding client worldviews: Investigating developmental counseling and therapy assumptions. *International Journal for the Advancement of Counseling, 19,* 220–247.

Welwood, J. (2002). *Toward a psychology of awakening: Buddhism, psychotherapy, and the path of personal and spiritual transformation.* Boston: Shambhala.

Winnicott, D. (1987). *Babies and their mothers.* Reading, MA: Addison-Wesley.

Answers to Self-in-Relation, Self-Esteem, and Other-Esteem Exercise

1. SE
2. SIR
3. OE
4. SIR
5. SE
6. OE
7. SE
8. SIR
9. OE
10. LSE
11. LSE
12. LSE
13. LOE
14. LOE
15. LSE

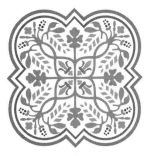

SECTION II
Skills and Strategies for a Developmental Practice

Developmental counseling and therapy (DCT) theory is summarized here, but the emphasis is on immediate practice. You will learn assessment and intervention skills and how to develop comprehensive multi-style intervention plans.

Chapter 4. Assessing Developmental Style. You will find that one of the most useful aspects of DCT is noticing how clients present their issues, concerns, and problems. Some are enmeshed in sensorimotor experience while others focus on concrete narratives and stories. You also find many reflective, formal-operational clients, but relatively few who think about issues through the dialectic/systemic style. You will examine this system as it applies to depressed clients. You will explore the relationship among DCT, Jean Piaget's cognitive theories, and Plato's Allegory of the Cave. By the time you have completed this chapter, you can expect to be able to assess your client's cognitive/emotional style in the here and now of the interview with some precision.

Chapter 5. Developmental Interventions and Strategies: Specific Interventions to Facilitate Client Cognitive and Emotional Development. Developmental strategies to facilitate vertical and horizontal development are presented. The assessment procedures of Chapter 4 are related to specific interventions to facilitate growth. The relationship of DCT to theories and strategies of counseling and therapy is explored through the holistic developmental sphere. Each strategy in this chapter can be used immediately in the counseling and therapy session with observable effect.

Chapter 6. Assessing Client Change: Creativity, Perturbation, and Confrontation. Counseling and therapy are presented as an opportunity to help clients create new ways of thinking, feeling, behaving, and making meaning. Basic to this process are identifying and synthesizing incongruity in clients. The Confrontation Impact Scale is presented as a way to identify client responses to your short-term and long-term interventions. Parallels between this scale and theories of death and dying are explored. Again, here and now usefulness of the model is stressed and you will be able to assess the effectiveness and impact of your interventions in the session.

Chapter 7. Developing Treatment Plans: DCT and Theories of Counseling and Psychotherapy. This chapter explores counseling and therapy theory and its relation to DCT. You will learn how DCT is applied in work with children through a case examination of child abuse and you will learn to develop treatment plans for children, adolescents, and adults. Style-shift theory and the need to change your counseling style to match that of the client are presented with practice examples. You will be familiarized with DCT's practical approach to integrating multiple theories into counseling and therapy treatment plans.

CHAPTER 4
Assessing Developmental Style

CENTRAL PRACTICE OBJECTIVE | Mastery and practice of concepts in this chapter will enable you to assess the four client cognitive/emotional styles through classification of transcripts and to identify client style in the here and now of the interview.

Empathic understanding of the client's worldview is essential to all counseling and therapy, and this chapter offers a way to become even more precise and clear in working with clients. Developmental counseling and therapy (DCT) shows how to assess client meaning-making style. With this knowledge, you can then match the language style of clients and help them expand their developmental competence. Through empathic use of assessment skills, you can facilitate the expansion of client development, and where appropriate, you can mismatch your style and help clients move to other ways of thinking of their issues. For example, in the early stage of counseling, it is important to clients with a concrete style to be exactly where they are; later you can mismatch styles to help them explore more abstract ideas.

This chapter expands developmental assessment with a detailed description of four client cognitive/emotional perspectives: two that represent the concrete world (sensorimotor and concrete operations) and two that represent abstractions (formal operations and dialectic/systemic thinking). All four perspectives offer us additional understandings of the world. No one perspective is necessarily "better" or "higher" than another. DCT stresses expansion and enrichment of cognition and emotion within all. In effect, "more possibilities" for thought and action are considered the goal. *Think of DCT as enriching possibility.*

Knowledge of and skill in the concepts of this chapter can enable you to:

1. Discuss the purposes of developmental assessment and its value for the interview and treatment plan.
2. Define the DCT developmental perspectives and assess client cognitions and emotions within the four major styles—sensorimotor/elemental, concrete/situational, formal-operational/reflective, and dialectic/systemic.
3. Apply developmental assessment with examples featuring depressed clients.
4. Discuss Piagetian theory and its relation to DCT theory and clinical and counseling strategies.
5. Discuss Plato's Allegory of the Cave and its relation to Piagetian and DCT theory.
6. Take theory into practice through reflective and practical activities designed to help you and also develop a personal portfolio of competence.

Appendices 1 through 5 at the end of the book will be important supplements to this chapter. There you will find additional information on classifying client cognitive/emotional styles and a full practice interview for rating.

INTRODUCTION: DEVELOPMENTAL ASSESSMENT

Each client makes meaning and organizes the world differently from everyone else. Our empathic task is to enter that world as well as we can and "walk in the client's shoes." DCT offers some relatively precise ways to understand *how* the client makes meaning and sense of the world.

In the design of appropriate interventions, it is most effective to conduct an assessment of client styles specific to a particular concern. You will find that most clients have a preferred cognitive/emotional style. That style may be sensorimotor/elemental, concrete/situational, formal-operational/reflective, or dialectic/systemic or some combination of these. The DCT style assessment can be done in the here and now of the interview and will enhance your understanding of the client's story. Matching client style in the interview could be called "precision empathy" as you can be more fully with the client. For example, if clients tell their story in a concrete fashion, you will have the skills to stay with them using concrete strategies. If they tell their story at the formal level, you also can match this style and thus help them tell their story using their preferred style.

At some point, you may wish to *mismatch* your style to help a client view the situation from a different perspective. Clients who have a concrete orientation could benefit from your helping them reflect on their issues from a formal-operational perspective. Clients who are very formal-operational and analytic, on the other hand, might benefit from a more concrete or sensorimotor perspective on their particular issue, thus helping them see their issues more completely.

The structured developmental assessment sequence, discussed in this chapter, has the added purpose of identifying *developmental blocks*—cognitive/emotional styles or modalities that block the client from functioning relative to a particular issue. For example, a client who has lost her mother in recent months may be able to talk about her through detailed examples of shared times together (concrete). She may tell you how she always depended on her mother for financial and material aid during times of transition (formal/pattern). The client may also describe her relationship with her mother and tell you how it was similar to and different from her relationships with other members of the family in recent years. She may remember as well her interactions with her mother when she was younger (dialectic). This same client may be devoid of sensorimotor emotion when talking about her loss. This splitting of affect and verbalizations reflects a block. The client is unable to express her feelings about the loss and may even verbalize her inability to cry even though she loved her mother dearly.

Developmental assessment procedures have been tested with many different counseling and clinical populations. Children, adults, and families with normal problems; agoraphobics; gay males; and several hospitalized populations have received extensive analysis (Hoffman, 1991; Ivey & Ivey, 1990; Gonçalves, Ivey, & Langdell, 1988; Kenney & Law, 1991; Marszalek, 1999; Marszalek & Cashwell, 1998; Myers, Shoffner, & Briggs, 2002; Rigazio-DiGilio, 1989; Strehorn, 1999). This research shows that counselors and clinicians can identify the cognitive/emotional style of clients and use this information to facilitate interaction in the interview.

The identification of preferred developmental styles as well as developmental blocks provides the counselor with important information for planning an appropriate and effective treatment. As we will see, the planning process is a natural outgrowth of the assessment itself. By using developmental and counseling therapy (DCT), counselors can ensure that treatment plans and interventions are intentional, thus significantly enhancing the potential for effective outcomes.

Listening to clients' thoughts, feelings, and meaning is essential throughout the developmental assessment process. Pay special attention to client *key words* and use them throughout the session. Mirroring body language at times can be useful, although it should not be overdone. The process of developmental assessment is best conducted with empathic understanding as the primary goal.

THE SKILLS OF DEVELOPMENTAL ASSESSMENT

Developmental assessment has multiple purposes. These include assessment of clients' presenting issues, selecting interventions, and treatment planning. The initial assessment, based on the clients' first verbalizations, is an attempt to determine preferred cognitive/emotional styles relative to the issue being presented. It is important in this context to note that *cognitive/emotional styles typically are issue specific.* For example, clients may present one issue, such as a work-related conflict, in a very concrete, detail-oriented manner, and another issue, such as problems with a partner, in a highly emotional manner. Some clients are able to function in all styles; others have one or more strong preferences that dominate their cognitions. Clients with developmental blocks will be able to process their experiences in some styles but not others. (See Box 4-1 for cognitive/emotional style definitions.)

(handwritten margin note: ★ Test ?'s (4). recognize where client is)

Box 4-1   Four Cognitive/Emotional Styles of Developmental Assessment[1]

Sensorimotor/Elemental: Focusing on the Elements of Immediate Experience	*Definition and strengths.* The client is able to experience emotions and cognitions holistically in the here and now and be in the moment. There is no separation of self from experience. You will often find a random expression of thoughts and feelings. Look for the ability to be in touch with the body, but expect a short attention span. At late sensorimotor style, some magical or irrational thinking may appear. *Emotions. Feelings* are experienced in the here and now rather than described or reflected upon. There is an emphasis on bodily experience. Crying, laughing, and catharsis of deep emotion represent this style. *Potential developmental blocks.* Clients may have difficulty in telling a clear, linear story of what happened. They will have real difficulty in reflecting on themselves and the situation. Behavior may tend to follow the same pattern—namely, short attention span and frequent body movement. There may be an inappropriate impulsive expression with tears, anger, or other emotions. *Example treatments.* Body-oriented work, imagery, relaxation training, medication, Gestalt exercises, metaphor, hypnosis.
Concrete/Situational: Searching for Situational Descriptions and Stories	*Definition and strengths.* The client gives concrete linear descriptions and stories about what happened, often with a fair amount of detail. Nonverbal clients, however, may give short yes and no responses. At the late concrete style, the client will display some causal reasoning, which is exemplified by *if/then* thinking. Moving to behavioral action is easier for this style. *Emotions.* Specific feelings will be named and described but not reflected upon. "I feel X because . . ." Some clients will have difficulty in naming emotion, but naming is basic to concrete emotional experiencing. This is an important step, but nonetheless a move away from direct here and now emotional experiencing.

[1]Most clients will present their issues in multiple styles, although one cognitive/emotional style will often be most prominent. The example treatments are focused on how one style may be most appropriate, but let us recall that most counseling and therapy works in several styles. For example, a psychodynamic dream analysis might draw out a concrete story of a dream, move to sensorimotor experiencing of a dream symbol, and then reflect on the dream in a formal-operational sense. Relatively few traditional theories, however, give primary attention to sensorimotor or dialectic/systemic experience.

(continued)

Box 4-1   *(continued)*

Potential developmental blocks. Clients may tell you detailed stories of their problems again and again, but be unable to see patterns in their behavior. This may be so even though they share many examples of the same patterned behavior. They will have difficulty in generalizing learnings with one problem discussed in the session to another that is obviously parallel to the interviewer. They often have difficulty in seeing a perspective other than their own.

Example treatments. Concrete narrative story telling, assertiveness training and many behavioral techniques, social skills training, rational-emotive behavior therapy, A-B-C analysis, reality therapy and Adlerians using "if . . . then . . ." problem analysis.

Formal-Operational: Reflecting on Patterns of Thought, Emotion, and Action

Definition and strengths. These people can talk about themselves and their feelings—sometimes even from the perspectives of others. Their conversations tend to be abstract. At the late formal style, these clients can recognize commonalities in repeating patterns of behaviors or thoughts. This is the type of client many counselors feel most comfortable with as they are often into analyzing themselves and their own identity.

Emotions. Feelings are reflected on and discussed rather than experienced. Patterns of emotional experience may be discussed.

Potential developmental blocks. Clients who present at the formal style may be good at pattern recognition, but have difficulty in giving concrete examples. They may reflect on themselves and situations, but they may fail to see the assumptions on which their thinking is based. They may be overly abstract and have difficulty in experiencing emotion at the sensorimotor style.

Example treatments. Reflecting on narratives and stories, most of Rogerian person-centered work, analysis of a Beck automatic thoughts chart or REBT thought patterns, psychodynamic dream analysis.

Dialectic/Systemic: Integrating Patterns of Emotion and Thought Into a System

Definition and strengths. Most people do not ordinarily make sense of their world from this perspective. A woman who realizes that sexism is the cause of her depression is using systemic thought. A Native American Indian or a Canadian Dene who realizes that systemic oppression leads to individual feelings of hurt and even depression is using dialectic thought. Multiple perspective taking and many alternatives are to be expected. The client is aware of systems of knowledge and is aware of how he or she is affected by the environment. Also clients will be able to challenge and reflect deeply on their own or others' style of thought and feeling.

Emotions. The client may be highly effective at analyzing and thinking about emotions. Emotions are often contextualized. A client may say "I'm sad about the loss of my parents in this accident, but proud of the life they led. In some ways I miss them terribly, but in my heart they are still there." The emotions change with the perspective taken.

Developmental blocks. The clients can "analyze it to death." Their ability to think constantly in new ways may result in intellectualization and distancing from the real problems. Some clients would rather think about the problem than do anything about it. There may be real difficulty in experiencing emotion at the sensorimotor style or even being able to name what they are feeling accurately.

It is possible to assess the cognitive/emotional style of clients from what they say in the interview, often from only 50 to 100 words. In this type of assessment, the clinician or researcher listens carefully to a selected segment of the interview and classifies the information into one of four cognitive/emotional styles. Further specifics may be obtained by classifying statements according to eight styles. This paradigm, described in Appendices 2 and 3, explains early and late aspects of functioning in each cognitive style. This greater specificity may be important for treatment planning and in-depth assessment. For the initial assessment, however, the four-style paradigm may be quicker and more useful.

A key DCT study with 20 hospitalized, depressed patients showed that independent raters could classify with satisfactory agreement (0.90) the presenting cognitive/emotional style of a client from the first 100 words he or she spoke (Rigazio-DiGilio, 1989; Rigazio-DiGilio & Ivey, 1990). The research also demonstrated that specific therapeutic interventions tied to such assessment affected clients' ability to talk about their problems using the specified developmental styles. It is not only possible to rate client cognitive/emotional style reliably, but we also find that clients talk about their issues at all levels, if satisfactorily encouraged to do so by their interviewers.

DCT stresses that recognizing cognitive/emotional style is an important part of any interview or treatment plan. Most experienced therapists and counselors learn, over time, that they must use concrete approaches with some clients and abstract approaches with others. The transcripts of prominent therapists reveal that they use developmental sequences in their sessions. DCT makes the learning sequences underlying much of counseling and therapy more specific and observable and provides a rationale for changing counseling interventions in an eclectic fashion as clients change, grow, and develop.

The first step toward integrating a developmental approach in your interviewing and treatment is learning to recognize client cognitive/emotional responses during the interview. This takes practice, but with experience and supervision, you will be able to access and assess a client's style during the initial phases of the interview. Then, with further practice and experience, you will find that you can apply this learning beyond the individual client and will be able to assess general family and group cognitive/emotional styles or the general tone or culture of an organization.

In Examples 1–4 following, sample transcripts of the first 50 to 100 words of four interviews are presented to give you practice in sharpening your developmental assessment skills. Refer to Box 4-1 for guidance in making your assessment or to Appendices 2 and 3, which provide further specifics. Box 4-1 presents the central dimensions for classifying the four developmental styles and the basic ways to determine the late stage of each style. Do not worry about distinctions between early and late categories until you feel comfortable with the four basic dimensions. If you have difficulty with the four styles, move back to two styles of observable concretes (behavior, action) and abstractions (ideas, concepts). As you make your assessment, recall that your assessment is based on only one question in one area. Remember that clients will tend to talk about their issues in different styles at different times.

Example 1. A 45-Year-Old Hospitalized, Depressed Client

Therapist: I would like you to say as much as you can about what happens for you when you focus on your family.

This question is important for two reasons: First, it provides the client with an open question that allows for many possible interpretations. Second, it is useful, as clients' issues are often related to their families. (The questions here are from the Rigazio-Digilio study cited earlier. The content of the conversations has been markedly disguised to maintain confidentiality.)

Client: I feel such love.

Therapist: Can you say more about that?

Client: My wife is wonderful. We have a loving and caring relationship. She has always hung in there with me throughout my hospitalizations. I feel very dependent on her. When I visit home I tend to rely on her a lot. She gets angry sometimes when I'm depressed, but for the most part, we get along fine. I sometimes feel that I never satisfy her.

Is the client primarily sensorimotor, concrete, formal, or dialectic/systemic?

Example 2. A 22-Year-Old Hospitalized, Depressed Client

Therapist: Could you tell me what occurs for you when you think about your family?

Client: What do you mean?

Therapist: Well, as you sit here, focus on any aspect of your family at all, any part of your family, and tell me what kinds of things just happen right here and now for you.

Client: What do you mean by family? Like my husband, my daughter, my husband's mother? I don't know what you mean.

Therapist: Who seems most in your mind today?

Client: Well, I guess my mother.

Therapist: Tell me more about what's on your mind.

Client: Well, she lives with us now to help take care of my daughter while I'm here. She came in yesterday for a visit and she got mad at me. It really hurt my feelings. (tears) I can't help it if I'm in here. She said that I was just faking and didn't want to take care of Jamie. Then I started to cry, and I said to her . . . (continues)

Is the client primarily sensorimotor, concrete, formal, or dialectic/systemic?

Client number 1 is formal. His comments are all abstract, with little in the way of concretes. He is able to identify some of his and his wife's patterns, although he may well be unaware of other patterns (such as his wife's seldom being satisfied with him) or unable to do anything about them. DCT would view this depressed patient as having several cognitive/emotional tasks. One of these is to think about the meaning of the patterns he and his wife share and how these affect his depression. This is a formal-operational, dialectic/systemic therapeutic task that may involve family therapy as well as individual work.

On the other hand, if this client is distanced from his emotions, he may need Gestalt exercises, relaxation training, and bodywork. If he becomes seriously depressed, treatment using drugs may be useful. If he is too abstract, the therapist may need to focus on the specific concretes of his conflict. Long-term depressed clients sometimes learn the jargon of therapy, talk very well at the abstract level, and, with the therapist's collusion, fail to examine themselves using other styles.

The second client is concrete. This type of client is often difficult for therapists to work with, as most of us are formal-operational, dialectic/systemic thinkers. Two key developmental tasks face this client. This brief interview segment suggests that the client is so mired in concrete description and experience that sensorimotor experiencing may be lost. Thus she may need the same type of body and experiential work required by the formal client above. In addition, this client needs to be able to reflect more on the self and recognize patterns. Within the concrete style, the client may benefit from skills training and problem-solving counseling, all aimed at resolving situational specifics.

Clients who think primarily in a concrete cognitive style typically do not move easily and readily to formal pattern thinking. (The next chapter provides specific guidance to facilitate change in cognitive/emotional style.) Thus, the therapist working with this type of client may need to operate for a period of time with a concrete orientation and listen to the detailed stories of the client. On the other hand, some clients can be very concrete but are able to process in other styles equally well. Listening to their concrete descriptions can be useful in understanding the way they construct meaning of the events in their lives, and the sequences of events, thoughts, and feelings that cause them difficulty.

If you are a primarily formal-operational person, you may find yourself bored, impatient, and "spacing out" (thinking about lunch or your last client) when you talk with a highly concrete client. Needless to say, this can jeopardize the relationship. If you are first willing to be with the client wherever he or she is at the moment and listen to the concrete details, you can later use the techniques and strategies of DCT to help broaden his or her understanding. The client with a concrete style, for example, may have real trouble in seeing repeating patterns. Don't move to discuss patterns until the client has first described several specific situations (early or middle concrete styles) and has shown some ability to engage in late concrete-operational reasoning (if/then causal thinking).

Example 3. A 35-Year-Old Client, Just Arrived at a Women's Shelter

Counselor: Could you tell me what's been happening?

Client: (tears) I couldn't take it anymore. He just reminds me of the devil. I don't know what to do. Where are my children? Are they OK? He hit me and hit me. I ran out of the house. Look at my arm. (Breaks down sobbing)

Is the client primarily sensorimotor, concrete, formal, or dialectic/systemic?

Example 4. The Same Client Three Days Later

Counselor: How is it for you right now?

Client: Better, but I'm still confused as hell. I find myself wanting to go back to him. When he's not drinking, he's fine. But he's beat me so many times, and this last time he started for the kids. I'm not sure where I should go.

Counselor: You're confused right now, wondering what to do?

Client: Yeah. I've been thinking about it all week. The counseling sessions have helped me put it together more, but I'm still not sure. If I go back, I can see a lot of trouble ahead. I know he won't go for family counseling. And I can visualize a lot of pain and more beating for me if I do. In that context, it makes no sense to go back at all. But when I think about it a bit more, I know he had an abused childhood himself and relationships are difficult for him. He needs my caring, and when things are good for us, they are really good. Then I think about how difficult it will be for me and the children on our own. Even though I'm a college graduate, I haven't worked for five years. I'm not sure I could support myself. It's very scary. And weirdly enough, a piece of me really wants to get back to him. I know I play into his abuse by being so dependent on him. I wish I didn't think so much. It just mixes me up.

Is the client primarily sensorimotor, concrete, formal, or dialectic/systemic?

The first interview represents a sensorimotor presentation of self common among people in crisis or experiencing trauma. They are close to the difficult situation and are often embedded in the emotional experience. The therapeutic task here is not to ask this woman concrete questions or to engage in formal analysis but simply to be with her and protect her in her moment of need. Housing and a safe relationship are what is needed. With some clients in crisis (for example, a rape survivor), it may be helpful to encourage them to talk about what happened from a formal-operational point of view, as this provides some cognitive and emotional distance from the trauma. Later, as appropriate, the counselor can move toward helping the client reexperience the event in both sensorimotor and concrete detail.

The second session with the same client is much more analytical. The client touches on several topics, each one of which seems to represent a pattern. When a client analyzes his or her situation in this manner, the distinctions between pattern and dialectic/systemic thinking often seem minimal. This client can be considered dialectic/systemic, since she looks at systems of operations. She is able to look at her situation from several perspectives and can recognize that her staying in an abusive relationship at times supports her husband's pathology. This ability to see a problem from several perspectives at once characterizes dialectic/systemic thought.

But the dialectic/systemic approach can also have drawbacks. In this interview, the client's self-analysis has safely distanced her from her deeper feelings; she can avoid the concrete specifics of what is likely to happen if she returns to her husband. The client would benefit from examining specific patterns of her behavior rather than considering multiple perspectives. She also could be helped to consider the sexism in the system in which she lives that bears on her husband's abusive behavior, and to look at the system of interaction in her family that may aggravate the difficulties in their relationship.

With each of these depressed clients, it is wise to start the interview matching the client's developmental style. But staying with that style throughout the entire session may not be enough. A more comprehensive interview and treatment plan may involve helping the client examine her or his difficulties from multiple developmental perspectives.

Now, let us broaden our understanding of DCT theory by relating it more closely to Piaget's theory. In this way, you can begin to understand how DCT provides a base for working with many types of clients from many theoretical perspectives.

EXPANDING DEVELOPMENTAL ASSESSMENT: CHILDREN, ADOLESCENTS, AND ADULTS

This section enlarges on the overview just presented. Here you will find examples of Piagetian thought with an emphasis on child and adolescent development. Elaborations of the DCT framework will then follow with more specifics of assessing children, adolescents, and adults.

Preoperational: Defining the Problem

Piaget's second stage of cognition is termed *preoperational* and covers roughly ages 2 through 7. The child learns to represent the world through language and to use some abstract symbols. Characteristic of this stage is egocentric, magical thinking, which denies external reality but functions well for the child. What Piaget terms preoperational, DCT terms late sensorimotor.

The word *preoperational* is another way of describing client problems, concerns, and issues. DCT points out that most, perhaps all, clients who come for counseling and therapy are preoperational in some way. If they were operating effectively with others and in their environment, they would not be clients and would not need the help of counselors and therapists. Thus, in this book clients and their problems are considered preoperational.

Our task as helpers is to aid clients in becoming operational and addressing their problems using sensorimotor, concrete, formal, and dialectic/systemic modes of thinking and action. The first part of this therapeutic task is to learn how to recognize the four styles in individual clients. Later, this assessment may be extended to families and groups.

Sensorimotor: Focusing on the Elements of Experience

The first Piagetian stage is the sensorimotor period (0 through 2 years of age); in this stage the child has little sense of self. A particularly striking example of this lack of separation of self might be a young girl who cries when seeing another child hurt. She is unable to separate herself from others. Another example might be a little boy having an angry tantrum during which he loses himself in total emotion. Typical of the sensorimotor period is a reliance on what is seen, heard, and felt—that is, immediate sensory and perceptual experience.

Sensorimotor functioning has many positives. When people can enjoy the closeness of a sensorimotor sexual relationship, sing and dance, experience the sun's warmth, swim and play baseball, and are conscious only of the moment, they are experiencing the best of what life has to offer. For example, to work through the grieving associated with serious loss requires the client to experience emotions with the emotionally deeper, sensorimotor style. One may say that there is more satisfaction in tasting an apple than in analyzing its chemical composition. Much of the helping endeavor focuses on getting clients in touch with this part of themselves.

People frequently handle an experience in their lives in an ineffective, embedded, sensorimotor fashion. Examples are an individual suffering the agonies of divorce or an adolescent out of control in an outburst of temper. Illogical and/or magical thinking may be common at such times. Such individuals may have difficulty separating themselves from others and display boundary problems. An example is, as family therapists term it, the overly enmeshed family. Clients can be so deeply affected by a traumatic experience, such as rape or an automobile accident, that they become, for a time, totally absorbed in their emotions.

A key to identifying clients who think and operate with the sensorimotor style is their immersion in the elements of experience. Clients who present with this style often talk randomly in disorganized fragments. This type of client usually has a short attention span. As interviewers, we can bring out this style of cognition by asking these clients to focus on the here and now and to note what is seen, heard, and felt in terms of direct experiencing. Think of children who are hurt or teased severely on the playground. They may be crying and they tell their story in random fragments. Adults, under severe stress, will often present in a similar fashion.

However, if a client has just experienced a major trauma, continuing to support sensorimotor focusing might be totally inappropriate. At such times, some clients need to be more concrete or formal and analytical to help generate some distance from the event. Later the therapist can return to the basics of the experience and help the client begin the process of working through the feelings.

Illogical and magical thinking can be considered sensorimotor in nature. For example, irrational ideas such as "She made me hit her"; "It's my fault—he wouldn't have abused me if I had been a better wife"; "I don't have a drug problem—I only take drugs when I need them"; and "I must be perfect" are common for those with the late sensorimotor orientation.

Nonverbal behavior of sensorimotor clients tends to be random as well. Movement is frequent with a certain jerkiness characteristic of this style. However, severely depressed clients who move very little are also classified as sensorimotor in that they are overwhelmed by their feelings. Depressed clients often have powerful feelings of weight or internalized sadness in their bodies.

Examples of Sensorimotor Style

Child. An example of a child with a sensorimotor style is the 7-year-old who has a fight on the playground, is crying, and talks about the situation in fragments. It is difficult to get a concrete, linear explanation of what occurred. The child *is* her feelings.

Adult. An example of an adult with this style is the otherwise well-functioning adult who is going through a divorce and is currently so confused and overwrought that she has difficulty staying on a single topic. A person who has just experienced racial or sexual harassment may respond internally with sensorimotor body hurt while simultaneously hiding what is going on inside. More complex behavior is found in the emotionally cold sociopath who has split feeling from thought. Similar patterns of separating thought and feelings may be found in the acting-out child or adolescent or those with other personality disorders.

Family. Families predominantly operating within the sensorimotor style tend to be chaotic in their functioning. The family reacts to the latest and strongest emotional event, and family interaction is thus guided by affect rather than reason. Families who underutilize this style tend to be less connected and less responsive to the feelings of others. Cultural differences particularly affect this dimension. Some Italian-American families tend to exhibit a great deal of sensorimotor affect in their interactions, whereas a British-American family may be more reserved. What is healthy behavior in one family may differ markedly from healthy behavior in another. It is important not to impose your definitions of what is culturally appropriate on individuals and families.

What is desirable for human development is a balance between the ability to enter into a full expression of feelings, as represented by sensorimotor experience, and the ability to become more concrete and analytical as the situation changes. Using only one style of cognition or emotion can be a problem.

Your personal experience. Think of a time when you were overwhelmed by a situation and by your thoughts and feelings connected with it. Relax and "get into" that problematic experience as much as you can. Summarize your thoughts and feelings below. Allow yourself to be random and free in developing a visual image of that time. Try to experience that image in the here and now. As you do so, ask yourself the following questions: What are you seeing? Hearing? Feeling? What is occurring for you in your body?

_____

_____

_____

_____

_____

_____

_____

_____

_____

_____

_____

_____

Concrete-Operational: Searching for Situational Descriptions

Erik Erikson says the developmental task of the elementary school-age child is to achieve a sense of industry versus inferiority. Young children achieve industry and capability by being able to operate concretely in the world. In elementary school, children learn to read, do elementary math, engage in basic sports, and participate for the first time in a peer group. The concrete-operational world is concerned with action.

Concreteness is an important counseling construct. We have learned that getting specific, concrete examples from our clients is critical if we are to understand them. We have many concrete approaches to counseling, including assertiveness training, instruction in basic living skills via social skills training, and the Adlerian approach of logical consequences. *ego strengthening*

Clients within this style tend to talk in very concrete terms about their problems, using many specific details. They may describe situations blow by blow, saying, "He said this, and then I said that." Clients in the late concrete orientation exhibit causal, if/then thinking. As interviewers, we encourage concreteness in our clients by asking "Could you give me an example?" There is little analysis and reflection in concrete thought. It is difficult for the concrete thinker to see patterns of thought, feeling, or behavior.

Clients using a concrete style tend to describe their emotions and feelings, often in the past tense, rather than experiencing them in the present. They may make such statements as "I felt sad" or "That hurt me because . . ." In skills-training programs on reflection of feeling, counselors and therapists are often instructed to say to their clients, "You feel (insert emotion)." This type of statement helps make the feeling present. To explore further, the counselor would say "You feel (emotion) because (insert cause of emotion)." This type of statement is representative of a late concrete-operational statement and will help move the client into that cognitive style.

Expect clients oriented to concreteness to be able to name emotions and perhaps reflect on their emotions, but have difficulty experiencing them. In helping a person work through a deep emotional experience, it is useful to move back and forth between sensorimotor and concrete modes. Alternately naming and experiencing emotions is basic to therapy. Formal-operational and more analytic clients may resist sensorimotor and concrete expression of feelings.

Concreteness is highly desirable for the individual or family constantly "up in the clouds" of abstraction or enmeshed in sensorimotor experience. The description of specific events can be helpful for both types of clients. However, too much concreteness can also be a problem, particularly for clients who keep repeating the same counterproductive behavior while failing to see the pattern. As with all other cognitive/emotional dimensions, achieving a balance is important.

Examples of Concrete-Operational Style

Child. Most children talk in very concrete terms. They may say very little (early concrete or late), or they may talk endlessly about small details of their experience (early concrete) or they may describe situations from an if/then perspective (late concrete). Perhaps the best way to identify concreteness is to ask a 10-year-old to tell you about a recent movie or TV show; the concrete description can be endless.

Adult. Adults do not differ much from children when they talk in concretes. Helping professionals need to move clients from the random, magical thinking of

Box 4-2   Assessing Developmental Style in Three Clients: Child, Adolescent, Adult

DCT Style	Child: Dealing With Teasing on the Playground	Adolescent: Talking About Examination Anxiety	Adult: Talking About a Parent's Death
Sensorimotor	(Crying, eyes full of hurt and anger, short of breath, and unable to tell a full story, except in fragments between breaths, but the general idea is "What's wrong with me?")	(Anxiously) So scared—I can't think. Things leave my mind. I feel like crying.	(Tearing/heavy sighing/deep breaths) It's just too much. (Choke) I can't say anything. I just hurt.
Concrete/Situational	The girls said I had funny shoes and cooties. I was just sitting there by myself and my shoes came untied. Maddy and Cara walked by and laughed at my old sneakers. They are rich and have Nikes. I looked away and felt like crying. Then they said, "You have cooties too!" Why don't they like me?	I felt very tense and anxious. I walked in and sat down—way in the back of the room. My pulse was going crazy. The exam was passed out and I just went blank. But, I had studied for hours and knew that material. I could answer only a few questions.	The funeral director showed us expensive coffins and urns. He told us how splendid a fancy funeral would be. My sister and I broke down in tears, but he just kept talking.
Formal/Reflective	(Later in the interview, after the counselor has focused on strengths) Yes, I am a good student. I read better than they do. I think they are unfair to me and they do it to other kids too.	It's a pattern for me. I used to do this in high school and now it seems to be getting worse in college. I always study and the more I study, the more anxious I seem to get. I've been noting lately that I seem even to forget to breathe in tense situations. It's almost a panic feeling.	As I think about it, I feel immensely angry about the situation. There we were, basically falling apart, and all he could think of was a big sale.

(continued)

the sensorimotor style to the specific concretes of the situation. These specifics give us an understanding of the client's world. The client who has just experienced an oppressive incident often needs to talk through the concrete specifics of their story. For example, a gay person or a disabled individual who has been discriminated against in some way often needs to share that story with an understanding listener.

Family. The clearest family example is the verbal family in which parents talk in the abstract while the young children, dealing in the concrete, wonder what is going on. Work with such families might focus on helping parents learn to talk and play

Box 4-2   (continued)

DCT Style	Child: Dealing With Teasing on the Playground	Adolescent: Talking About Examination Anxiety	Adult: Talking About a Parent's Death
Dialetic/Systemic	(After three sessions and some group work.) Now that I'm a peer counselor and have been in a friendship group, I want to help other kids have friends and stop all the bad things that happen in this school. (For the most part, children will not think in systemic terms unless prompted by the interviewer—counselors often need to intervene with teachers, set up small groups, and organize the school to work against oppressive events.)	(In a later session) The work with you has helped. I'm aware that several members of my family are anxious and they almost seemed to expect it of me. Now, I know that I can be my own person. The relaxation exercises and becoming aware of my thought patterns has helped. I think I have the tools for handling exams in the future.	With all the pressure, of course we broke down and over-spent. Fortunately, the funeral went well; at least there we feel good. On the other hand, the funeral industry is so crass. We need some type of regulation for people such as us who are faced with loss. It's a terrible system.

with children. Some families have a very concrete style; at the dinner table or in the interview they may give detailed linear descriptions of the day's events, with little accompanying analysis and reflection.

Your personal experience. Consider the specific situation you described above (when you felt overwhelmed) and write down the concrete, linear details. Describe the event in specific detail. What happened before the event? What happened afterward? Name the feelings you had. This linear presentation of specifics represents concrete thinking and emotion. If you can attach an if/then set of causal reasons to the specific situation, you will be describing the event in a late concrete-operational mode.

_____

_____

_____

_____

_____

_____

_____

Formal-Operational: Reflecting on Patterns of Thought, Emotion, and Action

The questions "Who am I?" and "What is my identity?" are particularly characteristic of formal thinkers and are often a special challenge for the adolescent engaged in defining the self. The search for a personal identity requires reflection on patterns and consistencies in the self. The formal thinker is well able to generalize and to synthesize several concrete situations into an overall pattern.

Piaget notes that the first abstract stage, the formal-operational period, starts between ages 11 and 17. In formal operations the individual learns to reflect on the self and to recognize patterns in the world. To develop a sense of self or a personal identity, an adolescent must have some formal-operational skills. Success in junior high or high school requires abstract, formal skills. However, most Piagetian scholars estimate that a quarter of the U.S. population never reaches full formal operations. They may be able to see some patterns, but cannot do so consistently. This poses an interesting challenge for the professional helper using DCT methods. DCT holds that with careful systematic questions, virtually all clients can see patterns in their thoughts and behaviors and many reach the dialectic/system orientation as well. Children and early adolescents often engage in a type of pattern recognition and reflection that is a form of formal-operational thought and feeling.

Much of counseling and therapy theory is formal-operational in nature. We are interested in self-actualization, changing patterns of cognition, reflecting on feelings, and discovering how present-day life patterns go back to childhood. If our clients are not ready to engage in formal operations, our formal theories must be adapted. A client with a concrete style may indeed need to have a better self-concept, but using abstract words to emphasize the importance of self-examination will most often be ineffective with this person. It is possible to build a positive self-concept in a more concrete way by focusing on specific things clients can do or have done that make them feel good about themselves.

The ability to be abstract and formal is not always positive. We all know individuals who talk a lot but are very short on action. A family or individual may analyze and talk about issues in a charming and interesting way, thus seducing the helper into thinking there is real self-awareness. Instead, these individuals may have learned to avoid coping with the real world and other people by using abstraction and analysis.

Critical to identifying the formal-operational mode is abstraction. One cannot see, hear, or feel abstractions. A self or a pattern is an abstract construct that exists only in the mind. (Recall the discussion in Chapter 1 on concrete versus abstract conversation.) When we talk in counseling and therapy about reflecting clients' feelings, it means we often are operating in the formal style. You may have had the experience of reflecting feelings to a concrete client and having the client, looking somewhat puzzled, reply, "Yes, that is what I just said." The ability to analyze and reflect on one's feelings and thoughts is critical to finding a sense of self and a personal identity. The ability to step outside and look at oneself is very useful. This type of emotional expression is very different from sensorimotor and concrete experience.

As counselors, we often encourage formal thinking when we ask, "Is that a pattern?" or "Do you feel that way often?" or "Does that happen in other situations?" If the client, adult or child, is able to recognize underlying patterns of behavior or

disagreement
realism vs optimism

emotions, he or she is operating in the formal mode. Young children are not usually believed capable of formal thought, but they do go through a form of pattern thinking that is structurally similar to adult formal thinking.

Examples of Formal-Operational Style

Child. Children exhibit a form of pattern thinking, as represented by such statements as "Daddy does that all the time," "That's the same as mine," or "I feel good about myself most of the time." These statements are, of course, not fully formal-operational in the Piagetian sense but they do illustrate that children are capable of a type of pattern thinking.

Adult. Examples of adult formal statements are "That seems to be a pattern of mine," "The two situations are very similar in that . . . ," "That's typical of my father," "As I think about my feelings, I find . . . ," "My reflection on that is . . . ," or "Comparing and contrasting the situations, I see . . ." A Muslim American who is racially profiled may feel angry and upset (sensorimotor) and first talk about a specific incident at an airport or with the police in detail (concrete). Later, when this client thinks about and reflects on the situation again, he or she may realize that Muslim Americans have experienced a *pattern* of discrimination or prejudice in other areas of their lives. Women, gays/lesbians, and People of Color become increasingly aware of patterns of sexism, heterosexism, and racism. What discriminates formal processing of these experiences from dialectic thought is that the client will reflect on his or her experiences and reactions to the prejudicial events. In the dialectic style, clients will begin to construct meaning of those experiences from multiple perspectives, not just their own.

Family. A professional family whose members tend to talk in abstractions represents an overly formal approach. The members may be able to analyze their issues but are unable to act on them or to change. They may talk about feelings rather than really experiencing them at the sensorimotor style. They may even be so deeply "into" reflection and analysis that you as an interviewer have a difficult time understanding what specifically happened to them.

There is also a late formal orientation in which the client integrates patterns of patterns. Successful therapy often helps the client integrate several patterns of thought and behavior into larger patterns or gestalts. For example, the client may have come to therapy with a vague sense of anger and discontent, blaming the spouse for difficulties in their marriage (a preoperational problem). The client may be blaming the spouse totally, exhibiting magical thinking characteristic of the later phases of this style. This larger pattern recognition also occurs when groups get together and share their experiences. Children of alcoholics (COA), war veterans groups, the Black and women's groups of the 1960s all help people see common patterns in their lives.

As counseling starts, the therapist typically will ask for concrete statements about the marital relationship. If all goes well, the client will then discover that there are certain situations that seem to repeat again and again. This is pattern thinking. The client may later discover that problems with a boss follow the same concrete behavioral sequences and patterns as do problems with the spouse. When the client begins examining interrelated, repeating patterns, he or she is moving into the late formal-operational stage. The therapist might look for patterns in the client's developmental history with his parents that are now repeating with the spouse and boss.

Your personal experience. Consider the situation when you felt overwhelmed. Has this happened in other situations? Is there a pattern? If so, what are some of your feelings about this pattern? What does the pattern imply about your own identity? Can you identify some repetitions of this pattern of thought and feeling in your own daily life now?

_____

_____

_____

_____

_____

_____

_____

_____

_____

_____

_____

_____

_____

_____

_____

_____

Dialectic/Systemic: Integrating Patterns of Emotion and Thought Into a System

Piaget also identifies post-formal thought, considering it a variation of formal operations. The most critical distinction between the two is the capability of the individual to step back, look at patterns, and reflect on the system of operations. Post-formal thinking and emotion require the capability for very abstract formulations. This style is exemplified by the adult who, having developed a sense of self, can step back and see the self and situation from varying perspectives. This ability to see one event from several perspectives is perhaps most indicative of post-formal cognition.

Counseling and therapy often seek to help clients take several perspectives on their problems. For example, some clients may have a very strong self-concept, but their self-view may be so rigid that they fail to see how they are hurting others

Patterns of patterns

very abstract ✓

in the family. A therapeutic task here, of course, is to help them change their cognitive/emotional style so they can see other points of view. DCT classifies this post-formal cognitive/emotional style as dialectic/systemic.

Thinking in the dialectic/systemic style requires one to step back to a third-order perspective and reflect on the systems of operations. Consider the following examples of different styles of thought on the issue of death and dying.

Sensorimotor. There is no perspective taking, no separation of oneself from others or from the situation. The response to a serious loss would be extensive crying and emotional catharsis—"I am my feelings." This may be the only style in which an individual genuinely works through grief and loss. Thus experiencing feelings in this style is a natural, essential part of grieving. Many clients who have experienced trauma have not yet explored their great sadness; the lack of sensorimotor exploration leaves the trauma unresolved.

Concrete-operational. The person is separated from objects or situations, but there is no awareness of one's emotional self. For example, "I feel sad" (said without emotion; early concrete) and "I feel sad because my mother died" (again a lack of emotion; late concrete). The person can talk about the experience, but in a manner devoid of feeling.

Formal-operational. The person is now able to step back and examine himself or herself looking at objects or situations. For example, "When I look at myself, I see myself feeling very sad about the loss" or "When my Grandma died, I felt sad, but I wasn't quite as upset as I might have been." There is a necessary distancing from the immediate impact of the death and an acceptance of the life process. However, this type of conversation is quite far from the actual feelings.

Dialectic/systemic. The person is able to reflect on the total system. Feelings may change in the context of varying systems—for example, "I felt overwhelmed and I cried a lot. I felt very sad about the loss. It's a pattern with me. I'm lucky now to be able to let some of it go. But I can think about it from another perspective. My mother was so full of pain from the cancer, that I get a feeling of relief about her death. I guess I learned from all this that life goes on. She lives in me. Sometimes I look at it one way and feel really sad, but at other times I know it was for the best." It would be difficult, perhaps impossible, to achieve this type of thought without first having gone through the other styles of grieving.

Another concept closely associated with the dialectic/systemic frame of reference is transformation. In the above example, the client was able to look at the situation from several perspectives and to transform the data into a new gestalt. Although such transformational thought is valuable, it is very intellectually abstract. Many clients prefer to stay abstract and may fail to deal with concrete reality or come to grips with the depth of emotional expression found within the sensorimotor orientation.

As helping professionals, we assist clients to think using the dialectic/systemic style when we help them consider a range of data and ask them such questions as "Can you look at your situation from another perspective?" or "How does all this look to you now that we've talked about it for a while?" or "How would you integrate all this?" Such questions encourage more complex, integrative thinking. When we ask clients to take another perspective on themselves or a situation, we are moving them toward the dialectic/systemic orientation.

Perspective matters!

Examples of the Dialectic/Systemic Style

Child. Children obviously cannot be expected to use dialectic/systemic thought. Nonetheless, when we help children see another child's perspective, we approach this dimension. "How do you feel when you are hit? . . . Now, how do you think Juan felt when you hit him?" Children are naturally empathic—witness the infant who cries when another child falls down in tears. We can build on this ability by encouraging children to talk about how other people might feel or think. Sometimes even "What would your mother say/think?" can facilitate elementary perspective taking.

Adult. The same strategies above with appropriate language changes will facilitate dialectic/systemic multiperspective thought. The effect of external systems on individuals may be harder to put across. For example, in your work with depressed clients, a real challenge can be to enable them to see that their sadness relates to a past history of family abuse, spiritual oppression, or a pattern of subtle racist or sexist acts in the workplace. It is natural in much of Western culture to attribute fault, blame, or causation to oneself. However, many times, internal psychological issues are the result of systemic issues. Is the problem to be attributed to the person or to the system? Most often, a reasonable balance of internal and external causation and attribution is most appropriate.

Your personal experience. Review your written responses where you used the sensorimotor, concrete, and formal styles. As you reflect on your various responses, how would you integrate them? What sense do they make to you? Can you now take another perspective, perhaps one different from the one you just arrived at? What stands out from your personal examination? How have varying systems affected who you are and how you think about these issues?

_____

_____

_____

_____

_____

_____

_____

_____

_____

_____

_____

_____

Now, let us turn to the philosophic aspects underlying DCT. In Chapter 1, we talked about Plato's philosophy as the search for the truth and new ways of thinking and being. As you engage in development assessment, recall that you are always working with a client's worldview deeply affected by that person's own definitions of what is truth and what is reality.

PLATO'S ALLEGORY OF THE CAVE

Plato's Allegory of the Cave presents the journey of a slave moving from chains to freedom. It is seen as a metaphor for the growth of consciousness and as the movement toward the light and truth. As you read the following summary of the Allegory, please refer again to Table 1.1 (p. 24)—a brief, visual outline of the stages of consciousness and how they might relate to Piagetian and DCT thought. Plato and Piaget both tend to emphasize "higher" forms of knowledge and thinking while DCT stresses that each consciousness style is important for a holistic approach to life.

The Sensory World of Images

Imagine a group of slaves chained together. Behind them is a candle throwing shadows on the wall in front of them. They cannot turn their heads. The only "reality" they see is ahead—the images or shadows on the wall. This has been their world and all their cognitions and emotions are based on these sensory impressions. The shadows have become reality to them.

Connections to Piaget and DCT: Piaget talks about children's magical thinking and distorted views of reality. For example, children may believe that their shadows "know where I am going and keep following me." DCT points out that adolescent and adult clients may also be embedded in sensorimotor emotion such as crying or deep sadness or they may come to therapy with confused thoughts or irrational ideas. Therapeutic strategies such as relaxation, guided imagery, and bodywork have a primary sensorimotor basis.

The Concrete World of Belief

One of the slaves is allowed to turn to the light and first reacts by wanting to return to the familiar and safer world of shadows. Eventually, however, he is rewarded with a new worldview or perception. What was seen before is now recognized as illusion. A new "reality" has been found and the slave believes that the light is the new truth. There is more in the cave than just shadows. He tells his fellow slaves about the candles and provides a concrete explanation for the shadows on the wall. The chained slaves, however, still see only the shadows and they deride his comments. *What you see is what you get!*

Connections to Piaget and DCT: Concrete-operational children are focused on observables and linearity. They are very good at storytelling and can supply many details. They have difficulty in seeing perceptions other than their own. DCT points out that many adult clients present their issues in story form with step-by-step concrete and detailed descriptions. Like the concrete children, they may have difficulty in seeing patterns of thought and in reflecting on themselves. Assertiveness training, concrete specific identification of thoughts and feelings, and the storytelling aspects of narrative theory are examples of concrete counseling strategies. On the other hand, taking behavioral action is often a strength of the concrete style.

The Reflective Formal-Operational World of Thinking

The slave "crosses the line" and is then taken outside the cave into the sunlight, which brings the pain of a new awareness He now realizes that his earlier beliefs about "reality" were naïve and limited. This new world is so full of possibility that he cannot see it all at once. He would rather return to the cave. He reflects on what he now sees. He encounters the abstract world of ideas.

Connections to Piaget and DCT: The person with the formal-operational style is able to reflect on operations and objects, develop patterns, and examine the self. You may think of the adolescent who discovers that he or she has a "self" and an "identity." This change can be difficult, stormy, and painful for the teen. DCT points out that much of counseling and therapy emphasizes reflection and thinking about things rather than direct experience. Cognitive-behavior and narrative therapy give this style of thinking considerable attention as clients look at their patterns of thought and behavior.

The Multiperspective World of Dialectic Thought

Plato's slave is then returned to the darkness of the cave and he tries to tell those remaining in bondage of what he has experienced and that what they see is only shadows. "They would laugh at him and say that he had come back with his sight ruined. . . . If they could lay hands on the man who was trying to set them free and lead them up, they would kill him" (quoted in Cornford, 1941/1982, p. 231). Plato points out that we live in a world in which there are many points of view, that we all need to examine ourselves as well as others, and that the interaction among many variables needs to be considered. The world is complex and varied and there is no final answer. *Noesis* is the dialectic, the study of multiple relations and systems.

Connections to Piaget and DCT: Piaget uses the term *post-formal operations,* which implies "thinking about thinking." Here we find a more "advanced" cognitive/emotional style that examines issues from multiple perspectives. In addition, sensorimotor, concrete, and formal/reflective thinking are seen as perspectives or points from which a person might develop an entire worldview. DCT's dialectic/systemic style continues in this tradition. The emphasis moves from "self" to "self-in-context" and systems (family, group, culture) become more important. Multicultural counseling and therapy and feminist therapy are two theories that focus on this area, although they recognize the importance of multiple styles of being.

SUMMARY

Clients come to us with a unique view of the world. It is our task to enter into their way of understanding the world. Before we intervene, we must learn how they think about themselves, their situations, and their problems. Developmental assessment is one part of developing empathy and helping us join the client where she or he is.

Piagetian terms are used here in new ways. A client who has a problem and some difficulty in operating on the self or situation is described as preoperational. *Clients present themselves for counseling in one of four primary cognitive/emotional styles: sensorimotor/elemental, concrete/situational, formal/reflective, and dialectic/systemic.* The four cognitive/emotional styles, in turn, can be subdivided into early and late styles. (Specific modes of identifying and classifying the eight styles can be found in Appendix 2.)

Sensorimotor style. Clients tend to talk in a random and disorganized fashion and tend not to separate themselves from their experience. Or they may be totally focused on a single emotional style. A severely depressed client is also illustrative of this cognitive/emotional style. At the late stage, there may be magical thinking and some beginning ability to be concrete. Key words: elemental, see/hear/feel.

Concrete style. Clients describe their situations and emotions in specific, linear terms, with many details. At the late concrete, there may be if/then causal reasoning. Key words: situational, specifics.

Formal style. Clients move to abstractions, talking about self and patterns of self or situations. They tend to reflect on feelings rather than experience them directly. If they move to late formal, clients consider patterns of patterns. Key words: reflection, self-reflection, patterns, patterns of patterns.

Dialectic/systemic style. Clients are able to operate on systems of knowledge and can take a multiperspective view. Complexity of thinking and extensive abstraction mark the dialectic/systemic style. At the late dialectic/systemic style, look for the ability to work with and reflect on systems of operations. Key words: post-formal, integrative, systemic, transformational, multiperspectives.

It is possible to identify the client's cognitive/emotional style and orientation, whether the client is a child, adolescent, or adult. The same assessment principles can be applied to family, group, and organizational counseling and consulting. Cultural variations, which will be elaborated in Chapter 6, are particularly important to consider when you are working with an individual from a group different from your own.

Plato's Allegory of the Cave. This story reminds us that cognitive/emotional development is not without pain or difficulty. As we grow and discover new styles of consciousness and other perspectives, we often have to give up old ways of thinking and being. Counselors and therapists need to anticipate resistance to change and development in clients.

Challenges: Clients, families, and groups present their issues in multiple styles. Do not allow yourself to become ensnared in assessment to the point that you blind yourself to the complexity of the human being before you. Also recall that the concepts of style and orientation presented here are metaphorical. Piaget himself pointed out that we could divide development into 4, 8, 80, or 800 styles and stages if we wished.

Research issues:

- Tape one of your counseling sessions and transcribe the interview, or obtain a tape of another counseling session or transcript of that session. Rate each statement in the interview according to the DCT classification system. Have a colleague rate the same interview and calculate your interrater agreement. How is your preferred style reflected in your counseling interventions?

- Think about some of your own interviews and counseling sessions. Note some times when the client's style preferences were the same as yours and some when they were different. By the end of the interview, especially when your client's preferred styles did not match your own preferences, did the client change? How?

- Classify one of your own past interviews using the DCT classification system. Have a colleague rate the same interview and calculate your own interrater agreement. Do your clients change the style of their cognitions through their interactions with you? You may find Appendix 2 helpful as you rate your own and your client's statements.

THEORY INTO PRACTICE: DEVELOPING YOUR PORTFOLIO OF COMPETENCE

You are the first focus in this series of exercises. What is your preferred style of helping? The exercises here are designed to help you identify and classify cognitive/emotional style. Two interview exercises focus on taking the theory to live practice sessions. Generalization and the ability to take theory home into practice is the focus of the next three exercises. A final self-reflective portfolio exercise asks you to reflect back on the chapter and indicate what the concepts mean to you personally. Theory is useless unless it has practical personal implications for you, the counselor or therapist.

Self-Assessment Exercise

Exercise 1. Your preferred style of helping

As we start your portfolio exercises, let's examine your own developmental preferences. Complete the DCT Preferred Helping Style Inventory (Appendix 5). What do your results say about your own preferences for working with clients in interviews?

_____

_____

_____

_____

_____

_____

_____

_____

_____

What kinds of clients will you be most comfortable working with? What cognitive/emotional styles may be more challenging?

_____

_____

_____

_____

_____

_____

We must always be aware of our own preferences, as clients will match our style rather than the other way around if we are not careful! When using DCT, it is important to learn the client's preferred styles and developmental blocks before mismatching with our own preferred styles. Of course, effective and ethical counselors choose their own style preferences only when these are in the best interests of clients, as discussed more fully in the next chapter, which explores treatment planning using DCT.

Identifying Client Cognitive/Emotional Style

Exercise 2. Identifying written client statements

Which cognitive/emotional style does each of the following examples represent? All of the following statements might be the first thing a client says to you. It is possible to identify reliably the cognitive/emotional developmental style of the client just by evaluating a few words or phrases. Also, remember that client cognitive/emotional style often changes throughout a single interview.

Sometimes it is hard to decipher print or understand intent and meaning or feelings without a typescript, videotape, or actual client interaction. In reviewing the following statements, refer back to the definitions earlier in the chapter of the four modalities, particularly Box 4-1. Remember that sensorimotor emotion is reflected in the experiencing of feelings in the here and now, whereas concrete experiencing of emotions refers to a more linear, factual statement of what was felt, when, and how.

Each of the cases below involves some mixture of developmental styles, as clients seldom present in just one style. Your therapeutic response affects how these clients talk about their issues, a point elaborated on in the next chapter. Circle the primary cognitive/emotional style(s) (S—sensorimotor, C—concrete, F—formal, DS—dialectic/systemic). At the conclusion of this chapter is an interpretation of the cases.

1. S C F D/S (age 16; ambitious high school student who has just done poorly on an examination, in tears) I just can't do it. I tried hard. I'm so confused. My dad will really get angry. (more tears) And my teachers are on me about it.

2. S C F D/S (age 35; parent talking about a problem with her 13-year-old) Sally and I just had an argument. I wanted her to wash the dishes and help for a

change. She said "No," with a very angry and nasty face. Then she ran upstairs. I ran right after her just as mad as she was. But she had locked the door. I just sat there and fumed.

3. S C F D/S (age 40; just working through a divorce) I just had another date. This is only the second person I've dated, but again I'm repeating that pattern. My perfectionism got in the way of my marriage. Even with the first person I dated, I noted that I started criticizing and making suggestions after the third time we went out. My perfectionism showed itself last night when I told my date that her car could stand some cleaning! How can I get rid of this pattern?

4. S C F D/S (age 63; just entering a new executive position) As I look back on my years with Carter Finance, I'm seeing so much. In my first years, I simply worked to make a living and didn't worry much about how the company was working either for me or against me. I just wanted the money. Then, when I was promoted to assistant head of the department, I started noticing that a lot of people had a pattern of not caring for the company. As I moved up in administration, I began to see how the company could be reorganized to meet personnel needs more effectively. And in the last few years, I've got a better handle on how the company relates to the external market. Each time I look at it, Carter Finance seems a bit different.

5. S C F D/S (age 24; documented problem of alcohol abuse and absenteeism on the job) I had a really great time last night. I really hung one on. St. James beer is the best. Just looking at the can makes me feel good. I love the sound of the tab popping open.

6. S C F D/S (same client as above) Yeah, I got drunk last night. Just before I went out, I found out that my wife had left me because I drank so much. I decided to hang one on. I went to my favorite bar and drank perhaps a six-pack of James. Then my friend and I went to another bar across town. (more details) At the end I didn't recall anything.

7. S C F D/S (same client as above) This is typical of me when I get upset. In situations where things don't go the way I want them to, I just have to get away. It's been a pattern for me throughout the marriage, too. Whenever Sue didn't pay enough attention to me, I threatened her by leaving. Then I'd go out and get drunk. I think I'm happier drunk than sober.

8. S C F D/S (same client as above) Drinking has been important in our family for generations. Drinking is a way we express ourselves. My Dad drank a good bit but was able to hold it. I understand Grandpa died of liver disease at 42. I understand people from our ethnic group have a higher probability of alcoholism than most people. As I look back on the pattern in the family over the years, I guess I have reason for concern.

9. S C F D/S (age 12; concerned about peer group pressures) If I don't dress better, others may not like me. I need to look good to keep up with other people. The way I look determines how other people see me. I've tried to talk to my parents, but they said the way I dress is fine. They treat me like a child!

10. S C F D/S (age 4; talking about father) Daddy took me to his office. He said he wanted to show me to his friends. He held me up in front of them. I put my face into Daddy's shoulder. He laughed. I felt good.

11. S C F D/S (age 15; in a dilemma about vocational choice) The career course is a bore. I know what I want to do. I want to be an actress. The tests they gave me suggested I should think about selling things. I don't want to be a salesclerk.

12. S C F D/S (age 45; during a family counseling session) My husband has a pattern of always telling the children what to do. Right now, look at him—so smug! He always thinks he is right. There is no way you can change him.

13. S C F D/S (age 23; gay male) I'm waiting for the results of my AIDS test. I'm scared and worried about what it might say (starts to shake and almost becomes teary).

14. S C F D/S (age 29; African American woman) At first, I thought it was my fault when I didn't get the promotion. I actually thought I ought to work harder. But later I realized that this is the fifth time that someone I've trained has been promoted over me. This office is really against People of Color.

Exercise 3. Assessing cognitive/emotional style for both client and counselor in a complete interview

Appendix 4 contains a full interview for practice in classifying client and interviewer responses. You can also categorize the helping leads of the counselor on the same four-style scale. You may want to draw on Appendix 2—The DCT Cognitive/Emotional Classification System to facilitate this task.

Toward Multicultural Competence

Exercise 4. DCT styles and cultural identity theory

Chapter 8 explores the relationship between DCT and multicultural counseling and therapy (MCT). One important concept in that chapter is cultural identity theory. As a pretest to help you anticipate that chapter, what DCT style might apply to the following client statements representing four ways of thinking about cultural identity? Answers to corresponding DCT styles will be found at the end of the chapter.

DCT Style	Cultural Identity Level	Example Identity Statement
	Preencounter	1. I don't see why people make such a fuss about color. Isn't everyone equal?
	Encounter	2. Now I see what is going on. It's oppression. I can't get into a restaurant and I'm angry about it.
	Immersion/emersion	3. Thinking about it, I'm proud of my race and really feeling good about my color. I feel better about myself and my people.
	Internalization	4. It's very complex. Oppression is clearly the central issue, but there are good and bad people of all races and colors. Those of us who want change need to work together.

Exercise 5. Examining yourself on multicultural issues

Multicultural Competency16. "Culturally-competent counselors and therapists become actively involved with minority individuals outside the counseling setting (via community events, social and political functions, celebrations, friendships, neighborhood groups, and so forth) so that their perspective of minorities is more than an academic or helping exercise." (Sue et al., 1996, p. 41)

If your body has not been there, the mind may have difficulty in understanding. DCT stresses the importance of helping clients see different frames of reference and experience their lives from several different perspectives. But rather than just think of multiple perspectives, we are asking you to encounter difference with a sensorimotor and concrete style. For example, Mary Bradford Ivey learned that she must get into the community if she was to obtain self-referrals for counseling from culturally different groups. She visited homes and attended community celebrations for over two years before enough trust was developed in the community for self-referral and full parent involvement. Sitting in your office and just seeing clients there is not enough. You cannot build trust with a community just by being in an agency or school.

To discover the depths of difference, we suggest that you visit a family, group, or community event different from your own background. If you are an African American or White American, attend a Native American Pow-wow or other cultural celebration such as a Mexican fiesta. The goal is to encounter different cultures directly. You may engage in volunteer work in a community different from your own. You might attend a Black church or a Mass in Polish or Spanish or visit a synagogue or mosque. Such experiences are essential if you are to expand your view of multicultural issues.

What was the sensorimotor experience? What did you see, hear, feel?

_____

_____

_____

_____

_____

Describe your experience in concrete and specific terms. Tell a story about the event.

_____

_____

_____

_____

_____

What are your formal reflections of your experience? What new patterns did you observe? How did these affect your conception of yourself?

_____

_____

_____

_____

From a systems frame of reference, how might people in this culturally different group come to think and behave similarly to and differently from you? And, perhaps most important, reflecting on your reflections for this exercise is only a small beginning.

_____

_____

_____

_____

_____

Interviewing Practice Exercises

Exercise 6. Identifying client cognitive/emotional style in a role-played situation

Find a volunteer partner with whom to practice identifying cognitive/emotional style. Each can take turns identifying client style. Following is a list of interview openers and questions with space where you can take notes on the client's answer. Identify the client's developmental style and your evidence for making that assessment. Evidence usually consists of specific verbal behaviors of your partner/client. However, recall that nonverbal cues can be useful in your developmental assessment. Follow standard ethical procedures in the session.

An alternative to this exercise is to divide into groups of four. The first individual acts as client; the second, as interviewer; the other two are observers. The interviewer asks the first question and, by using listening skills, draws out data. The session is stopped after about 50 to 100 words are spoken by the client, and the entire group discusses the cognitive/emotional style of the client. Once the discussion is complete, the interviewer becomes the client, and one of the observers asks the second question. Again, the cognitive/emotional style is examined. Continue rotating through the questions until there is some feeling of comfort about being able to identify client style on the spot.

Write down key words and thoughts of the client in the space provided. Then identify the cognitive/emotional style, using specific evidence to back up your decision.

1. Tell me about a time when you were late with an assignment.

_____

_____

S C F D/S Cite specific evidence for your decision below.

_____

_____

2. When you hear the words *alcohol* and *drugs*, what comes to your mind?

_____

_____

S C F D/S Cite specific evidence for your decision below.

_____

_____

3. Tell me about an interpersonal conflict you had in the past.

_____

_____

S C F D/S Cite specific evidence for your decision below.

_____

_____

4. What occurs for you when you think about leaving home for the first time?

_____

_____

S C F D/S Cite specific evidence for your decision below.

_____

_____

5. What happens for you when you focus on your family?

_____

_____

S C F D/S Cite specific evidence for your decision below.

_____

_____

6. Almost all of us have at some point faced some form of discrimination or intolerance. Please tell us about your experience and how you felt.

_____

_____

S C F D/S Cite specific evidence for your decision below.

_____

_____

7. Formulate your own question.

_____

_____

S C F D/S Cite specific evidence for your decision below.

_____

_____

8. Formulate another question.

_____

_____

S C F D/S Cite specific evidence for your decision below.

_____

_____

Exercise 7. Group practice in cognitive/emotional styles

Given that client cognitive/emotional style can be identified, let us turn to a more complex observation process: the identification of both client and counselor cognitive/emotional style in a role-played session. Do not expect to be immediately proficient in this type of rating skill. With practice over time, you will develop increasing skill. Obtain appropriate permission and use standard ethical procedures.

Groups of three or four are required for this type of practice, which is similar to microcounseling practice sessions (see Ivey & Ivey, 2003).

Step 1: Divide Into Practice Groups
Get acquainted with each other informally before beginning. Use standard ethical procedures agreed upon by your class or workshop.

Step 2: Select a Group Leader
The leader's task is to ensure that the group follows the specific steps of the practice session. It often proves helpful if the least-experienced group member serves as leader first.

Step 3: Assign Roles for the Practice Session

- *Role-played client.* The role-played client will be cooperative, talk freely about the topic, and not give the interviewer a difficult time. In later practice sessions, it is critical that difficult problems or clients be selected.

- *Interviewer.* The interviewer will ask one of the questions above (including any question the interviewer and the client agree to beforehand) and practice drawing out the client in conversation about the selected topic. The interviewer should feel free to use his or her natural style and theory of helping.

- *Observer 1.* The first observer will fill out the feedback form in Box 4-3, summarizing observations on the client's cognitive/emotional style.

- *Observer 2.* The second observer will fill out the feedback form, summarizing observations on the interviewer's cognitive/emotional style.

Step 4: Plan the Session

- The interviewer and client must first agree on the topic. Please use the list of topics in the earlier practice exercise for this group session. The interviewer may wish to facilitate client talk with his or her own natural style of interviewing.

- The client may wish to think through how he or she wants to talk about the agreed-on topic through the session.

- The two observers can examine the feedback forms and be ready to classify each client or interviewer statement. You will find that it is possible to list the main words of the client; this will help in reconstructing the interview for the discussion period.

Step 5: Conduct a 5-Minute Interviewing Session
The interviewer and client will discuss the issue for 5 minutes while the observers keep track of their progress and classify the statements of each. It is helpful to videotape and/or audiotape practice sessions.

Step 6: Provide Immediate Feedback and Complete Notes (5 Minutes)
This is a highly structured session, and there is often immediate need to personally "process" and discuss the session. In particular, it is helpful for the interviewer to ask the client "What stands out for you from this practice session?" Allow yourself some time to provide true personal reactions to the practice.

The interviewer needs the same opportunity to reflect on what happened. The client may ask for these personal reactions to the session. This change of role can be useful to both. At this point, the observers should sit back and let the participants take control. Use this time to complete your classification and notes.

Step 7: Review the Practice Session and Provide Feedback (15 Minutes)
It is important in giving feedback to allow the person receiving the feedback to be in charge. Thus, the interviewer should be the person who asks for feedback rather than getting it without having asked. At this point, the observers can share their observations from the feedback form. Feedback should be specific, concrete, and nonjudgmental (that is, avoid saying "That was terrific" or "That was terrible. You should have . . ."). Pay attention to the strengths of the interview.

You will find that classification of client and counselor cognitive/developmental style is not easy when you focus solely on single comments, because most people talk in multiple styles. Thus, in the first stages of learning, allow yourself time and be satisfied with the ability to note the clearest examples of each style. Later you will be able to recognize cognitive/emotional style and shifts in style automatically.

Generalization: Taking Developmental Assessment Home

Many ideas are presented in books and in workshops designed for the professional practice of counseling and therapy. Most of these books are left on the shelf, unused, to gather dust and then are forgotten. The question for you at this point is whether you will incorporate the concepts of developmental assessment into your daily life and into regular interview practice.

To "take developmental assessment concepts home" requires some commitment to action on your part. In effect, ideas and abstractions are presented here. Ultimately, it is your concrete practice and action that counts. Following are some activities that have been found especially useful in ensuring that these basic ideas are used.

Exercise 8. Personal observation of individuals in daily life

A beginning step toward useful generalization of developmental assessment is to observe those you come into contact with in daily life. With what cognitive/emotional style are friends and family members talking to you? At what cognitive/emotional style are you answering? Do they talk about issues at several styles or at one style? Do they move through developmental progressions (for example, starting with concretes and then moving to formal abstractions)?

Can you notice mismatches between the cognitive/emotional styles of two or more individuals? You may find considerable misunderstanding and conflict between a concrete and a formal approach to problem solving. Plan to observe at least one person per day during the coming week. Do not hesitate to observe yourself now and then. Summarize your observations using the feedback sheet in Box 4-3.

Exercise 9. Observation of a family, group, or organization

Following the same method and format as above, observe a group. You will find that there is a general "tone" of a family, group, or organization that can be assessed as one of the cognitive/emotional styles. Different members of the group will have different ideas about the interactions of the group. Record your observations using an adaptation of the form in Box 4-3.

Exercise 10. Taking developmental assessment to the interview

Each day, listen carefully to one client in a helping interview. You will find that it is possible to make a general assessment of cognitive/emotional style in the overall way a client conceptually approaches a particular problem, concern, or issue. Also learn to note the way a client approaches issues stylistically. The client may have an overall formal approach to thinking about the problem but, on prompting from you, may move at times to the concrete style. This type of client may have some difficulty working in the sensorimotor style. Most clients need to develop their basic

| **Box 4-3** | Assessing Developmental Style Feedback Sheet |

Instructions: First, write down the main words of the client or interviewer statement. You'll find that you can obtain a fairly close record of the actual interview as it progresses. Do not, however, expect your numbering system to exactly match other observers'. Most important is getting a few key words so that the interview can be reconstructed. If you are working with audio or video, you may wish to replay the session step by step for more precision. Second, classify both client and interviewer's statements. Over time, and with practice, this way of observing will become easier and more natural for you.

Circle the developmental style used by client or by interviewer.

1. S/M C F D/S _____
2. S/M C F D/S _____
3. S/M C F D/S _____
4. S/M C F D/S _____
5. S/M C F D/S _____
6. S/M C F D/S _____
7. S/M C F D/S _____
8. S/M C F D/S _____
9. S/M C F D/S _____
10. S/M C F D/S _____
11. S/M C F D/S _____
12. S/M C F D/S _____
13. S/M C F D/S _____
14. S/M C F D/S _____
15. S/M C F D/S _____
16. S/M C F D/S _____
17. S/M C F D/S _____
18. S/M C F D/S _____
19. S/M C F D/S _____
20. S/M C F D/S _____
21. S/M C F D/S _____
22. S/M C F D/S _____
23. S/M C F D/S _____
24. S/M C F D/S _____

(Continue on a separate sheet of paper.)

concrete skills. Others have allowed themselves to become so abstract in the formal and dialectic/systemic areas that they have lost touch with reality.

Again, provide specific evidence that you have been able to assess the cognitive/emotional style of your own clients.

_____

_____

_____

_____

Portfolio Reflections

Exercise 11. Your reflections on developmental assessment

What stood out for you from this chapter? What sense do you make of what you have just read? What are your key points? Record your thoughts here and in a Portfolio Folder in your computer.

_____

_____

_____

_____

_____

_____

_____

_____

REFERENCES

Cornford, F. (1982). *The republic of Plato*. London: Oxford. (Original work published 1941)

Gonçalves, O., Ivey, A., & Langdell, S. (1988). The multilevel conception of intentionality: Implications for counselor training. *Counseling Psychology Quarterly, 1*(4), 377–387.

Hoffman, L. (1991). Developmental counseling for prekindergarten children: A preventive approach. *Elementary School Guidance & Counseling, 26*, 56–67.

Ivey, A. (2000). *Developmental therapy: Theory into practice*. North Amherst, MA: Microtraining. (Original work published 1986)

Ivey, A., & Ivey, M. (1990). Assessing and facilitating children's cognitive development: Developmental counseling and therapy in a case of child abuse. *Journal of Counseling and Development, 68*, 299–305.

Ivey, A., & Ivey, M. (2003). *Intentional interviewing and counseling: Facilitating development in a multicultural world* (5th ed.). Pacific Grove, CA: Brooks/Cole.

Jankowski, P. J. (1998). A developmental-constructivist framework for narrative therapy. *Family Therapy, 25*(2), 111–120.

Kenney, D., & Law, J. (1991). Developmental counseling and therapy with involuntary mid-life career changers. *Journal of Young Adulthood and Middle Age, 3,* 25–39.

Marszalek, J. (1999). The gay and lesbian affirmative development (GLAD) model: Testing the validity of an integrative model of gay identity development theory and Ivey's developmental counseling therapy model. *Dissertation Abstracts International: Section B. The Sciences & Engineering, 59*(11–B), 6107.

Marszalek, J., & Cashwell, C. (1998). The gay and lesbian affirmative development (GLAD) model: Applying Ivey's developmental counseling therapy model to Cass' gay and lesbian identity development model. *Journal of Adult Development and Aging: Theory and Research, 1*(1), 13–31.

Myers, J. E., Shoffner, M., & Briggs, M. (2002). Developmental counseling and therapy: An effective tool for understanding and counseling children. *The Professional School Counselor, 5,* 194–202.

Rigazio-DiGilio, S. (1989). *Developmental theory and therapy: A preliminary investigation of reliability and predictive validity using an inpatient depressive population.* Unpublished doctoral dissertation, University of Massachusetts, Amherst.

Rigazio-DiGilio, S., & Ivey, A. (1990). Developmental therapy and depressive disorders: Measuring cognitive levels through patient natural language. *Professional Psychology: Research and Practice, 21*(6), 470–475.

Strehorn, K. C. (1999). Examining services to postsecondary students with learning disabilities through the use of Ivey's developmental counseling and therapy (DCT) model. *Dissertation Abstracts International: Section A. Humanities & Social Sciences, 59*(7–A), 2367.

Sue, D. W., Carter, R., Casas, J., Fouad, N., Ivey, A., Jensen, M., LaFromboise, T., Manese, J., Ponterotto, J., & Nuttall, E. (1996). *Multicultural competencies: Individual and organizational development.* Beverly Hills, CA: Sage.

Answers to Chapter Exercises

Identifying Client's Cognitive/Emotional Style

1. S—overwhelmed by emotions; frequent topic jumps; some concrete elements as well.
2. C—concrete description here.
3. F—relatively advanced formal; able to see a variety of repeating patterns.
4. D/S—able to operate on systems and see complex relationships.
5. S—emphasis on direct sensory experience; a certain amount of concreteness present as well.
6. C—description with no analysis.
7. F—words such as *pattern* or *typical*, which are characteristic of formal thinking.
8. D/S—multiperspective thinking; ability to operate on systems.

(The final four are more complex and are mixtures of varying styles.)

9. C and F—almost any response can be classified into more than one grouping. (Children just about to enter adolescence present with a mixture of formal and concrete thought.)

10. C—although primarily still in SM, pieces of conversation are clearly concrete; examples of childish formal thought evident in such statements as "Daddy is always like that." (Most young children are able to see and name patterns in their parents' behavior.)

11. C and F—a mixture is characteristic of clients about to make critical transformations. (Our therapeutic task usually is to start at the concrete style and get things clear before we move to the pattern thinking required at the formal style.)

12. F—particularly clear example of how formal thinking can be preoperational and a problem. (Some clients are so involved in identifying people and patterns that they are unable to see concrete change or the systemic nature of the event.)

13. S and C—Even if we are firmly concrete or formal, there are events that can reduce us to sensorimotor experiencing.

14. D/S—early on the client acted formally, but now has moved to dialectic awareness.

Toward Multicultural Competence

Style 1 because the individual is expressing what in multicultural counseling and therapy is termed an embedded style of consciousness. This can appear in People of Color or White individuals. What occurs is a relative lack of awareness of the issues and an acceptance of the status quo.

Style 2 because the individual, whether White or of Color, has encountered the reality of oppression and racism and wants to take concrete action.

Style 3 because the person is thinking/reflecting about the self and the situation.

Style 4 because we see the beginning of multiple perspectives.

CHAPTER 5
Developmental Interventions and Strategies

Specific Interventions to Facilitate Client Cognitive and Emotional Development

CENTRAL PRACTICE OBJECTIVE | Mastery and practice of concepts in this chapter will enable you to apply specific DCT questioning strategies with many types of clients and to adapt the strategies for your work utilizing many theories of counseling and therapy.

Assessment leads directly to specific treatment strategies in developmental counseling and therapy (DCT). You assess client cognitive/emotional style and then, using specific skills and strategies, you facilitate personal growth and/or change. You'll find the DCT strategies discussed here helpful with many types of clients—a child who has a friendship problem, a teen searching out sexual identity, an adult working through a difficult divorce, or a depressed client in an inpatient situation.

As an integrative metatheory—a theory about counseling and therapy—DCT offers ways to assess client cognitive/emotional patterns, match interventions to client needs, and draw from traditional theoretical approaches in establishing treatment plans. It will also give you a rationale for selecting various interventions to help clients who may present with varying cognitive/emotional styles and developmental issues and blocks. These interventions may be strength-based, operating from a wellness perspective, and based on strengths identified in the DCT assessment. As we will see in later chapters, personality disorders also may be conceptualized and successfully treated using the wellness perspective combined with DCT assessment and interventions.

Developmental counseling and therapy can be described as an integrative, learning-based theory about human growth and change. As clients develop, they follow identifiable patterns. The preceding chapter showed how to identify the various cognitive and affective styles. Given variations in the developmental styles of our clients and the fact that a single client will often present her or his issues using multiple styles, we as professional helpers need to have an array of skills and theories available so that we can change what we are doing in the moment in synchrony with changing client needs.

Knowledge and skill in the concepts of this chapter can enable you to:

1. Utilize specific questions and interventions to facilitate client cognitive and emotional development in the interview. (These DCT interventions can themselves form the basis for treatment.)
2. Understand traditional therapy and counseling theory from a cognitive/emotional developmental perspective. (DCT uses a learning framework for integrating seemingly competing theories of counseling and therapy.)
3. Apply DCT strategies and traditional theory to the many developmental tasks faced by our clients.
4. Apply the concepts of this chapter in real life through reflection and practice exercises and develop a portfolio of competence. Special attention is paid to practicing the DCT questioning strategies.

INTRODUCTION: YOUR INTERVIEWING STYLE AND THEORY DEEPLY AFFECT HOW CLIENTS RESPOND

Basic to the developmental counseling and therapy model is the premise that the actions and thoughts of the therapist affect how the client thinks about and discusses issues in the interview. At one point, it was fashionable for therapists to think they are totally objective and never influence what their clients say or do.

But, you cannot *not* affect the client's world. The very fact that you are in an interview with a client changes the client's way of experiencing the problem. DCT talks about mutual influence issues in counseling and therapy. Data clearly indicate that clients talk about what their therapists reinforce. For example, a classic study examined how a single client changed language and thinking as she worked with three different prominent therapists—Albert Ellis, Fritz Perls, and Carl Rogers (Meara, Shannon, & Pepinsky, 1979). Close examination of the client Gloria in the well-known film *Three Approaches to Psychotherapy* showed that she quickly learned to follow the language system of three different therapists. In this case, Gloria talked like Carl Rogers when talking to Rogers, used language similar to Albert Ellis when talking to Ellis, and spoke a more Gestalt-oriented language when she was talking to Fritz Perls. The therapeutic conversation is a mutual influence process in which both you and the client are influenced, and it will change your language.

It is clear that different theoretical approaches affect the way clients look at and discuss their issues. Similarly, the specific actions in terms of questions and listening skills that you use in the session impact what the clients will say next—and, eventually, how they construct their solutions to problems and concerns.

This chapter first explores specific questioning strategies of developmental counseling and therapy. We then turn to the more general question of how theories and strategies of counseling and therapy can be examined from a developmental perspective.

DEVELOPMENTAL QUESTIONS AND STRATEGIES FOR VERTICAL AND HORIZONTAL DEVELOPMENT

For each of the four cognitive/emotional developmental styles (sensorimotor, concrete, formal/reflective, and dialectic/systemic), specific developmental questions and strategies have been generated that help clients talk about their issues within their own cognitive/emotional frameworks. But working within the client's zone of comfort is not always appropriate. The DCT questions can also be used to help the client explore issues from a new point of view. For example, a person who discusses concerns primarily within a concrete orientation may benefit from a review of these same issues from a formal/reflective orientation. An over-intellectualized client using a formal/reflective or dialectic/systemic style may learn to experience things more deeply through a sensorimotor style. The counseling or therapy task, then, is both to work in the client's presenting style (horizontal development) and also to help the client move to new styles of consciousness (vertical development).

Horizontal Development

Individuals and families cannot grow and progress effectively unless a solid developmental foundation has been established. DCT stresses that it is important to help clients expand their understanding of issues and problems within their primary cognitive/emotional style. Thus, expanding the client's sensorimotor functioning may be needed before moving to concrete and formal understandings. Similarly, it is important to help abstract formal/reflective or dialectic/systemic clients to expand their cognitions and emotions within their usual styles before helping them progress to sensorimotor and concrete styles. In short, first meet the client where he or she "is," and then later mismatch styles and help clients look at themselves in new ways.

Vertical Development

Vertical development involves moving "up" to reach more complex ways of thinking or "down" to build more solid foundations. Higher is not necessarily better. Vertical development involves helping a client expand developmental potential at other levels or styles than where he or she started. Often, vertical development will be facilitated by returning to basic sensorimotor and concrete cognitions and then moving sequentially to formal and dialectic/systemic orientations.

To facilitate horizontal and vertical development, DCT interventions are often focused on specific questions. See Box 5-1 for the basic list and Appendix 3 for a more detailed presentation. Questions are sometimes controversial in the helping process. Specifically, some authorities state that questions come from the interviewer and do not represent the client's perspective. Furthermore, questions can be used to control the session and disempower the client. DCT points out that the questions presented here are open and actually facilitate clients' talking about their own issues as they see, hear, and feel them in more depth. What happens with DCT systematic intervention procedures is that clients and families do talk about issues from their own personal experience and they learn how to gain new perspectives on themselves, but always within their own frame of reference. It would be possible, of course, to facilitate client discussion in each of the developmental styles through less directive means. For example, note how the transcript of Carl Rogers (presented later in this chapter) facilitates client discussion within varying cognitive/emotional styles. (For a more detailed discussion of this important issue, see the discussion of holistic issues and dialectics in Ivey, 1986/2000, Chapters 6 and 7.)

open ended ?'s

Box 5-1	Developmental Strategies Questioning Sequence (Abbreviated)
Opening Presentation of Issue	"Could you tell me what you'd like to talk about today?" "What happens for you when you focus on your family?" Obtain story of from 50 to 100 words. Assess overall functioning of client on varying cognitive-developmental levels. Assess client cognitive/emotional style. Use questions, encourages, paraphrasing, and reflection of feeling to bring out data, but try to impact the client's story minimally. Get the story as he or she constructs it. Summarize key facts and feelings about what the client has said before moving on.
Sensorimotor/Elemental	"Could you think of one visual image that occurs to you in that situation?" "What are you seeing? Hearing? Feeling?" It helps to locate the feeling in the body. Elicit one example and then ask what was seen/heard/felt. Aim for here and now experiencing. Accept randomness. Summarize at the end of the segment. You may want to ask "What one thing stands out for you from this?"
Concrete/Situational	"Could you give me a specific example of the situation/issue/problem?" "Can you describe your feelings in the situation?"

(continued)

Box 5-1 *(continued)*	
	Obtain a linear description of the event. At late concrete operations, look for if/then causal reasoning. Ask "What did he or she do? Say? What happened before? What happened next? What happened after?" Possibly pose the question "If he or she did X, then what happened?" Summarize before moving on. For affective development, ask "What did you feel?" The statement "You felt X because . . ." helps integrate cognition with affect at this level.
Formal/Reflective	"Does this happen in other situations?" (or) "Is this a pattern for you?" "Do you feel that way in other situations? Are those feelings a pattern for you?" Talk about repeating patterns and situations and/or talk about self. Ask "What were you saying to yourself when that happened? Have you felt like that in other situations?" Again, reflect feelings and paraphrase as appropriate. Summarize key facts and feelings carefully before moving on. "As you look back at the situation you just talked about, what are your thoughts/reflections?"

Dialectic/Systemic/
Integrative
	Begin by summarizing all that has been said. Ask "How do you put together/organize all that you told me? What one thing stands out for you? How many different ways could you describe your feelings and how they change?"
	In addition to providing an integrated summary of what has been said, these questions serve the following functions: They enable the counselor and client to
	
	    a. see how reality is co-constructed, not developed from just a single view
	    b. obtain different perspectives on the same situation and be aware that each is just one perspective
	    c. note flaws in the present construction, co-construction, or perspective
	    d. move to action and test out new insights in daily life
	
	As we move toward more complex reasoning, several options are open. Before using any of them, summarize what the client has been saying over the entire series of questions.
	
	Integration: How do you put together/organize all that you told me? What one thing stands out for you most?
	
	Co-construction: What rule were you (they) operating under? Where did that rule come from? How might someone else (perhaps another family member) describe the situation? (Feelings can be examined using the same questions.)
	
	Multiple perspectives: How could we describe this from the point of view of some other person or using another theoretical framework or language system? How else might we put it together using another framework?
	
	Deconstruction and action: Can you see some flaws in the reasoning or in the patterns of feelings above? How might you change the rules? Given these possibilities, what action might you take?

Along with the specific questions, DCT strongly recommends extensive use of listening skills, such as encouragement, paraphrasing, reflection of feelings, and summarization. A high level of empathy, helper genuineness, and respect are needed or the systematic questioning procedures can be reduced to meaninglessness. *The questions, particularly with the sensorimotor style, can be quite powerful and moving to the client.* At times, new insights gained by the client can be extremely unsettling. Use these procedures with care, according to the needs of each client. Seek clinical supervision periodically when using these concepts.

Let us begin to examine these strategies using a simple and straightforward exercise. All of us have had to leave home or separate from someone or some area. For practice, take the topic of leaving and separation and work through the following set of questions. Imagine that a counselor is asking you the questions. Write down your answers or speak into an audiotape recorder. As a first step, you are asked to think about yourself and a developmental transition, such as an issue of separation. (This issue could be the first day of school, life at camp as a child, the loss of a loved one, leaving home for college or a major trip, or divorce.) After you have written your response, you can assess your own initial cognitive/emotional style on this issue (note that different issues in your life are likely to be thought of and discussed from varying developmental styles).

In completing this exercise, you will have worked with questions with the four central cognitive/emotional styles. You may find that you have taken four different perspectives on the same issue. Even in a brief exercise such as this, people will obtain a valuable new way of looking at an old situation. One of the major goals of many approaches to therapy and counseling is helping clients take a multiperspective point of view of their problems.

The questions below are not new. They are part of the vocabulary and skills of most effective counselors and therapists. What DCT offers that is new is the observation that these questions can be arranged in a systematic sequence similar to that of Piaget's stages of learning. This learning sequence can be applied more consciously in the interview. Rather than moving through each style by having the client answer one or two questions, it is better to help clients develop sufficient understanding at each developmental style before moving on.

The DCT questioning strategies can help you focus your interventions more precisely and systematically. They will also help you recognize when clients are not responding. A common problem in therapy is the client who talks about emotion but does not deal with it. You can use the DCT model questions to encourage the client to explore emotions using cognitive/emotional styles different from the one he or she seems most comfortable with.

As you work with the following and provide your own answers, note carefully how the specific sequence questions lead you to think about the issues using different cognitive/emotional styles.

1. *Initial cognitive/emotional style.* Could you tell me what occurs for you when you think of a time of leaving or separating? (e.g., leaving home, breaking up a relationship, graduating, moving, divorce)

_____

_____

_____

_____

Using what you have learned about developmental assessment, within what style did you present your discussion about leaving and separating? Circle one of the following and summarize evidence justifying your decision.

Sensorimotor

Concrete

Formal

Dialectic/systemic

Cite specific evidence below.

_____

_____

2. *Sensorimotor.* Think of a specific time involving leaving or separation. Can you get a specific image in your mind of that time of leaving? (The more specific, the better.) Most of us have a single, key visual, auditory, or kinesthetic image or recollection of important life scenes. Describe what you see. What do you hear? What do you feel—in particular, what and where do you feel this in your body? (The location of a felt body sense can be especially helpful.)

_____

_____

_____

This overlapping focus on see/hear/feel can be very powerful in helping clients recreate their past experiences and these techniques should be used, with sensitivity, ethics, and caution, in practice sessions and with your clients. Emotion is easily stirred by this simple exercise if an adequate foundation of trust and understanding has been previously established.

Expanding horizontal development with the sensorimotor style can include deeper emphasis on images from the past and present, Gestalt exercises, imagery techniques, and a wide array of therapeutic alternatives (which are discussed later in this chapter).

3. *Concrete/situational.* Could you give a specific example of a time you separated from someone or left an important place in your life? Describe in detail what happened and/or tell me a story about it. How do (or did) you feel about the separation?

_____

_____

_____

Concreteness is an important counseling construct. One of the best ways to cope with overly abstract clients is to ask them for concrete, specific examples of issues. When we obtain these specifics, our understanding often changes.

Expansion of development in this style demands that the therapist be willing to encourage and listen to a number of concrete stories and examples. It is in this sometimes frustrating but nonetheless important type of work that the formal and more pattern-oriented counselor often becomes impatient and moves too fast.

4. *Formal/reflective.* Does this relate to other situations involving leaving? Is this a pattern? Have you felt this way before? How do you feel when you look at these things in this way? What are your reflections on this incident?

_____

_____

_____

_____

Many counselors and therapists prefer the reflective formal style. We tend to like to work in the abstract world of ideas, with an emphasis on self-understanding and repeating patterns of thought and action. Expansion of thinking with clients who use this style, of course, can be highly beneficial. Instead of solving just one concrete problem, the client solves many problems by recognizing a common pattern.

5. *Dialectic/systemic.* Select one of the following questions: (1) Looking back on your responses earlier, what stands out for you? How would you integrate what you have learned? (2) Where did this come from? How might your thoughts and feelings about leaving have originated in your family of origin? (3) From how many different perspectives could you talk about what leaving means for you? (4) How might your ethnic or racial background affect the way you think about leaving and separation?

_____

_____

_____

_____

Dialectic/systemic questions help us think about our thinking patterns. Questions used in this orientation help us integrate past thinking into new perspectives. With this style, we begin to see how our emotions, concrete behavior, and formal thought patterns have been influenced by the systems we operate and live in. *Self is now seen as self-in-system, self-in-relationship, person-in-community.*

THE DCT QUESTIONING SEQUENCE WITH FAMILIES, CHILDREN, AND ADOLESCENTS

The DCT questioning sequence has also been found clinically useful in work with families. By making minor changes in the DCT sequence (such as the following), helpers can encourage families to view their issues from varying cognitive/emotional perspectives. For example:

You said your husband was insensitive. Could you give me a concrete example of that? (Concrete)

When he did that, could you get a specific image in your mind? What did you
  see/hear/feel? (Sensorimotor)
Is this a pattern for the two of you? (Formal)
Where did that rule come from in your family of origin? (Dialectic/system)
You say you have a lot of conflict. Could the family give me a more specific example
  of that? (Concrete)
Is there a single image that the four of you could come up with that summarized the
  conflict? What do you see/hear/feel? (Sensorimotor)
Does that happen elsewhere in your family? Is that a pattern? (Formal)
Is there a rule underlying those patterns? Where did you learn those patterns? Is
  there a flaw in that rule? (Dialectic/systemic)
How does your family style relate to your cultural background? How does being
  White/Person of Color, gay/lesbian, or your spiritual orientation relate to how
  your family functions? (Dialectic/systemic)

Those who work with children and early adolescents will find it useful to adapt these
assessment and questioning techniques. With the excited or overstimulated child,
simple, clear focusing on single elements of sensory experience ("What did you see?"
"Hear?" "Feel?") will often help the child calm down. Do not expect a clear linear
story from young children until you have allowed them to present the experience in
their own way. Then it may be possible to draw out the concrete linear details of
what happened.

With older children and adolescents, use of late concrete, causal questions can
be especially effective ("*If* you get mad when you are teased, *then* what do the other
kids do?"). You can follow up by early formal pattern reflective questions ("Does that
happen a lot?" "Have you gotten mad before in other situations?"). If challenged
sufficiently and patiently, these youngsters can be encouraged to learn formal ways
of thinking about themselves and their interactions.

Note that the questioning process for moving children and adolescents to new
styles of cognitive/emotional development is very similar to that used in adult counseling. What is important here, however, is the helper's willingness to move more
slowly and build a more solid sensorimotor and concrete foundation before attempting to encourage late concrete or formal thinking patterns.

In-classroom observations of effective teachers reveal that they use systematic
questioning and teaching styles similar to DCT, even though they may have not
heard of DCT. Less effective teachers tend to use random sequences of learning that
fail to take into account children's and adolescents' cognitive/emotional styles.
Surviving as a teacher at both elementary and secondary levels demands that one
match one's teaching strategy to the cognitive/emotional styles and abilities of the
learner. We have all had the frustrating experience of listening to some teachers who
are so abstract, formal, and analytical that we simply cannot understand them. These
teachers might have been more effective if they had been willing to provide more
concrete examples.

The systematic questioning strategies of DCT are useful in work with children,
adolescents, and adults, both in counseling and in the classroom. Thus far the discussion has focused on cognitive and emotional development. Where does emotion come
into this picture? With some clients, emphasis on the emotional aspects is needed if
they are to become aware of and fully understand their emotions (see Box 5-2).

Box 5.2   The Cambodian Trauma: Interview Excerpts Using DCT Questioning Strategies

The following interview is a highly distilled summary of an actual interview conducted by a counseling student. The questions listed below were used by the student interviewer as they are presented below, but spaced over a full hour. The essence of the actual client responses, using the client's key words, are presented as well. The situation has been changed slightly to disguise identities, and permission was obtained to use this material.

Opening statement and question

Student interviewer: I understand that you would like to share some of the things that occurred for you during the Cambodian Holocaust. Only share what you feel comfortable with. Could you give me a general idea of what you'd like to talk about today?

Client: I remember—the Vietnamese invaded Cambodia. There were a lot of shootings between the Khmer Rouge and the Vietnamese soldiers. My parents were returning home when they invaded. It was a terrible time. . . (The client continues with her story of this difficult experience.)

Sensorimotor question

Student interviewer: What were you seeing? Hearing? Feeling? (These questions were presented over a longer period of time.)

Client: I heard the sound of big guns. Explosions were glowing at night like Fourth of July celebration. I saw the Khmer Rouge walk in front of my home. I was really scared and very cold. I saw big horrible eyes staring at me. Even right now I get a feeling of fright, right here near my heart. (Note the potential power in the sensorimotor area. Always use care and do not move too deeply too fast. Work with a full sense of ethics and appropriate supervision.)

Concrete question

Student interviewer: Could you tell me the story of how you got to this country?

Client: One day my mom went to the river to wash clothes. She saw the Khmer Rouge calling her. She returned to the place and called me and my dad. We all escaped on that day. My mom cut the banana trees and tied them together like a raft. She put our belongings on and we got across the river. My mom was four or five months pregnant. I knew how to swim, but my dad did not. He had to wait and cross in a very crowded fisherman's boat. The next day, my mom went back home to get rice and she saw many people being killed by the Khmer Rouge. My mom just grabbed rice and swam back. . . . It took a long walk, but we got to Thailand to live in a refugee camp. We got accepted to live in the U.S. and now we are here. It was very frightening and I feel kind of numb now. (Needless to say, the story was far more detailed and the student interviewer used extensive paraphrasing, reflection of feelings, and summaries during this process.)

Formal question

Student interviewer: I hear that you felt fright and numbness. How does that affect you now?

Client: It comes and goes, but like now, I feel it all again. Every time I see blood or think of the story, I do not feel well. I think you call it a pattern. What I try to do is to think

(continued)

Box 5-2 *(continued)*

of good things and avoid the bad, but sometimes the bad thoughts come in anyway. What does help is thinking of wonderful Mom and that we were lucky to get away from the Khmer Rouge. (This self-reflective response summarizes several issues discussed by the client.)

Dialectic/systemic question

Student interviewer: How do you organize that powerful experience now?

Client: Well, first I kind of shared my story as we escaped with our lives. I returned to Cambodia about ten years later and went to the place where people were killed. The Khmer Rouge tortured and killed people like animals. When I got there, I thought about all the evil they did. Many people know about the Holocaust and the Nazi concentration camps, but not many people know about us Cambodians. I believe that many escaped prisoners survived, but they did not talk about their story or write about it. We learned in Cambodia to be quiet and not to be noticed. In Victor Frankl's story of the Holocaust, he talked about life in a concentration camp and what it was like. Cambodians have the same story as him, but nobody knows about it. (This segment was briefer, but here we see the client examining the larger system and how it affects individuals and families.)

FACILITATING EMOTIONAL DEVELOPMENT

No affect without cognition; no cognition without affect.

Affective development cannot really be separated from cognitive development. DCT views emotion as a special form of cognition that is always attached to experience and thought. Sensorimotor cognitions and affective cognitions are particularly difficult to separate and are often one and the same. Other forms of emotional expression and development are equally important for full adult development, but experiencing the richness associated with sensorimotor emotional experience is especially important.

Questions that bring out sensorimotor affective and cognitive experience have been reviewed in the preceding section. For example, "What are you seeing? Hearing? Feeling?" A here and now emphasis is also key to sensorimotor experience. It is often helpful to anchor emotions in specific parts of the body. Most clients are able to recognize a specific part of their body where the emotion seems to be felt. Both negative and positive emotions can be anchored in this way.

With clients using a late sensorimotor style, it is sometimes helpful simply to provide names for emotions that clients cannot quite describe. Posing questions such as "Do you feel X?" or reflecting feelings and naming the unspoken emotion are also useful skills.

With the early concrete style, the task is to draw out the linear specifics of a problem or situation; the focus here is more on naming emotions that may be attached to various parts of the story. Again, the naming of emotions may be useful as are simple reflections of feelings (e.g., sad, glad, mad). Emotions also tend to be all good or all bad, with relatively little shading of expression.

When working with the late concrete style, search for causal relations: "Do you feel X because . . . ?" Skill-training programs all focus on reflecting feelings using concrete language (see Carkhuff, 2000; Egan, 2002; Ivey & Ivey, 2003). The causal reflection of feeling can be useful in helping a client understand the basis of emotional experience.

With clients who operate within the formal style, the more abstract notions of Rogers's person-centered therapy (1961) are illustrative. Whereas concrete skills-training programs focus on identifying and clarifying feelings, the formal approach to emotions is to examine emotion itself. This abstract form of emotional reasoning is much used in counselor and therapist training programs. For some, such analysis of emotion makes the therapy process more cognitive than emotional. Reflecting on feelings can be a way for a client and/or a therapist to avoid direct contact with the power of emotional reality.

Despite their pitfalls, formal, more analytic approaches to emotions are an important part of any treatment program. Using these approaches, clients learn how to examine their emotions and discover underlying patterns of how the self relates to past emotional experience (see Box 5-3).

Box 5-3   Enlarging Treatment Options Through the Sensorimotor: Bodily Awareness, Locating and Naming, and Discovering Meaning

You will find it helpful for both yourself and your client to use awareness of bodily sensations as clues as to what might be occurring in the here and now of the session.

Focus first on positives: Counselors and therapists all too often emphasize problems. We strongly recommend that the first work you do with this exercise focus on strengths and positives located in the body. Before dealing with negative feelings still residing in the body, be sure that you have a reservoir of strengths in both yourself and your client. You'll find that you have positive memories that are located in your body. Once you have a foundation of positives, then you can deal more effectively with problems and concerns. The strengths often serve to alleviate difficulties and sometimes even provide solutions.

Bodily awareness: "Pay attention to the subtle feelings and sensations in your body when things are happening that could trigger feelings. All emotions have a physical sensation connected to them if you take the time to look for it" (Freeman, 2003, p. 51). It is best if you begin with yourself and start to notice what occurs for you during the day. You'll also find that your clients' thoughts and actions affect not just your mind, but your body as well. Start noticing what occurs in your own body when you work with clients. Give special attention to positive feelings in your body. For example, think of a hero, family member, or friend who represents a particular strength to you. Focus on that person and note where that positive feeling is located in the body.

Locating and naming: Once the feeling is located in a specific part of the body—the heart, the hand, the chest, and so on—name the emotion that appears to be associated with that body part. Working positively, you may feel a warmth in your heart as you think of someone who cared for you or strength in your arm when you, yourself, stood up for something important. Sometimes you may find

(continued)

Box 5-3   *(continued)*

that you are counseling a client and suddenly discover you have stopped breathing or your fist is clenched. Pay attention to that body part and then name the feeling(s) associated with it. You may find that a client's story literally takes your breath away in amazement or fear (breathing stops) or that your clenched fist is a sign of anger prompted by the client. What words would you use to describe that feeling in your body? Focus your early work on just being able to locate bodily feelings and naming them.

Discovering meaning: Focus on that feeling in your body and allow it to be there. With a focus on your bodily feelings, relax and allow yourself to drift freely and notice whatever comes into your mind. Do not censor; just allow the thoughts to come. Very often you will discover what is behind the here and now situation. You may, for example, find that the client reminds you of someone you knew in the past. The client may have reminded you of your own difficult experience. Body memories are strong, and with discovery of how present-tense bodily feelings relate to the past, your feelings may become even stronger. You may develop insights to why your body reacts as it does. Let the client find the meaning, not you. Therapists who name clients' feelings and outline meanings for them are, we believe, acting inappropriately.

Implications for interviewing practice:

- *Ethical and practical caution:* Used irresponsibly by a counselor or therapist, this type of sensorimotor work can be upsetting to a client. It can lead to false memories. Before moving into this type of work, let the client participate fully; do not lead the client.
- *For the interviewer:* Becoming sensitive to your own body reactions to clients will help you become aware of overreactions to the clients and serve as an indicator of problematic countertransferential situations. This same awareness can help you understand your clients' feelings more fully in the here and now of the session. In addition to reflecting their feelings, you can draw on your own body experience to understand what is occurring for them. At times, you will discover that your own body is a mirror of the clients' experience.
- *For the client:* You can educate your clients to notice their own body feelings. Many of these feelings go back to early childhood experiences, both positive and negative. In this way you gain useful therapeutic information. Focusing on here and now body experience is the foundation. Often feelings can be overwhelming, but if clients are in tune with their body sensations, they will be able to monitor their behavior, name and control feelings, and stop outbursts more easily. They can also note strengths in their bodies and then act on this knowledge.

Examples of counselor approaches to emotion for the first three styles follow:

Client: I feel very guilty about my parents. I've ignored them for years. They made me very angry early on, but perhaps now is the time to make amends.

Counselor: (using sensorimotor affect) Take that feeling of guilt. (pause) Where is it located in your body? What image comes to your mind? What do you see? Hear? Feel?

Counselor: (using concrete affect) You feel guilty because you've ignored your parents for years. You felt angry before, but now your feeling is one more of *caring*? (The counselor here names the unsaid feeling but uses a questioning tone of voice so the client can define the feeling.)

Counselor: (using formal affect) You seem to have a pattern of feeling anger toward your parents that now seems to be changing. You're becoming aware that your feelings are changing over time. As that happens, how do you feel about yourself in this process? (focus on internal self and affective development) You have some mixed feelings about your parents, which seem to center on guilt and anger, but at the same time, I hear you striving for something more. Could you go further with that? (focus on complexity)

The dialectic/systemic approach to emotional development is the most complex. The central focus is on examining and, at times, encouraging the client to experience varying emotional reactions to the same situation. Much of the emotional work in the prior three styles is oriented toward identifying and clarifying emotions. The primary purpose of dialectic/systemic approaches to emotion is to encourage understanding of the complexity, context, and developmental history of emotional experience. As one encounters this complexity, it is easy to become lost in abstractions and intellectualization. Dialectic/systemic thought and emotion can enable us to integrate the other three styles in a more holistic emotional experience in which the client both experiences and reflects on feelings.

There are multiple possibilities for exploring emotion with the dialectic/systemic style, as illustrated below.

Approach 1: Emotions develop over time. As I hear it, your feelings about your parents have changed over time. Could we explore that change in emotion? First, let's look at how you felt as a child toward your parents, then how you felt during at your teenage years, and finally, let us look at your feelings now that you are older. What events happened at each stage leading to those changes?

Approach 2: Transference issues. When you mentioned guilt, you looked at me questioningly. Could you go back to that moment and tell me how you felt and what you were thinking just as you said that? Do you have any fantasies about what I was thinking and feeling? (Other issues between the client and the counselor could be explored in the same fashion. Here the client learns that he or she is repeating old issues in the here and now of the interview with the therapist.)

Approach 3: Family systems. Your feelings and thoughts were generated in a family context, perhaps out of some family rule or rules. What rules did your family operate under? Specifically, can you identify some things that are important in your family that showed up in repeating messages you got as a child? What was your role in the family? How did your family relate to the extended family? The neighborhood and community?

Approach 4: Multicultural. As you look back and reflect on your experience as a (man/woman, Person of Color/White, heterosexual/gay/lesbian, spiritual person), how does that background affect how you feel about yourself? How might those feelings change if you came from a different background? You are Latino and gay—how might those two cultures view your personal life differently and what feelings does that bring out in you? You say that constant racial harassment has made you angry and is one of the reasons you have tension headaches and high blood pressure. What are some others feelings you have as you think about your family and your health?

Obviously, there are many possible forms of dialectic/systemic approaches to emotional understanding. In all the above approaches, the client learns how to consider emotional experience in a broader context. This type of complex exploration of emotions can be beneficial, but clearly, complexity is not necessarily better unless accompanied by sensorimotor experience and concrete action.

Think about your own parents and your feelings toward them. Can you identify sensorimotor images and feelings, concrete emotions surrounding a specific situation, patterns of feelings, and how all these feelings might change in context?

Can you develop an image of your parents when you were younger? What do you see? Hear? Feel? Can you locate that feeling in your body? (Sensorimotor)

_____

_____

Describe a specific situation that occurs to you in relation to your parents. In sequence, what happened? Name the feelings you had at that time or now. Can you write the causal statement, "I feel X because . . ."? (Concrete)

_____

_____

Did those feelings occur in other situations with your parents? Was there a pattern? (Formal)

_____

_____

Over time, as you view the image, the situation, and the pattern, do the meanings change? Can you see varying perspectives in which you might feel differently at different times? (Dialectic/systemic)

_____

_____

Following is a discussion of counseling and therapy theories and how they may be used to facilitate client cognitive and affective development. You will find that the questions and concepts presented thus far in this chapter can be useful additions to your work in other theoretical orientations.

COUNSELING AND THERAPY THEORIES AND DCT

The changing "seasons" of human development are summarized in the developmental sphere of Figure 5-1. The four cognitive styles are represented as circular movement through the life space. The effective therapist meets the client where he or she is, using developmentally appropriate interventions, expanding client developmental potential before attempting to move vertically (either "higher" to the next stage or deeper, returning to foundation styles).

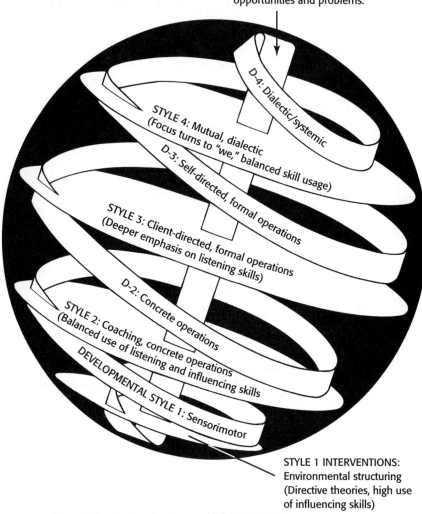

And with each problem solved, each developmental task met, you and the client must return to the beginning or to another level to work on other developmental opportunities and problems.

D-4: Dialectic/systemic

STYLE 4: Mutual, dialectic (Focus turns to "we," balanced skill usage)

D-3: Self-directed, formal operations

STYLE 3: Client-directed, formal operations (Deeper emphasis on listening skills)

D-2: Concrete operations

STYLE 2: Coaching, concrete operations (Balanced use of listening and influencing skills

DEVELOPMENTAL STYLE 1: Sensorimotor

STYLE 1 INTERVENTIONS: Environmental structuring (Directive theories, high use of influencing skills)

Example theories/applications:

Style 1: Body-oriented therapies (medication, meditation, exercise, yoga) and here and now strategies (imagery, Gestalt empty chair, focusing)

Style 2: Concrete narratives/storytelling, assertiveness training, thought stopping, automatic thoughts inventory, skills training

Style 3: Reflection on any of the above, person-centered theory, psychodynamic theories, cognitive work

Style 4: Multicultural counseling and therapy, feminist therapy, intergenerational family therapy, social action in community

Figure 5-1   Developmental Sphere. (Reprinted by permission of Lois Grady.)

Note especially the core of the developmental sphere and how it returns to the beginning. Having achieved so-called higher or more complex levels or styles of consciousness is not the end of development. We always return to the beginning as we face new challenges and new developmental tasks. There is no end to development. Each cognitive/emotional style brings new richness to human experiencing.

Higher consciousness is not necessarily better. Recall the flower . . .

Consider the following from *Developmental Therapy* (Ivey, 1986/2000, p. 111). Which is the "higher" consciousness?

Sensorimotor	Seeing and experiencing a flower
Concrete	Placing the flower in an arrangement
Formal	Writing a poem about the arrangement
Dialectic	Analyzing the poem about the flower (or analyzing the analysis of the poem about the flower)

Have we arrived at the "end" only to begin again?

The sphere also gives us another way to think about the whole person. The words *fully rounded* come to mind. If a person or family is to reach developmental potential, they need a balance of sensorimotor, concrete, formal, and dialectic/systemic cognitive and affective understandings. Imagine a distorted sphere heavy at the top with abstract cognitions but spindly at the bottom, having little sensorimotor or concrete foundation. Or think about a pear-shaped sphere, heavy on the bottom but thin on the top.

The developmental sphere also shows us that different theoretical approaches seem to relate better to some client developmental styles than others. For example, if the client is very concrete, a formal person-centered approach may be ineffective and a behavioral intervention may be needed.

The developmental sphere suggests that counseling and therapy theory can be organized into four basic types. As you review this abbreviated list, circle those theories and methods with which you personally feel skilled. Underline those you would like to add to your repertoire. Finally, since the list is incomplete, you may wish to add theories and techniques you believe are representative of this cognitive/emotional style.

Sensorimotor Theories and Techniques

Counselors and therapists tend to use structuring methods such as imagery, behavior modification, and Gestalt exercises. Drug therapy and the structuring of environment (as in a psychiatric hospital) are another type of sensorimotor orientation. An increasingly important aspect of sensorimotor work focuses on the body using breathing exercises, relaxation training, nutrition, and exercise. Bodywork is an important part of public health, both mental and physical (Dubbert, 2002).

List additional skills, techniques, and theories.

_____

_____

_____

Concrete Theories and Techniques

behaviorial

The therapist operates more as a coach and may use behavioral methods such as thought stopping, assertiveness training, and life-skills training. Reality therapy, structured problem-solving methods, decisional counseling, and vocational placement exemplify methods of this style. The late concrete style is represented by the logical-consequences concepts of Adler and Dreikurs, and the "A-B-C" analysis of logic used by Ellis in his rational-emotive behavior therapy.

List additional skills, techniques, and theories.

_____

_____

_____

_____

Formal Theories and Techniques

Rogerian
client-centered
more philosophic

As client thinking patterns mature, counselors tend to use formal modes of treatment (such as cognitive, person-centered, psychodynamic approaches, and logotherapy). Most counselors and therapists are formal thinkers and thus often feel most comfortable with these theories, even though many of their clients may be using a more concrete style that may not allow them to understand what the counselor or therapist wants them to do.

List additional skills, techniques, and theories.

_____

_____

_____

_____

Dialectic/Systemic Theories and Techniques

Social phenomena

Therapists and clients using this style often operate in a more mutual fashion. The individual begins to use data to form multiple perspectives and sees the self as operating in a world of complex systems. Feminist therapy is an example of this approach, in that women are encouraged to note how much individual "pathology" results from a sexist system. Multicultural counseling and therapy and much of traditional family therapy are in this mode. Social justice action in the community to attack systemic issues of oppression can be an important aspect of treatment for many. For example, a woman who has been raped may participate in activities to prevent violence against women (Ivey & Collins, 2003). A school counselor may decide to change a school system whose policies are failing to respect students. At another level, issues of transference and countertransference in the psychodynamic tradition are also illustrative of the dialectic/systemic style.

List additional skills, techniques, and theories.

_____

_____

_____

_____

At this point, you may want to review the above list and your additions; they represent your own evolving eclectic or metatheoretical approach to counseling and psychotherapy.

We need to match our therapeutic style to the developmental needs of the client. One of the most basic tenets of DCT theory is that we need to assess client cognitive/emotional style and then use a language system that matches the client. Theories and strategies for change matched to individual style fit best within the cognitive/emotional framework of the client. A formal/reflective client will likely respond most easily to the reflective or analytic style of person-centered, cognitive, or psychodynamic therapy. A client using a concrete style will often have difficulty with formal strategies and may prefer concrete storytelling, assertiveness training, or other behavioral techniques.

Mismatching and style shifting can be helpful. The therapist, while matching the theoretical framework to client cognitive/emotional style, also needs to include appropriate mismatching. For example, after a client who is formal/reflective has generated a good sense of self, it may be wise to add Gestalt exercises to enhance sensory experience and assertiveness training to provide concrete action skills. This type of mismatching challenges clients to expand their developmental potential to other styles of being.

We should not stereotype different theories or their advocates. Effective therapists of many different persuasions appear to follow the systematic, sequential, developmental sequences suggested here. Person-centered therapy is considered predominantly formal in nature as it focuses on patterns of the self. However, Rogers does therapy using multiple styles, as illustrated by this excerpt from *On Becoming a Person* (Rogers, 1961, p. 93).

Therapy Transcript	*DCT Analysis*
Mrs. O: I have the feeling it isn't guilt. (pause, she weeps) . . . I can't verbalize it yet. . . . It's just being terribly hurt.	Here, Mrs. O *is* her feelings. There is no separation of self from emotion. This sensorimotor experiencing is important in working through issues.
Rogers: M-hm. It isn't guilt except in the sense of being wounded somehow.	Rogers searches for a deeper meaning in the client's emotional experience.
Mrs. O: . . . often I've been guilty of it myself, but in later years when I've heard parents say to their children "Stop crying," I've had a feeling, a hurt . . . why should they tell them to stop crying. . . . who can feel more adequately sorry for himself than	The meaning-oriented reflection moves Mrs. O partially away from her deep emotional experience and we see her thinking about others rather than herself. She has moved almost instantly to reflective formal operational thought, although she still is crying. The power in the child metaphor shows when she talks

the child. . . . I thought they should let them cry. And feel sorry *(for the child)* too.

. . . that's something of the kind of thing I've been experiencing. . . .

about how similar this is to her own experience—being bottled up and not being allowed to experience emotion.

Rogers: That catches a little more the flavor as if you're really weeping for yourself.

Rogers responds holistically here as he helps clarify that she is crying for herself and makes a useful formal operational connection, while still maintaining a sensorimotor base.

Mrs. O: Yeah . . . and there's the conflict. Our culture is such . . . that one doesn't indulge in self-pity.

Mrs. O returns to a more fully formal operational pattern and approaches dialect/systemic thought. The example here is a particularly beautiful one of a therapist working at multilevels to facilitate client growth.

Depending on the specific developmental task of the client, suitable treatment interventions may vary. Our very human clients are too complex to "wrap up" with a few quick words and concepts. Objections could be made by other theorists to Rogers's work with Mrs. O. Fritz Perls (Gestalt therapy), for example, might object to Rogers's taking Mrs. O so quickly to intellectual generalizations. Gestalt therapists often prefer to develop a more comprehensive foundation in sensorimotor experiencing before turning to analysis and issues of meaning. The goal of both Gestalt theorists and cognitive behaviorists would be behavior change in addition to cognitive growth.

In practice, many theorists and practitioners follow a common sequencing in the therapy process. Effective helpers seem to ground their work in sensorimotor experience, examine concrete action, and then reflect on patterns of experience. This learning sequence seems to undergird many different therapies. Some less effective practitioners unconsciously may try to force or allow their clients to work within only one cognitive/emotional style. Then when clients do not improve or change, they label the client resistant or lacking motivation for change.

As a final step in this chapter, let us explore how to integrate DCT practice and theory using the many alternative modes of helping available in the developmental sphere.

MOVING CLIENTS THROUGH DEVELOPMENTAL STYLES USING VARYING TREATMENTS

A client facing divorce must work through a variety of developmental tasks. Before the divorce, her or his overall cognitive/emotional style may be complex formal and reflective. During the divorce, the client may be able to think effectively on the job. But when it comes to dealing with the emotional and concrete aspects of divorce, the same person may be totally nonfunctional. Sophisticated perspective taking may be lost. In many ways, the client working through divorce is preoperational.

Following is a list of some of the developmental tasks faced by a person going through divorce (or the end of any long-term relationship). Some of the tasks are primarily concrete (finding a place to live); others are sensorimotor (allowing oneself to cry and grieve); still others are formal (learning to reflect on oneself and why the relationship ended).

Circle the required style(s) for each task as you see it. Use the space to make notes about your family member, yourself, or a friend or client as any one of these faced the task of breaking up a long-term relationship. How effectively did they (or you, working through your own separation) move through these tasks? (See the answers on p. 168.)

Key: Sensorimotor = S; Concrete = C; Formal = F; Dialectic/systemic = D/S

1. S C F D/S Obtaining a lawyer _____

2. S C F D/S Driving to find new housing _____

3. S C F D/S Experiencing a new community
   and developing a new support system _____

4. S C F D/S Finding a new job _____

5. S C F D/S Allowing oneself to experience
   sadness and anger in the here and now _____

6. S C F D/S Thinking about how to
   plan to live on less money _____

7. S C F D/S Anxiety about a forthcoming new date _____

8. S C F D/S Telling the story of your
   separation to your new date _____

9. S C F D/S Working out at the gym and running _____

10. S C F D/S Planning nutritional meals _____

11. S C F D/S Enjoying the tastes in a nutritional meal _____

12. S C F D/S Gaining a positive self-concept _____

13. S C F D/S Relating with family of origin _____

14. S C F D/S Other _____

15. S C F D/S Other _____

Few people going through divorce handle all these developmental tasks effectively. Some of the above problems are best solved by concrete methods, such as direct advice and decision making. Other problems require formal therapies and family systems approaches.

The person going through a major separation must also deal in sufficient depth with emotional experience. When working with the sensorimotor style, you may see a client overwhelmed by the situation. Crying, random behavior, and even the adult version of the 2-year-old tantrum may occur. The purpose of sensorimotor functioning may be to deny emotions. Furthermore, a treatment plan may involve other sensorimotor modalities, such as meal planning and an exercise program. Expansion of such sensorimotor foundations is an example of horizontal development.

Moving to concrete operations, clients going through a major separation may be unable to act. They may need concrete advice about what they should do next to find housing or a lawyer or to make adequate financial arrangements. At times, even the individual who has always carefully planned ahead finds that the concrete specifics of a divorce are simply too much to handle. Direct decisional counseling is often helpful at this point.

If a solid foundation of concrete and sensorimotor experience has been developed, the divorcing client may be able to move vertically and recognize repeating patterns of behavior and thought that caused the marriage breakup. Divorce can lead to massive self-examination, and here person-centered and psychodynamic theories are most helpful. However, some divorcing clients will use formal analysis as a way to avoid critical expression of deeper feelings and taking concrete action.

When using the late formal style, the client may be able to recognize that he or she is repeating with a dating partner the pattern played out in the divorcing relationship. Here the client can examine patterns of patterns, often through some type of psychodynamic formulation.

When we turn to the more complex dialectic/systemic style, the client may become more aware of context. Women may see divorce as a gender issue related to male oppression (and men may feel the same way but may view oppression from another perspective). An important goal for therapy is helping this type of client move to a more multiperspective frame, perhaps through systems formulations such as family therapy or feminist counseling.

Another type of dialectic/systemic reasoning may appear when the client notes that one of the critical issues in the divorce was perfectionism, a trait that has been "in the family" for generations. Family systems thinking integrated in the interview can be especially helpful. Or you may wish to engage in couple and/or family counseling and work with a larger group.

Finally, examination of transference and countertransference patterns in psychodynamic work requires dialectic/systemic thinking, as the nature of therapist/client relationships is explored. In the later stage of psychoanalytic treatment, clients and their therapists will use this form of reasoning as clients discover that they are repeating their past pattern of relationships in relating to the therapist. For example, clients going through divorce will often relate to their therapists as they related to their ex-spouses. The ability to reflect on oneself and one's system of relationships requires highly advanced abstract thinking. Full psychoanalytic treatment is seldom successful unless the client is highly verbal and abstract.

No matter how sophisticated the thinking pattern, there always seems to be something more to learn, experience, and understand. Thus, as we reach the so-called highest style of dialectic thinking, we may note that the core of our being returns us to the beginning. Once we solve our problems, no matter how complex our thinking, we find ourselves needing to return to beginning sensorimotor awareness and concrete action. You must take the sophisticated awareness of the intellectual dialectic style (the world of abstractions and ideas) back to concrete awareness and action, or no movement or growth will occur.

The outline of varying styles of treatment corresponds with the increasingly eclectic orientations to helping. However, DCT suggests that eclecticism can be informed by a broader, neo-Piagetian theory of learning. DCT is compatible with existing modes of helping and adds a rationale for much of eclectically oriented approaches to helping.

SUMMARY

A smooth blending of both horizontal and vertical development is recommended by DCT. Thus, the specific questions and recommended DCT interventions can be adapted and integrated into the practice of many other helping theories. The specifics of the model include (1) assessing the developmental style of the client, (2) matching your theory to the specific needs of the client, (3) changing your approach as the client grows and develops, and (4) modifying and adapting your theory of choice (if working with a single theory) as your client changes.

Counseling and therapy theories can be organized according to the four developmental styles: (1) sensorimotor/elemental: bodywork, experimental awareness, and environmental structuring theories are oriented toward sensorimotor growth; (2) concrete/situational: narrative exploration in storytelling, assertiveness training, and problem-solving approaches are examples of concrete methods; (3) formal/reflective: reflection on narratives and stories, person-centered, and psychodynamic orientations are related to formal operations; (4) dialectic/systemic: feminist therapy, African American or gay consciousness raising, family systems, and social justice community action are examples of the dialectic/systemic style.

Each therapeutic system also operates using multiple styles. Different theories of counseling and therapy seem to be more effective with some styles than others. However, each theory in some way devotes some attention to each of the styles. Very little attention is given to the dialectic/systemic area in any theory.

DCT offers specific questioning sequences oriented toward the four developmental styles. These interventions can be used by themselves as a treatment alternative, or they may be integrated into various types of counseling and psychotherapy practice.

Emotional development cannot truly be separated from cognitive development. When one moves to a developmental model and discovers the power of sensorimotor experiencing, it is easy to forget the value of emotional experience within the concrete, formal, and dialectic/systemic styles. The last, in particular, needs more attention in counseling and therapy, as it provides an integration of emotion missing from concrete and formal approaches to emotion currently popular in counseling and therapy.

Human experience is so complex that no theory (including this developmental model) is sufficient to describe all events. The core of the developmental sphere shows us that we constantly return to the beginning for further exploration of new developmental tasks.

Challenges: Experience has shown that questioning, particularly on issues of imaging, and facilitating sensorimotor horizontal movement are very powerful. A sophisticated counselor commented, "I always thought I was good at feelings. Now I know that I was only using a formal style. In the sensorimotor, I experience a deeper form of emotion that I have been trying to escape from much of my life." Many participants in DCT training have experienced real, powerful emotions when using the visualization techniques suggested here. Always work within professional ethical standards and with a suitable consultant or supervisor.

We must always focus on the client and the way the client makes sense of the world. You can practice staying within the client's world by using her or his key words and main ideas. We all need to watch that we don't take over and dominate the session. While clients may agree with what we say, they may lose their own experience. The danger lies in inaccurately assessing a developmental block, thus leading to an inappropriate treatment plan. In learning DCT, the more effectively you can stay out of the client's way, the more the client can pursue meaning and find new personal solutions.

Research issues: One desired outcome of successful counseling and therapy may be increased cognitive/emotional complexity. For example, a client may discuss problems in a formal pattern. Successful therapy might include interventions aimed at the sensorimotor, concrete, and dialectic/systemic styles. Specifically measuring attainment of these styles is possible. Consider an interview at the beginning and at the end. Does the client's cognitive/emotional style change on a specific topic during that session? Over a period of sessions? What specific interventions and leads on the part of the therapist contributed to that change?

THEORY INTO PRACTICE: DEVELOPING YOUR PORTFOLIO OF COMPETENCE

Self-Assessment Exercise

Exercise 1. What theories and strategies do you favor and what have you mastered?

Examine your own conception of helping. What theories and methods do you find most helpful? Sort out your conceptions of helping using the following format. Underline the specific skills and theories you have mastered that seem to be appropriate with varying developmental styles.

Sensorimotor: _____

_____

_____

Concrete: _____

_____

_____

Formal: _____

_____

_____

Dialectic/systemic: _____

_____

_____

Exercise 2. Reflections on your present theoretical and practical strengths

Do you find yourself able to work with all developmental styles, or are you stronger at some styles than at others? Does the assessment in Exercise 1 lead to new goals for the future?

_____

_____

_____

_____

Identifying DCT Strategies

Exercise 3. Classifying developmental strategies

With your present knowledge of and experience with DCT, you may find it helpful to examine the interview in Appendix 4. This interview is designed so that you can classify both counselor and client statements. You will find a transcript of a session that will give you practice in assessing counselor and client statements as to developmental style. This practice will help you learn to recognize client developmental styles in the here and now of the interview and will also help you start monitoring your own questions and interventions.

What developmental style do you manifest most often in your interviewing interventions? If you have a transcript or tape of your work from the past, review it again and classify your own work.

Toward Multicultural Competence

Exercise 4. Gender awareness

Since the arrival of the women's movement, most women have a fairly deep sense of what it means to be a woman. Men, on the other hand, may be less aware of what their gender means to them. Heterosexual people tend to be unaware of themselves as heterosexuals, whereas most gay/lesbian/bisexual/transgendered people are deeply aware of the centrality of sexual orientation and power. Most groups who are in power have less awareness of themselves and may see "culture" and "race" existing only in others.

Ask these questions of yourself and share them with a colleague.

Concrete narrative or story: Can you recall a story in which you experienced yourself as a man or woman—ideally for the first time? Recall that story and put a few words here to summarize it.

_____

_____

Sensorimotor: Select a single aspect of that story. What are you seeing? Hearing? Feeling?

_____

_____

Formal: Can you reflect on that story and your feelings and notice any issues related to power or control or lack of same?

_____

_____

Dialectic/systemic: How does your gender relate to your degree of power in society? What other multicultural factors relate to this issue in terms of power or lack of power? How does the general social system within which you live affect all this?

_____

_____

Interviewing Practice Exercises

Exercise 5. Specific questions and goals for each developmental style

Applying developmental questions can be made easier by practice with the sequence and its variations. Box 5-1 contains an abbreviated developmental strategies questioning sequence that has been found useful in early practice. A more expanded set of questions oriented to eight styles can be found in Appendices 2 and 3.

Ask a partner to role-play a client. Sit down with the Box 5-1 list of questions in your lap. (Don't try to memorize the questions at this point.) Go through each stage, step by step. After you have gone through the series, exchange roles and go through them again. It is often helpful to share the questions openly with the volunteer client.

Stop after each step in the interview and discuss with your client what has just happened. Were you and your client able to achieve the goal of that particular interview segment?

In this exercise, it is particularly important to share information with your client. Tell him or her what is about to happen and what your goal is. Then together, evaluate whether the goal was achieved. Mutual sharing of goals and methods with your client is a useful counseling strategy in itself. We tend to overmystify our techniques. Many clients appreciate an openness about our purposes and may be more willing to take risks if they understand what is going to happen and what we are looking for.

Exercise 6. Group practice in cognitive/emotional strategies

Follow the agreed-on ethical procedures for your practice session.

Step 1: Divide Into Practice Groups
Get acquainted with each other informally before beginning.

Step 2: Select a Group Leader
The leader's task is to ensure that the group follows the specific steps of the practice session.

Step 3: Assign Roles for the Practice Session

■ *Role-played client.* The role-played client will be cooperative, talk freely about the topic, and not give the interviewer a difficult time.

- *Interviewer.* The interviewer will work through the developmental strategies, going through all styles without stopping. It is wise to have the list of questions available and to refer to them throughout the session.
- *Observers 1 and 2.* Both observers will fill out the same feedback form (Box 5-4) summarizing their observations. Does the client talk about issues as predicted in the questioning sequence? Does the counselor enable the client to reach the specific criteria for discussion within each developmental style?

Step 4: Plan the Session

- The interviewer and client need first to agree on the topic. The interviewer may wish to facilitate client talk using his or her own natural style of interviewing. A useful topic for this session may be procrastination or an interpersonal conflict in the past or present.
- The client may think through how he or she wishes to talk about the agreed-on topic throughout the session.
- The two observers can examine the feedback forms and be ready to complete the form for the most valuable feedback.

Step 5: Conduct a 15-Minute Interviewing Session
The interviewer and client will go through the specific stages while the observers keep track of their progress and note whether the interviewer has been able to reach goals. It is helpful to videotape and/or audiotape practice sessions.

Step 6: Provide Immediate Feedback and Complete Notes (5 Minutes)

- Again, it is helpful for the interviewer to ask the client "What stands out for you from this practice session?" Allow the client time to provide true personal reactions to the practice.
- The interviewer needs the same opportunity to reflect on what happened. The client may ask the interviewer for his or her personal reactions to the session.
- At this point, the observers should sit back and let the participants take control. Use this time to complete your classification and notes.

Step 7: Review the Practice Session and Provide Feedback (15 to 30 Minutes)
The interviewer should be the person who asks for feedback rather than getting it without having asked. The observers can share their observations from the feedback form (Box 5-4). As usual, feedback should be specific, concrete, and nonjudgmental. Pay attention to strengths of the interview. Just as with clients, trainees will grow and develop from getting feedback on what they do right.

Generalization: Taking Developmental Questions Home

The question now is how to take the concepts of developmental strategies for horizontal and vertical development into your daily life and into practice. Following are some activities that can be especially useful in ensuring that these basic ideas are used practically.

Exercise 7. Personal practice with others in your daily life

A beginning step toward useful generalization of developmental assessment is to practice these skills with those you come into contact with in daily life. When

Box 5-4   Feedback Sheet With Criteria for Each Style

1. **Opening presentation of issue.** How does the client organize and describe the problem?
Check all that apply: ___ S/M   ___ CO   ___ FO   ___ D/S
Specific evidence for this assessment:

_____

_____

2. **Sensorimotor.** Were the following accomplished? Check all that apply.
___ Client was able to describe a single image of the situation/problem/issue.
___ Client described what was seen in sensory terms (ideally, in present tense).
___ Sounds were described.
___ Feelings were discussed that were closely related to or integrated with cognition.
___ Random elements of the situation were presented.
___ Client located feelings in the body.
Cite specific evidence for this assessment:

_____

_____

_____

3. **Concrete.** Were the following accomplished? Check all that apply.
___ Client described a specific example of the situation/problem/issue.
___ Concrete details were presented.
___ Linear sequences, with cause-and-effect thinking, were presented.
___ More than one situation was presented, but not seen as a pattern.
___ Feelings such as "I felt X" or "I felt X about Y" were presented.
Cite specific evidence for this assessment:

_____

_____

_____

4. **Formal.** Were the following accomplished? Check all that apply.
___ Client discussed two or more situations and recognized similarities.
___ Client discussed repeating patterns of behavior, thought, or action.
___ Client engaged in analysis of self or situation.

(continued)

Box 5-4   (*continued*)

____ Client noted repeating patterns of feelings across situations or within the self.

____ Client was able to move to late pattern thinking and analyze patterns of patterns or repetitions of behavior or thought.

Cite specific evidence for this assessment:

_____

_____

_____

5. Dialectic/systemic. Were the following accomplished? Check all that apply.

____ Client was able to present an integrated summary of the above data.

____ Client was able to demonstrate multiple perspectives on the integrated summary.

____ Client was able to demonstrate that the situation or belief was co-constructed in a complex relationship.

____ Client was able to confront contradictions and flaws and engage in deconstruction of patterns or behavior.

____ Client was able to map out a reasonable plan of action and commit to this plan.

____ Feelings were discussed from multiple perspectives.

Cite specific evidence for this assessment:

_____

_____

_____

What did this interviewer do right in the session? Identify specific strengths of the interviewer.

_____

_____

_____

_____

Was the interviewer able to use the systematic questions with a sense of empathy, caring, and respect? Was the interviewer attuned to the client's or family's needs in this session?

_____

_____

_____

_____

friends or family talk to you about issues, what cognitive/emotional style are they using? When a friend or a family member has a specific issue, ask permission to go through the developmental strategies questioning sequence. Share the sequence with the person and discuss each style as you work through it.

You will find that your understanding and ability to communicate with children is improved when you use the DCT framework. The simple language and concepts of the sensorimotor and concrete styles are basic to communicating with children. With practice, you will find that children can engage in a type of formal pattern thinking. DCT proposes that early adolescents particularly can benefit from encouragement from adults in learning formal pattern thinking.

It is particularly important to recall in this exercise, and in the following exercise, that sensorimotor questions and imaging procedures are powerful and can easily cause tears and deep emotional experiencing. Use these skills ethically, with sensitivity and care.

Summarize your impressions of this experience and obtain specific feedback from your friends or family members about their reactions.

Exercise 8. Observation and practice with a family, classroom, group, or organization

Observe a group in interaction. Note the cognitive/emotional style and the communication style of the family members, teacher, students, and group members. What impact do leaders and key family members have on the group?

Using the same method and format as above, obtain consent of a classroom, group, couple, or family. Let them know before you start the purpose of your interview and show them the questions. Take them through the questioning sequence and report on (1) the cognitive/emotional style of the group and its members, and (2) what happened as you went through each of the four styles. (You may want to add some more extensive questions from the Standard Cognitive/Emotional Developmental Interview in Appendix 3).

Again, be particularly sensitive to and aware of ethical and professional issues surrounding sensorimotor imaging. Report on your observations and obtain feedback from the group members.

Exercise 9. The acid test: The interview

It will be most helpful if you can find a recent audiotape or videotape of your own interviewing style and theory. Listen to this tape and classify yourself and the client as to developmental style. Particularly note the developmental style of your questions and the style at which your client responded to them.

What has been your theoretical orientation? Is it primarily concrete, formal, sensorimotor, or dialectic? Undoubtedly, regardless of your theory of choice, you function with your clients at several developmental styles. Discuss the above issues and present specific examples from your own work illustrating how you operate using multiple styles.

Finally, carefully employ the skills presented in this chapter with one client in counseling or therapy per day. Again, you may want to inform your client what you are about to do before you start and why it might be beneficial to her or him. As you become more acquainted with the value of the conceptual and practical developmental model, you may find yourself using the concepts in your interviews.

Portfolio Reflections

Exercise 10. Reflections on developmental strategies and the interview

What stood out for you from this chapter? What sense do you make of the exercises and how will you use them in the interview? What are the key points you want to remember from this chapter? Record your thoughts below and in your Portfolio Folder.

_____

_____

_____

_____

_____

_____

_____

_____

_____

_____

REFERENCES

Carkhuff, R. (2000). *The art of helping* (8th ed.). Amherst, MA: Human Resources Development Press.

Dubbert, P. (2002). Physical activity and exercise: Recent advances and current challenges. *Journal of Counseling and Clinical Psychology, 70,* 526–536.

Egan, G. (2002). *The skilled helper* (7th ed.). Pacific Grove, CA: Brooks/Cole.

Freeman, J. (2003, May). The four steps to emotional literacy. *Natural Awakenings,* 51, 57.

Ivey, A. (2000). *Developmental therapy: Theory into practice.* North Amherst, MA: Microtraining Associates. (Original work published 1986)

Ivey, A., & Collins, N. (2003). Social justice: A long-term challenge for counseling psychology. *The Counseling Psychologist, 20,* 3–11.

Ivey, A., & Ivey, M. (2003). *Intentional interviewing and counseling: Facilitating client development in a multicultural world* (5th ed.). Pacific Grove, CA: Brooks/Cole.

Meara, N., Shannon, J., & Pepinsky, H. (1979). Comparisons of stylistic complexity of the language of counselor and client across three theoretical orientations. *Journal of Counseling Psychology, 26,* 181–189.

Rogers, C. (1961). *On becoming a person.* Boston: Houghton Mifflin.

Answers to Cognitive/Emotional Style Rating Practice (p. 157)

1.	C	8.	C
2.	C	9.	S
3.	D/S	10.	F
4.	C/F (depends on the job requirements)	11.	S
5.	S	12.	F
6.	F	13.	D/S
7.	S		

CHAPTER 6
Assessing Client Change
Creativity, Perturbation, and Confrontation

CENTRAL PRACTICE OBJECTIVE

Mastery and practice of concepts in this chapter will enable you to facilitate change by perturbing and confronting client discrepancies and incongruities in a supportive fashion. Equally important, you will be able to assess the impact of your confrontation on client change processes using the Confrontation Impact Scale.

This chapter is about change and how we can measure change in the here and now of the interview. Clients come to us stuck and immobilized, repeating again and again ineffective behaviors, thoughts, and feelings. Our task is to listen carefully and then provide alternatives so that they can work with their issues and problems more effectively. Often we need to confront clients and perturb the status quo. This chapter provides a framework for assessing where clients are in terms of their attitudes toward change and, as well, a system for examining behavioral change.

Creativity underlies client change—we need to help clients create new ways of thinking, feeling, acting, and finding meaning. Much of creativity comes from noticing contradiction and incongruency—and then perturbing/confronting the clients supportively to help them let go of old ways of being. The flexibility of cultural intentionality requires the creative spark as we all learn to generate new alternatives in our multicultural context.

Knowledge of and skill in the concepts of this chapter can enable you to:

1. Define and discuss cultural intentionality as a major goal for counseling and therapy.
2. Understand how creative processes can be used in the interview to facilitate creation of new ways of thinking, behaving, and feeling.
3. Identify and utilize five types of confrontation approaches to perturb clients and encourage developmental growth.
4. Employ the Confrontation Impact Scale to assess developmental change in the here and now of the interview and as an outcome measure for the success of your sessions.
5. Expand your understanding of the change processes through seeing how cognitive and emotional change occurs in death and dying theory and in responding to traumatic life issues.

INTRODUCTION: CULTURAL INTENTIONALITY

Cultural intentionality provides us with a goal for change and the creation of new ways of thinking and behaving. Counselor intentionality optimizes our potential for effective helping interventions and reminds us of the importance of flexibility and the need to be creative as we work with our clients (Ivey, D'Andrea, Ivey, & Simek-Morgan, 2002; Ivey & Ivey, 2003; Miller, 1997; Schmidt, 1994). In turn, cultural intentionality is also a goal for our clients. Consider this brief definition and its relevance for both counselors and clients.

> Culturally intentional individuals can think in new ways and generate new behaviors flexibly. Multiple approaches rather than "single solutions" are characteristic. Listening to feedback and the consequences of past actions leads to further adaptive change. In addition, cultural expertise requires the ability to work within the cultural framework or varying multicultural frameworks.

Intentionality involves creativity—the willingness to take new perspectives, generate new behaviors, and find new meanings in old situations. Intentionality brings purpose for the creative process, and the development of intentionality in our clients provides us with a goal as we seek to facilitate change in our helping interviews. Development, either horizontal or vertical, requires creativity—the generation of new possibilities.

Clients in therapy need to be perturbed and confronted with their contradictions and inconsistencies in thoughts, feelings, and behaviors—and in their ways of making meaning. Out of this perturbation comes creative synthesis and growth. Creativity, whether in children or adults, is the transformation of previously existing structures into something new. Confrontation and perturbation move clients to new ways of organizing and viewing the world.

The word *New* is perhaps as central to this chapter as cultural intentionality. You will find us speaking of the "creation of the *New*" in various ways throughout. The theologian Paul Tillich (1964) talks about creation of the New as bringing restoration and fulfillment. Creation of the New could be described as a close variation of cultural intentionality, but the word focuses perhaps even more clearly on finding novel, original, fresh, and innovative ways of thinking, feeling, behaving, and creating meaning. Our task is to help clients find the New within themselves. Questioning and confrontation are basic to this process.

CREATIVITY, INTENTIONALITY, AND THE NEW

Creativity is necessary for generating the New and learning how to cope with the challenges we face in life.

What do you see in Figure 6-1? Take some time and record your initial impressions below. What occurs for you when you focus on the picture?

_____

_____

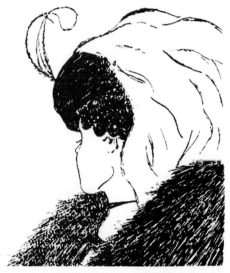

Figure 6-1   A Figure to Figure. (Originally drawn by W. E. Hill and published in *Puck,* November 6, 1905. First used for psychological purposes by E. G. Boring, "A New Ambiguous Figure," *American Journal of Psychology,* 1930.)

At first glance, some people see an older woman, whereas others see a younger woman. Take some time with the picture until you can see both.

Lack of intentionality can be described as "stuckness"—seeing only one way of doing things. Lack of intentionality is illustrated by the individual who sees only one person in this picture. Many people find it difficult to see both women, especially at first. "Multiple seeing" requires you to let go of previous impressions and restructure old information in new ways.

If you look again at the picture of the two women and relax, you can perhaps see the two images alternating: first, the older woman, and then the younger woman. With a little more relaxed concentration, it is possible to see both at once. This is multiple seeing. Work with the drawing and attempt to see both women at once. For many people seeing both at once requires creativity and the ability to create New ways of seeing and thinking.

Why is the woman with the large nose and jutting chin generally seen as an older woman whereas the woman with a smaller nose is seen as young? Some of this judgment is created by cultural and sexual stereotypes. Such stereotypes cause us to define beauty in terms of youth while lack of attractiveness is often associated with advanced age. In actuality, our cultural background defines beauty for us. With plastic surgery and economic advantage, one can never be sure which person is old or young. Moreover, age is actually an arbitrary criterion for defining beauty, which truly does lie in the eye of the beholder. To her 75-year-old husband, a 74-year-old wife may truly be beautiful!

Multiple seeing is another way to describe intentionality. The pieces of the picture remain the same, but as we construct ideas about the picture in our mind, we see many different things. The ability to see the same picture or client simultaneously from multiple perspectives is invaluable in counseling and psychotherapy.

The next section describes the mechanism of creativity and offers some specifics on how the counselor can provide useful environments most likely to facilitate client growth.

THE PRIMARY CIRCULAR REACTION: CHANCE AND DELIBERATION IN CREATIVITY

Piaget describes the mechanism of creativity as the primary circular reaction, the active repeating of results that were first achieved by chance (Piaget, 1952/1963). This description is important, as it demystifies the creative process and creation of the New. The following are key points of the primary circular reaction:

A. Chance variation in behavior or thought is basic to creativity. Creativity happens; the moment of discovery cannot be planned. Although we may systematically examine the picture of the two women, there is something beyond this deliberate search—an inevitable "aha" experience when we see a new perspective.

B. Human beings tire of the old and search for the New even though at times they may not know what they are searching for. We also may find the New through mistakes, oversights, and surprises. We can enhance our experience of the New by placing ourselves in an environment that facilitates the creative spark.

C. Discovering new thoughts and behaviors through chance is not enough. A child learning a new skill or a client engaging in a new behavior needs to repeat actions actively and with conscious intent. While creativity may not be planned, planning and action are required to reinforce the new skill or learning. This conscious repetition helps us establish and maintain new behaviors and ideas. What began as chance becomes systematic and deliberate.

This primary circular reaction may be illustrated more concretely by the example of how infants learn. The infant is in a crib with a rattle suspended overhead. Small infants reach out randomly. They have not yet learned that they can affect things in their environment. With enough random reaching (and with the rattle being close enough), the child will eventually knock the rattle by chance. Often, merely touching the rattle will increase the activity level of the child (feedback from the primary circular reaction). If the rattle is again touched by chance, the child gradually becomes able to reach for and touch the rattle deliberately.

Although the environment provided by the parents (the suspended rattle) gives the child the opportunity for learning, learning occurs only within the child. We cannot teach; however, we can provide opportunities for learning. In this example, chance behavior in a facilitative environment is followed by the active repeating of the experience.

We can apply the same principles to therapy.

A. The client comes to us stuck, or immobilized. The client has old, assimilated structures that result in this immobility. Our task is to provide an environment that allows for development of movement. Our support and rapport are important parts of the change process.

B. The client reaches out, and almost by chance, one of our interventions is useful and the client accommodates the new experience.

C. We then deliberately seek to help the client repeat the experience so that the learning will become more fixed and easily assimilated by the client. When this learning has occurred, the client has assimilated something new.

Piaget described the twin processes of assimilation and accommodation, which together provide the background for developmental change. In summary form, assimilation can be described as our past learnings. We have assimilated and integrated a representation of the world. These assimilated representations (ideas about the world) form the lens through which we look at the world. People who have rigidly assimilated patterns are unable to take in or accommodate new data; they find change difficult. Accommodation is the process through which we absorb and incorporate new information from the environment. The two processes need to be balanced. Too much accommodation results in continual change and no stability, whereas too much assimilation results in stagnation. (A detailed elaboration of these concepts and their implications for the practice of counseling and therapy can be found in Chapter 2 of Ivey's [1986/2000] *Developmental Therapy.* In that chapter, information processing theory is joined with Piagetian concepts and broadly applied to developmental processes.)

As counselors, we like to think that our conscious efforts, derived from our careful theoretical study, are what change the client, what help the client develop and grow. But ask a client what was the most helpful aspect of a session. It rarely is your brilliant intervention. More likely clients will tell you that it was some small thing you did, perhaps unintentionally, that was most helpful. Often, through interaction with you, individuals or families generate on their own the creative spark that gets them moving.

A family coming to therapy may present only their narrow perception of reality. The therapist offers a different view—a separate reality, so to speak. A family already has important structures that can be recombined in a new, more effective way. Through "mixing" with the therapist, the family can examine and reconstruct feelings, meanings, and behaviors.

Can you think of a special moment of creative insight you have had—a time when you created something new? This moment could involve the understanding of a complex concept, the learning of a new skill, or the generation of a new idea. What was the creative moment?

_____

_____

_____

What in the surrounding environment may have helped spark the new learning? Creation usually does not come without some form of external stimulus or support.

_____

_____

_____

The primary circular reaction stresses the importance of deliberation and practice to "fix" the new idea or skill. How does this dimension of the creative process apply to your experience?

_____

_____

_____

New constructions, perceptions, and behaviors occur in and belong to the client. However, you as counselor or therapist can provide an environment that can facilitate growth and development and the deliberation that helps stabilize the new creation.

PERTURBATION: PROVIDING AN ENVIRONMENT FOR CHANGE

Discrepancy, incongruity, and paradox rule the lives of many clients. There may be discrepancies between a real self and an ideal self, a present behavior and a goal behavior, rational and irrational ideas, or between a problem and a desired solution. Clients come to us with many unresolved conflicts and contradictions.

Our task is to provide clients with an environment conducive to expansion, transformation, change, and developmental growth. We can do this by applying skills, strategies, and the multitude of theoretical approaches available to us. Any one of many approaches may "perturb" the client and encourage change.

Perturbation is an important term in Piagetian theory. Essentially, the word means to disrupt the status quo, to break homeostasis, to produce a sense of unease. Perturbation is very similar to the counseling term *confrontation,* which means to point out discrepancies or incongruities in the client's thinking or behavior. The skill of confrontation can be used to perturb the client's equilibrium and open the way for the client to construct new knowledge, thoughts, and behaviors. *growth*

Questioning skills are basic to the confrontation/perturbation process. Mark van Doren was a world famous Columbia University professor, known for his teaching skills. His student, Thomas Merton, the spiritual philosopher, was even more famous. Merton comments on his superb teacher (1999, pp. 139–140):

> Most of the time he (van Doren) asked questions. His questions were very good, and if you tried to answer them intelligently, you found yourself saying things that you did not know you knew. He had "educed" them from you by his question.
>
> Do not think that Mark was simply priming his students with thoughts of his own, and then making the thought stick to their minds by getting them to give it back to him as their own. . . . The results were sometimes quite unexpected . . . casting thoughts that he had not himself foreseen.

Your task is first to listen carefully, then note how the client constructs or makes sense of the problem or personal issues. Then through careful confrontation and questioning skills, help that client find a new way of thinking or being. Some theorists and practitioners seek to put their ideas into the client's head. Careful listening, questioning, and perturbation will help the client make sense of the world in their own way. DCT strives to increase personal uniqueness, while simultaneously encouraging clients to think more fully about themselves as beings-in-relation, persons-in-community.

Both support and challenge are needed to facilitate change. We can usually best confront clients if we have first built with them a relationship of trust and understanding. Direct confrontation is not the only challenge we can offer. Effective perturbation can result from reframing and interpretation and from good questioning and good listening skills. Once clients have been effectively perturbed, returning to a supportive counseling style may help them maintain their new learnings more effectively.

Thus far we have examined Piaget's theories as they apply to clients. It is also useful to examine Piaget's questioning style. Piaget was constantly asking children questions or setting up situations that perturbed the status quo. The questions he asked are not just assessment and information-gathering techniques; they are also treatments in themselves. Questions are interventions that challenge the status quo, perturb the individual, and create an opportunity for change.

By asking questions such as the following, Piaget (1972) perturbed, or confronted, the child's conception of reality. He did not give sufficient attention to the effect his questions had in the evolution of the child's thought processes. Consider the following questions he asked:

- When you go for a walk in the evening, does the moon stay still?
- What makes the clouds move?
- How does this bicycle work?

Here are several more examples (Piaget, 1965):

- Is it fair to keep children waiting in shops and to serve the grown-ups first?
- A father had two boys. One of them always grumbled when he was sent [to fetch] messages. The other one didn't like being sent either, but he always went without saying a word. So the father used to send the boy who didn't grumble on messages oftener than the other one. What do you think of that?
- If someone hits you, what do you do?

When a child is perturbed with a contradiction, even if he or she has never thought of it before, there is a natural effort to resolve the contradiction and develop a new synthesis. Children present many interesting and amusing ways to resolve the various contradictions that are posed to them.

Bill Cosby, the popular comedian is well known for his ability to interview children. Early in his career, he worked with Art Linkletter, a radio and television personality popular during the 1950s. Linkletter was able to draw out fascinating pearls of wisdom and amusing anecdotes from children. Following are some examples from his book *Kids Say the Darndest Things!* (1957). Note how his questions perturb the children and move them to creative solutions. Here again, we see how the interviewer affects the changing cognitions of the child interviewee.

Linkletter: Where does the sun go at night?

Child: Behind the clouds?

L: Then where does the moon come from?

Child: Well, naturally, it gets too hot back of the clouds when the sun goes there, so the moon *has* to come out.

L: What does the saying "a wet blanket" mean?

Child: It's the blanket the baby lies on.

L: What does the expression "The grass is always greener in the other fellow's yard" mean to you?

Child: That's easy. He's using better fertilizer than you are.

Cosby, Linkletter, and Piaget represent effective interviewers. Their questioning techniques perturbed children and thus help us better understand children's cognitive processes. In the three examples from Linkletter, the meaning-making process of each child takes varying forms. The explanation of where the sun goes is characteristic of magical, late sensorimotor thinking, whereas the responses to the two sayings represent a charming form of concrete thought.

Can you recall similar examples of childish meaning making in your own life or perhaps with children you have known? Can you identify clients you have had who present unusual or magical modes of meaning making? If you have difficulty recalling a specific incident, remember your belief in Santa Claus or a similar figure. Children (and parents) often dream up clever ways to explain Santa's behavior. Write down some of these thoughts and memories.

_____

_____

_____

_____

How did you, your child, or your client change faulty or magical thinking processes? Assuming you no longer believe in Santa, what happened when you changed your thinking about his reality?

_____

_____

_____

_____

How can you use this example of the change process from magical meaning making to concrete reality in your own counseling and therapy process—particularly when you deal with children, adolescents, and adults who may use a form of magical thinking?

_____

_____

_____

_____

Clients have varying forms of meaning making. They may engage in magical thinking, they may be overly concrete, or they may be overly abstract and formal. Our task is to facilitate cognitive development. We can do this through our questioning techniques (as described in earlier chapters), by using an array of theoretical techniques, and through the counseling skill of confrontation.

PERTURBATION, INTERVIEW CONFRONTATION, AND THE CREATION OF THE NEW

Counseling and therapy rely on perturbing clients' ways of thinking and behaving. Therapeutic theory is oriented toward understanding the client's world and then promoting change through varying forms of perturbation. A Rogerian may perturb through careful listening. The therapist, through accurate mirroring of the client's words, may be able to perturb the client and thus motivate her or him toward positive movement. The behaviorist may perturb by environmental change or assertiveness skills training. The rational-emotive counselor may perturb by challenging illogical thought patterns.

A review of research on helping skills interventions found that only 1% to 5% of interviewer statements could be classified as confrontations (Hill & O'Brien, 1999). But these confrontations can be what leads to new thoughts, feelings, and behaviors. They perturb client status quo and may even make clients uncomfortable at times. Thus, it is usually important to support your clients before you challenge them. Timing of confrontation is also crucial. Evidence suggests that the more rapport you have with your clients, the more able they will be to hear the confrontation (Sharpley & Sagris, 1995). In early work with psychiatric inpatients, Ivey (1973) found that confrontation used too early could disturb the therapeutic process. Moreover, confrontation should be used sparingly to assure success when it is used.

Families also need to be perturbed. The family may consider the bulimic, anorexic, or acting-out teenager to be the problem but fail to see how parental difficulties and family enmeshment contribute to the situation. Minuchin often begins his interviews by asking the family to define why they have come to therapy (Minuchin, Wai-Yung, & Simon, 1996). The family then talks about the anorexic daughter, for instance, as the problem, and the anorexic agrees with this definition. Minuchin's first intervention is simple but profound. He carefully and respectfully summarizes each family member's problem definition and then redefines it by saying that the family has the problem, not the individual. This interpretive reframe offers a new view that perturbs the family system of thinking. The reframe then becomes the focus of the remaining therapy sessions.

The questioning skills presented in Chapters 4 and 5 are oriented toward perturbing clients and encouraging them to find new meanings in their old structures. Much as with Piaget and Linkletter, the skilled use of questions helps clients learn to look at themselves and the world differently.

You will also find that other skills and interventions in the interview help perturb the client to new ways of thinking. Thus interpretation and reframing, feedback, skilled use of directives and advice, plus other skills and strategies are important in helping confront/perturb clients and find new ways of thinking and being. Simply listening and responding to clients carefully through paraphrasing, reflecting feelings, and summarizing often help them to reflect on what they said. Effective therapists know that listening skills by themselves form the foundation of all confrontation.

The skill of confrontation is another way to challenge and perturb clients who are stuck and repeating patterns of thought and behavior (Ivey & Ivey, 2003). The counselor first observes the client's conflict and the incongruities, discrepancies, and mixed messages in the client's statements and behaviors. These observations are then fed back to the client in a clear, concise, nonjudgmental manner. Following are examples of confrontations a helper might use when working with a client having difficulties with love relationships:

- On one hand, you say you love your spouse, but on the other hand, you continue with your lover. How do you put that together?
- As I hear you, you seem to be saying two things. First, you say you love the tenderness, yet this very tenderness seems to frighten you. What sense do you make of that?

- I hear you saying that that doesn't bother you, but your fist is closed tightly right now as if in anger.

Each of these statements actively focuses on perturbing the client's verbal or nonverbal discrepancies. Questioning techniques tend to be confrontive and the focus is on incongruity. In using questioning approaches (such as Piaget's), the therapist controls the direction of the interview. However, the technique of confrontation focuses on the client's statements as they reflect his or her worldview. By paraphrasing and summarizing these observations, the therapist can help the client generate new ideas.

It is best to think of confrontation as *supporting while challenging* (Ivey & Ivey, 2003). It is important to listen carefully and empathically. We need to hear the client's story fully. Like Piagetian perturbation, confrontation tends to be most effective in a relationship characterized by rapport and understanding. While listening and rapport remain central, some clients need direct, sometimes even dramatic confrontations. For example, the acting-out, alcoholic or drug abusing, or sociopathic client who simply can't hear your confrontation often requires a stronger statement. But, even here, supporting while challenging and effective listening remain important.

There are six basic types of observations that are helpful in noting incongruities and contradictions—namely, discrepancies or conflict:

- Between two verbal statements (between any of the four DCT styles)
- Between statements in the interview and actions outside the interview (formal/concrete or concrete/concrete)
- Between statements and nonverbal behavior in the interview (between any of the DCT styles and sensorimotor behavior)
- Between two nonverbal behaviors (sensorimotor)
- Between two or more people (any developmental style)
- Between any of the above and the context (dialectic/systemic)

Once having observed the discrepancy, it is useful to feed back your observations to the client. Using the phrasing "On one hand . . . , but on the other hand . . ." is a very useful way to communicate observations nonjudgmentally. By adding an open question such as "What sense do you make of that?" or "How do you respond to what I observed?" or "How do you put that together?" you encourage the client to make a new synthesis. If you move your hands as if balancing the contradiction, you increase the sensorimotor impact of the question.

With families, you can use similar language. In addition, you may add such questions or suggestions as "Can you help your daughter/son figure this out?" or "How do you think your mother and father will react to that?" or some other modified form of circular questioning in which you encourage family members to present their views more clearly. These questioning procedures help families bring out "hidden" secrets that are often well known to all but never discussed openly.

The counselor in skilled confrontation captures the essence of the client's problem, feeds it back clearly and concisely, and tries to help the client resolve discrepancies. Effective confrontation and perturbation aids problem resolution. Questioning and confrontation perturb clients and encourage them to generate new meanings and behaviors.

The primary circular reaction described earlier consists of the following three parallel dimensions in counseling and therapy:

A. The client comes to us stuck or immobilized. Our task is to provide an environment that allows for client development.
B. The client reaches out, and almost by chance one of our interventions is useful.
C. The counselor and the client then deliberately seek to repeat the experience so that learning occurs.

Providing an environment that allows for development may involve careful listening, the judicious use of counseling theory and strategies, skilled questioning techniques, and/or constructive confrontation/perturbation. All three approaches encourage client development and movement toward the New. The client is the primary meaning maker in the client-counselor relationship, and he or she reaches out to us. It is not unusual for beginning counselors, and sometimes those with years of experience, to try several interventions before one works, seemingly by chance. At this point, we try to repeat the chance learning experience so that new learning is fixed and becomes part of the client's new way of being. Therapist and client together have created the New. Alternately, a skilled counselor may assess a client accurately and provide an intervention that works, at which point the client is able immediately to create the New. We have found that the process of selecting interventions that work is greatly enhanced through the use of the developmental counseling and therapy model. In fact, one of the greatest strengths of the model lies in the provision of this road map to effective treatment.

Confrontations and perturbations can be cognitive, affective, or behavioral. Behavioral change can lead to cognitive change, and thus behavioral confrontation may be effective as a first approach. Blending cognitive and behavioral confrontations can be especially helpful, for often the discrepancy is between thought and action—saying one thing but doing another.

It is possible to assess the effectiveness and impact of your interventions. Let us now turn to specifics of assessment in the session. You'll also find that the Confrontation Impact Scale has implications for long-term evaluation of your counseling and therapy interventions.

THE CONFRONTATION IMPACT SCALE (CIS): EVALUATING THE EFFECTIVENESS OF OUR INTERVENTIONS

When confronted, clients have a variety of responses. Ideally, they will respond actively to your confrontation, generate new ideas, and move forward. However, they may ignore or deny the fact that you have confronted them. Most often, the confrontation will be acknowledged and absorbed as part of a larger process of change.

You can assess the impact of your confrontation on your client by using the Confrontation Impact Scale (CIS). The CIS has some practical implications for the practice of counseling and therapy in that it enables the therapist to assess the impact of interventions in the here and now of the interview. In addition, this assessment helps the therapist keep the interview on track and note client growth potential. An outline of the CIS (adapted from Ivey, 1993) is found in Box 6-1.

Box 6-1   The Confrontation Impact Scale[1]

You will find that virtually every helping lead you use, whether a question, reflection of feeling, or directive (whether you intend confrontation or not) leads to a client reaction that can be located on this five-point scale. Clients will sometimes deny your question or confrontation; at other times, they will recognize it. When things are going well, clients will transform their concepts into new ideas, thoughts, and plans for action.

For example, the counselor may confront a client considering divorce with this comment: "On one hand, you still seem to care for your spouse, but on the other hand, I see an underlying anger as well."

Level 1: Denial	The individual may deny that an incongruity or mixed message exists or may fail to recognize it. (For example, "I'm not angry about the divorce. It happens. I don't feel anything in particular.")
Level 2: Partial Examination	The individual may recognize a part of the discrepancy but fail to consider other dimensions. (For example, "I care, I really care. How can I make it alone?" Here the client fails to deal with issues of anger and frustration.) Alternatively, the client may move into full anger. Anger is often a level-2 response, since it covers up deeper sadness and hurt.
Level 3: Full Examination But No Change	The client may incorporate the confrontation fairly completely but make no resolution. Much of counseling operates at this level or at level 2. Until the client can examine incongruity, stuckness, and mixed messages accurately, developmental change will be difficult. (For example, "I guess I do have mixed feelings about it. I certainly do care about the marriage. We've spent years together. But I sure am angry about what has happened.") The client may also acknowledge feelings of hurt and sadness underlying the anger. An honest experience of anger as part of a complex relationship is an important level-3 goal.
Level 4: Creation of New Dimensions	At this level, the individual is able to gain a new understanding of the total picture. There is not a major restructuring but rather a gradual progression toward larger Gestalts at level 5. (For example, "As I hear you, I realize that it makes sense to have mixed feelings. We had many good things. I wonder if part of my anger is about the loss of a dream that went sour and really represents my fear of loss.")
Level 5: Development of New, Larger, More Inclusive Constructs, Patterns, or Behaviors	A confrontation is most successful when the client recognizes the discrepancy, works on it, and generates new thought patterns or behaviors to cope with and perhaps resolve the incongruity. (For example, "I like the plan we've worked out. You've helped me see that mixed feelings and thoughts are part of every relationship. I've been expecting too much. I'm having dinner tonight with my spouse, and we are going to have to develop a new way of thinking about the meaning of the relationship. The divorce may still be necessary, but I need to look at it a new way. I'm sad about the idea of a breakup. It is a loss that I may not really want.")

---

[1]A paper-and-pencil measure of the Confrontation Impact Scale was developed by Heesacker and Pritchard and was later replicated by Rigazio-Digilio (cited in Ivey, 2003). Factor analytic study of over 500 students and a second study of 1,200 revealed that the five CIS levels are identifiable and measurable dimensions.

The following is an exercise that will give you experience using the Confrontation Impact Scale of Box 6-1. Classify the following client responses by circling the appropriate level. (Correct responses are listed at the end of this chapter.)

Counselor statement: You say you are feeling OK about your father's lack of interest in you and that you've worked through your problems with him, but just as you said that, your voice tone went down, your body slumped, and you looked very discouraged. (Confrontation between the formal verbal presentation and the unspoken, body-response sensorimotor style)

Classify the five following possible client statements using the CIS.

1 2 3 4 5   "No, no such thing. I didn't do that. I didn't move at all."

1 2 3 4 5   "You're right, I have worked through most of my problems. Things are moving the right way."

1 2 3 4 5   "Hmmn. I did say that, but you say my body and voice changed when I talked about Dad."

1 2 3 4 5   "Wow! I guess I haven't worked things through as fully with him as I thought."

1 2 3 4 5   "Your feedback is helpful. I have been wondering lately if things were really as good as I hoped. Just hearing that from you helps me recall something that happened that week. I need to work a lot more on this."

Counselor statement: You've been late for work three times in the last week; the boss has talked to you about her concern and says she is about to let you go. (Concrete confrontation)

Classify the five following possible client statements using the CIS.

1 2 3 4 5   "Yeah, you've got it. I'm worried that the boss has about had it with me."

1 2 3 4 5   "I have so much to do, getting the kids ready. I guess I need to plan things better with them."

1 2 3 4 5   "As you said that, I just realized that this is a pattern for me. I get a good job; start off well, then somehow it starts to fall apart. I think we need to work hard on that pattern."

1 2 3 4 5   "Yeah, and as I think about it, the boss was pretty sympathetic with my family issues at first. I wonder if I have pushed her too far."

1 2 3 4 5   "That's not what I said. The boss is out to get me."

Counselor/family interaction: The therapist's observations of a family have been centered on the mother's over-involvement with her physically disabled 6-year-old son to the point that the mother is constantly watching him and helping him. The therapist asks the child to move from one chair to another, and the mother moves toward the child to help, saying, "Wait Mikey, let Mommy help." The therapist says, "Irene, how have you decided that Mike needs help?" The mother replies, "Well, the chair is high, and Mikey is nervous here in this environment." The therapist says, "Let's see if you are right. Mike, can you get down from that chair and get up into this one?" Michael looks at his mother but does what is asked.

The therapist says, "Let's be sure that was not luck. Please do it again." Michael succeeds again. The therapist then says to the mother and father, "Your wife thought your son Mike needed help, but in fact, he was able to do this on his own. Could you two talk about what this all might mean?" (Multiple-level confrontation— Mikey moving to the chair is sensorimotor and concrete; asking parents to talk together is formal.)

Classify the five following possible client statements using the CIS.

1 2 3 4 5   (mother) "Mikey was able to get into the chair, but you forced him. He mustn't be pushed so hard."

1 2 3 4 5   (father) "That's what I've been telling you, Irene. Mike can do lots of things if you'll just let him. Didn't you see what happened?"

1 2 3 4 5   (mother) "Well, perhaps, but it makes me so nervous." (Starts to cry)

1 2 3 4 5   (father) "Could it be that both of us worry about Mike so much that we don't give him a chance to do what he actually can do?" (Mother, drying eyes) "Well, maybe what the therapist is saying to us is 'Hold back a bit. Mikey can do more things on his own.' "

1 2 3 4 5   (mother continues) "I guess I'm so much like my own mother. She was always hovering over me. How I hated it. Could I be doing the same thing with Mikey?" (Tears)

Recycling and the CIS: Do not expect all your clients to move through the Confrontation Impact Scale in the step-by-step fashion discussed above. Some clients may move very quickly from denial to transformation when an important insight comes to them. At other times, clients will discover that advances in cognition and emotion can be made only with regression to earlier stages from time to time. With difficult experience, the whole process may start all over again as new discoveries are made.

The CIS as a measure of longer-term change: You will discover that the five levels of the CIS are also useful in assessing change over a full set of interview sessions. For example, the client may be an alcoholic who starts by denying the problem and then, gradually, over several sessions engages in partial examination, then bargaining and recognizing the problem. Real change, of course, happens at levels 4 and 5 when the client stops drinking.

Things that cannot be changed: Many of your clients will present issues that will simply require them to live with contradiction. Jean Vanier described this reality with honesty and grace (cited in de Waal, 1997, p. 13):

> In our times there is a danger of thinking that everyone may become perfectly healed and find perfect unity in themselves and others. This type of idealism is rampant everywhere. New therapies engender more and better illusions. And each day new techniques are born which will bring about this long-awaited healing. Personally, I am more and more convinced that there is no perfect healing. Each human being carries their own wounds, their own difficulties of relationships and their own anguishes. It is a question of learning to live day after day with this reality and not in a state of illusion.

When a client has gone through a major trauma such as rape or war, or lives with a severe illness such as cancer, diabetes, or multiple sclerosis, the issues lie deep and often will stay in the client's mind throughout life. Breaking through denial and reaching higher levels on the Confrontation Impact Scale seem necessary and wise, for it is essential to recognize fully that you indeed do have a problem. Level 4 is often defined as accepting what one has to deal with and living with it relatively effectively. There is no cure for life and we all encounter difficulties that will stay with us. Transcendence, level 5, may occur, but it usually requires a large change in meaning-making structures. Often, service to others is a route toward transcendence. The woman who is a rape survivor or the person who lives with cancer may find wholeness through working in the community and social action to bring about awareness of women's and/or health issues.

Always recall that our field is indeed about change. But some things cannot be changed. Paraphrasing Alcoholics Anonymous, "Help me to change the things I can and accept those I can't." This is useful advice for both you and your clients.

DEATH AND DYING THEORY: PARALLELS WITH DCT CHANGE ASSESSMENT

Elisabeth Kübler-Ross expanded the world's consciousness in her classic work *On Death and Dying* (1969/1997) in which she explored, with great sensitivity and understanding, five stages individuals work through when they face death and dying. Kübler-Ross's five stages have interesting parallels to the five levels of the Confrontation Impact Scale (see Box 6-2). Both the CIS levels and the five stages represent creative changes in understanding and consciousness. The content and objectives of the two, of course, are markedly different, but these parallels may offer some interesting ideas for helping clients deal with many complex life issues.

Box 6-2	**The Confrontation Impact Scale and Five Stages of Death of Dying**	
Level/Stage	Confrontation Impact Scale	Five Stages of Death and Dying
1	Denial of the incongruity or the problem	Denial and isolation—"It can't happen to me."
2	Partial examination	Anger—"What have I done to deserve this?"
3	Full examination of incongruity without change	3a. Bargaining—awareness of issue, but still not full acceptance
		3b. Depression—emotional awareness of the issues
4	Creation of new dimensions	Acceptance—living with what one has to live with
5	Development of new, larger, and more inclusive constructs	Transcendence—moving beyond acceptance

grief

Kübler-Ross's five stages of death and dying can be summarized as follows:

1. *Denial and isolation.* When first told they are terminally ill, many people respond with immediate denial: "It can't happen to me" or "The lab tests must be mixed up." Sometimes they simply are unable to hear what the physician has just said. Some seek out faith healers and claim that the illness has been cured. Others may isolate themselves. A cancer patient, on finding she had cancer of the hip, told her family, "Don't tell anyone I am in the hospital." Kübler-Ross notes that people generally move rapidly from full denial to at least partial recognition of their condition. But some patients go to their death denying the reality of the situation, and their families may do the same.

   Kübler-Ross is careful to respect all the ways individuals and families cope with death and dying. For some, avoiding the truth can be an effective and even beautiful defense. However, there are cases when both the individual and the family are aware of the nearness of death and never share their knowledge with one another, seeking to "protect" each other from worry. They thus deny themselves a chance to discuss openly what is happening.

   The Confrontation Impact Scale's first two levels are "denial" and "partial examination." Clients who cope with either mild or serious difficulties use language in many ways similar to those described by Kübler-Ross. A person who has suffered rape may deny the issue for years or may think that the rape was her or his "fault." An abused woman may deny the importance of the emotional or physical beating and continue in the relationship.

2. *Anger.* Denial is soon replaced by a realization of the reality of the situation. This realization is coupled with often unreasonable anger at the situation, the family, the physician, and the hospital staff. The angry person facing death is not an easy person to be around or sympathize with. Busy nurses may avoid these people and respond to them angrily.

   Underlying anger in most people is deep fear, hurt, and sadness. It is safer to be angry than to acknowledge one's fear and hurt. Anger is often a defense against pain. A young husband became immediately and irrationally angry when his bride of two weeks burned her finger on the stove. He calmed down fairly quickly and took her to the emergency room, where she received minor medical attention. Talking about the incident with his therapist the next week, he came to realize that he so loved his wife that he couldn't bear even a relatively small injury to her, since it represented potential loss and eventual death. The young husband, due to a difficult childhood, was terrified of loss and could cope with his fear of loss only through denial and anger. As he began to understand his anger, he broke into tears.

   Breaking through denial of alcholism in the family, the fact that one's partner is abusive, or that one has been consistently lied to often results in anger. Sometimes such anger becomes a lasting part of the person's being. For example, if one suddenly finds that one's spouse or lover has been unfaithful, the anger that erupts is lasting. At some point, however, moving beyond anger to acceptance of the situation will likely be healthier for the client. Anger is not a healthy emotion and holding onto anger can be physically damaging.

So it is with those facing dying and death. Kübler-Ross (1969/1997) presents a lengthy interview with a dying nun, who is full of anger (pp. 73–79). The woman was resentful of the nuns who cared for her. The interview revealed that the nun's anger went back to her early childhood, when she had been expected to be a "good girl." She was furious that Hodgkin's disease was the reward she got for being good. The resentment and anger toward her family and her anticipated early death were transferred to her caregivers. Through the interview, the nun gained more peace and felt more acceptance of her condition. This interview reveals that patience and understanding are a necessary part of therapy if one is to help a client develop new understandings and meanings.

As counselor or therapist, you are not the target of your client's anger, hate, or love. People facing crisis become very much in touch with basic feelings. Responding to internal cues, they may appear angry with therapists and helpers but are really reacting to the immediate crisis or to past life history. Those who work with victims of trauma (rape, incest, child abuse, serious accidents) will often encounter manifestations of anger similar to those described by Kübler-Ross.

In terms of the Confrontation Impact Scale, anger as described here is usually a level-2 response, since it covers deeper, underlying issues. Anger may be described as a displacement of real feelings and thus a partial examination of issues. However, at the same time, the open discussion of honest and useful anger can be beneficial and represent level 3 on the CIS.

3. *Bargaining.* Kübler-Ross likens this stage to the child who is told, "No, you cannot have the toy." The child stomps off and is angry, but may soon return, saying, "If I am very good, can I have the toy?" Adults facing death do something similar: They attempt to postpone the inevitable. This stage is relatively brief, since the fact of terminal illness does not change, and there is no one to bargain with in person. The dying person may try to bargain with God: "If I become a better person, then will you let me live?"

As mentioned above, this stage is brief and may not appear at all. In this stage, the person displays a magical way of thinking similar to what DCT terms the *preoperational problem.* Continuing the parallel with the five levels of the Confrontation Impact Scale, the bargaining stage is late level 2. The individual is trying to work on issues but has not yet confronted them directly.

Many of your clients will try to bargain away their problems by presenting excuses for themselves or for the one who may be hurting them. The bargaining style is particularly characteristic of some women who are seriously abused. After an abusive incident (even if repeated several times), the male may indicate regret and apologize profusely. The abused partner wants to believe it is true and continues in the relationship, making a hopeless effort to please her partner.

4. *Depression.* Loss and life's difficulties make all of us sad and depressed. Whether it is poor grades, an automobile accident, or a divorce, most of us feel sad about the event but may take some time before reaching the stage of depression. We may deny ("The professor must have scored the exam wrong"), become angry ("Why didn't you watch where you were going?"), or bargain ("If you'll stop

beating me, I'll do a better job around the house and we won't have to get divorced"). But ultimately, reality comes to us and we must acknowledge our deep hurt, frustration, or sadness.

Facing separation and loss and the resulting natural sadness and depression is something many people cannot bear. A woman who remains with an abusive man may deny anger and spend most of her thinking time bargaining, while simultaneously becoming more and more depressed. Older individuals who lose friends and physical capacity are particularly susceptible to depression.

Those facing death deal with one of life's ultimate tragedies. Thus, sadness and depression are necessary and important parts of grieving. When we work with depressed clients in therapy, we know that reassurance and encouragement are of little use. Similarly, it does not help much to tell the depressed patient that "it is all for the best."

Depression and sadness, then, are real parts of life, and we must allow the individual and the family to experience these feelings fully but not be overcome by them. To illustrate this stage, Kübler-Ross (1969/1997) presents an interview with Mr. H. (pp. 88–108). Severely depressed, Mr. H. thought he would not be able to talk for more than five minutes. He had lost hope; his father had died following a similar operation with the same surgeon. He talked about his feelings and then later explored his disappointments in his own life, particularly in his marital relationship. He was reviewing his life, searching for meaning in it, and had not been able to share his thoughts and feelings with his wife.

Mr. H.'s wife was described as a powerful, busy woman who felt that "life will go on the same" with or without her husband. Kübler-Ross met with her and helped her understand her husband's feelings. Her view changed, and she was able to reframe the situation and appreciate his good qualities. She was able to share herself and some of her caring with her husband for the first time in many years. His depression passed, and he went to his death peacefully.

The stage of depression described by Kübler-Ross may be viewed as a level-3 response on the CIS. Depression is often a full awareness of sadness and loss. Death is indeed something to be sad about. Unless one allows oneself to grieve and be sad, one remains enmeshed in denial, anger, or bargaining.

Depression and sadness are necessary, but if they become a focus, as happened with Mr. H., these feelings can become a serious problem. A level-3 response such as depression, when continued too long, becomes a form of level-1 denial and isolation. Kübler-Ross helped this couple transcend depression, bringing husband and wife together in a new synthesis, a more creative way of being. They could accept the situation as it was and view it from a new perspective.

5. *Acceptance.* The fifth stage of death and dying is acceptance—living with the inevitability of death. Some describe this as finding meaning in death and reviewing the positives in one's life; others look forward with enthusiasm to an afterlife. Whatever the person's approach, acceptance can be described as a physical sigh—a letting go, a recognition of the inevitable, a joining of oneself with the physical and spiritual environment. "Ashes to ashes, dust to dust" is not a joyful statement but it is a realistic statement of what *is*.

As one of Kübler-Ross's patients described it: "Acceptance should not be mistaken for a happy stage. It is almost void of feelings. It is as if the pain had gone, the struggle is over, and there comes a time for 'the final rest before the long journey'" (p. 113). Some people continue in denial to the end; others fight until the last; others may remain in deep depression. Thus, the period of acceptance may not be experienced at all by some. Still others, facing a slow, lingering death, may have a long period of acceptance. Each individual is unique and will work his or her way through the stages of dying differently.

Individuals who move to the stage of acceptance appear to do so most easily if they are supported and encouraged to experience the other developmental stages of the dying experience. Particularly, they need to express anger and rage, as well as their fears and sorrows, and to discuss their past victories and defeats, thereby finding meaning in their lives. Again Kübler-Ross (1969/1997) presents an excellent interview (pp. 120–137) in which she helped a couple toward an acceptance of death.

In this case, the couple had been arguing, failing to understand one another and some of the positives they had shared in their time together. Kübler-Ross helped them work through their separate needs in the death and dying process and gradually come to a more satisfactory resolution. This is particularly important as it reminds us that death and dying are not just individual issues—they are issues for the entire family.

Similarly, issues of denial and anger can be part of a family therapy process. Any time there is a traumatized individual, there is usually a traumatized family as well (Figley, Bride, & Mazza, 1997). Not only does a family need to learn to accept death and dying, but they need also to recognize that a teen does have a serious alcohol or drug problem, that a father's loud talking is actually verbal abuse, or that the 97-pound daughter is indeed anorexic. One of your most important therapeutic tasks with a family is to help them move from denial of a problem to acceptance that a problem exists. With acceptance comes the possibility of transcending and coping with the problem through creative new solutions.

Acceptance of what *is* may be equated to level 4 on the CIS. Nothing new can be done, but remarkably, something new—acceptance—has been added to the client's experience. The individual has transcended the very real sadness of dying by simply accepting death. Kübler-Ross describes a 76-year-old woman with terminal liver cancer. The woman offered her son and daughter-in-law ceramic figurines she had prized throughout her life. They refused the gift, saying she should continue to enjoy them, as she would be "around for a long time" and should "keep fighting." She died two months later, never having had the chance to explore the meaning of her life or to share her feelings with her loved ones. The woman was at the acceptance level; her son and daughter-in-law were still in denial. The family missed a chance to transcend the death experience and share their love and concern.

For many clients in therapy, nothing can be done about the circumstances of their lives—for example, an abusive childhood, the loss of an arm in an accident, the birth of a child with severe cerebral palsy, or the loss of a job at age 55. At another level, failure in school, the breakup of a promising relationship, or being rejected by a social club are also depressing events. Clients often react to all these events by denying that they have happened, by becoming angry, or by trying to bargain their way out of them before they come to acknowledge their sadness and depression and accept the continuing hurts and problems that are part of life. Though the objective circumstances cannot be changed, how the client makes meaning of events is a matter of choice.

True transcendence of death is described by Kübler-Ross as hope. Love, faith, hope, and charity are difficult mystical concepts that defy real description, but they represent the moment of opportunity in which individuals and families move beyond themselves and see themselves in relationship with others and perhaps even as part of the cosmos.

The parallels between the five levels of the Confrontation Impact Scale and the Kübler-Ross stages are not perfect. Each construct was developed for a different purpose. Kübler-Ross provides a philosophical perspective. DCT and the CIS offer a more technically oriented way to relate the stages of death and dying to the general issue of loss that is so often the topic in the helping interview.

Death forces us to confront life's major incongruity. In dealing with death, we have the opportunity to confront the meaning of life and construct the New. Piaget's theory of equilibration provides a framework that helps explain the relationship between the CIS and Kübler-Ross's stages. To illustrate this concept, Piaget describes how a child develops new ways of thinking when confronted with a stimulus. The child's learning may involve denial of data, partial accommodation, a balancing of new data with the old, or what Piaget calls the "gamma solution" in which a new totality or schema is generated out of the old.

However, the death and dying framework just reviewed does not give sufficient attention to level 5 of the Confrontation Impact Scale. Here we see major ongoing change. The rape survivor has worked through many issues and become active in counseling and helping other men and women who went through the same experience. The abusive wife has likely left her husband and started the active construction of a new life. The alcoholic client has moved from acceptance and identification of the problem to stopping drinking and participating in Alcoholics Anonymous.

Just as children must constantly construct the New when they face life's challenges, so must those facing such major issues as death and dying or trauma. Clients confronting less difficult developmental tasks also must construct the New if they are to continue growing.

A holistic view of the five stages of death and dying: Just as with the CIS, do not expect all people to work through issues of loss and death and dying in the linear step-by-step fashion described here. Some may never move beyond denial and bargaining; others may start with acceptance. Furthermore, with time and experience in dealing with the disease or loss, a client who apparently had reached acceptance and perhaps even transcendence may recycle back to so-called earlier stages. In short, the loss model is an important contribution, but it never should be considered absolute.

CHANGE: A LOSS OR AN OPPORTUNITY?

Psychotherapy and counseling are about development and change. As we work through the developmental tasks of life, some changes bring about joy whereas others are painful. At times we need to work through the pain so that we can later experience joy and rebirth. As noted earlier, the theologian Paul Tillich talks about creation of the New as bringing restoration and fulfillment. But this does not deny the pain that sometimes must be endured before growth and development can be fully established.

Change does not always come easily to us or to our clients. Many clients hold onto old ineffective ways of thinking and behaving because they feel safer with these than they do dealing with the rigors of change. The major points in dealing with change thus far include the following:

1. Change is a creative process that can occur by chance or by deliberation.
2. Piaget's primary circular reaction provides us with specific information on how change and new ideas are incorporated in the individual.
3. Perturbation and confrontation are intimately related. A task of the professional helper is to perturb or confront clients and facilitate their movement to new levels of cognition, affect, and behavior.
4. Five levels of client response to counselor interventions and perturbations may be identified through the Confrontation Impact Scale.
5. Kübler-Ross's stages of death and dying have interesting parallels to the CIS. Clients facing serious loss seem to follow her stages, and this process may extend beyond death and dying issues.

In this section we extend these five points to the exploration of the change process in general. It appears that many clients in the process of growth experience a loss before they are able to encounter the joy of the creation of the New. Recent thinking in organizational development provides some helpful linkages to consider.

Change in organizations does not come easily, and much management literature focuses on resistance to change. Bolman and Deal (1990, 2000) conclude that change often involves feelings of loss to employees in a company or institution. An example of a change that relates to feelings of loss would be the wholesale firings and staff reductions that occurred because of the Wall Street investment scandals that resulted in layoffs of thousands of workers. Here, it is easy to see that management decisions can result in feelings of loss for both those given pink slips and those who remain with the company.

Organizational development consultants often seek to change procedures in a business or governmental agency. Bolman and Deal (1990, 2000) note that when a change agent moves too fast, without due consideration of the client's perspective, resistance is likely to grow. (This is also true in individual or family counseling and management consultation.) Changes in management and culture in organizations represent loss for many individuals. They must give up their old "comfortable ways" of doing things. Bolman and Deal state that change agents need to recognize the employee's and client's needs to work through and mourn their losses in a supportive atmosphere. Organizations and employees may say that they want change, but when actually faced with it, they may begin a process of grieving and loss that may build up resistance to positive change.

We, as professional helpers, need to be aware that even though most clients say they want change, many of them resist doing something new. Resistance to change is parallel to denial, partial examination, and bargaining as represented in the Confrontation Impact Scale or in the Kübler-Ross death and dying framework. Whether you are working with resistance or denial, your task is to help clients break through this initial phase so they can enter into new phases of growth and enjoy the more positive aspects of development.

For example, a depressed client may say he or she does not want to continue in the cycle of sadness relating to feelings of depression. However, when confronted with the possibilities of the world and the many challenges that must be faced daily, some depressed clients will return to clinical depression as safer and more comfortable than going through the agony of behavioral change. Similarly, a child diagnosed with a conduct disorder must give up many, many things if he or she is to learn how to get along more successfully with peers, parents, and teachers. This process is especially clear in substance abusers. They may recognize the need for change, but giving up drugs or alcohol and facing the difficulties of daily life can represent a serious loss for them. It is sometimes easier to hide behind our symptoms of depression, conduct disorder, or substance abuse than face the real issues of life.

Often when you propose change to your clients via a Gestalt, Rogerian, behavioral, or family systems intervention, they will behave very much like those clients described by Kübler-Ross or Bolman and Deal. Denial can be so complete that you may find that clients don't even hear what you have just said in a normal vocal tone. Alternatively, they hear you and deny your point through skillful argument ("I'm not an alcoholic. I can stop anytime I wish.") Others may move to a level-2 type of anger or bargaining in which they work on only part of what you have said. Even if clients agree with your intervention, they may simply become depressed once they recognize the truth.

Often, we think of depression and sadness around our interventions as a level-3 response on the CIS. For some clients, there is a real need to mourn and feel sad about knowing that change must come. Giving up old habits is not always comfortable, and many clients will sit still and do nothing about change. They may prefer to obsess and grieve about the problem and make no move to correct it. An obsessive client may become aware of the need to loosen up and learn a new interaction style but may spend most of the time grieving about the need for change and leaving old, safe, and predictable habits. It is at this awareness level (3 on the CIS and stage 4 of Kübler-Ross) that suicide becomes a real risk for seriously depressed clients, for they have allowed themselves to see more fully how very bad they feel. In addition, they may fear the changes they need to make to enable themselves to feel better.

We work through the Kübler-Ross and CIS stages by moving to acceptance and action at stage 5 and levels 4 and 5, respectively. We think about our old behavior in new ways and implement new action oriented toward change. Here, change can be difficult and painful, but the possibilities for growth, rebirth, and development often make this part of the process more joyful. At this point, the client or family may begin to reinterpret past pain as a useful prelude to the possibilities of the future. Despite successful movement and the creativity inherent in positive change, the process for many represents loss and will be painful throughout. It is not enjoyable for an alcoholic or a borderline client to confront deliberately a history of family abuse.

Your ability to be warm and empathic and supportive is critical as you help clients and families move through the change process. Our culture tends to think of change and development as positive processes, which indeed they are. Yet, we have given insufficient attention to the need to support those who seek change. Confrontation, perturbation, and skillful interventions are not enough. It is important that you, the change agent, be there with clients and support them throughout the process. In addition, you will want to recruit family members, coworkers, and friends at times to support clients who are working through change issues. Particularly useful in this process are support or action groups, such as Alcoholics Anonymous, an eating disorders support group, or Mothers Against Drunk Driving.

For practical purposes in the individual or family session, you can use the CIS and adaptations of the Kübler-Ross framework to indicate how clients are moving in the interview. With some practice you will be able to note whether clients are denying your intervention, bargaining with you, or accepting what you say. Your ability to observe client response to your interventions may enable you to provide the necessary balance of support and challenging confrontation needed by the client.

The creation of the New can indeed be joyful, but many clients will see change as loss and need your support to help them move to new ways of thinking and behaving. In the long run change will be useful and joyful, but the process will be much less painful if the counselor, therapist, or change agent is fully attuned to the needs of the individual, family, group, or organization. A useful goal may be to help the client think of change as a process of gradual illumination of possibility.

SUMMARY

Counseling and psychotherapy are concerned with creativity and cultural intentionality. The primary circular reaction is basic to the creation process. Clients come to us stuck and immobilized, unable to create something New in their lives. Their repetition of unsatisfactory and stuck behaviors, thoughts, and feelings is what leads most, perhaps all, clients into the helping relationship. The culturally intentional interviewer is creative and has many alternative actions to assist clients toward creative problem solving.

The interviewer provides an atmosphere for the creation of the New. In therapy, clients will reach out to us through the behavior and language they use in the interview. Their behavior and language are directed by the past, but clients now interact with a new set of environmental contingencies: you and your behavior and language. The therapist's task is to provide an environment that perturbs clients' current levels of functioning, to move them toward change and renewed developmental progression. We perturb by using theoretical and practical therapeutic interventions (behavior modification, rational disputation, Gestalt exercises) or through interviewing skills such as questioning, reframing, and confrontation. Those interventions that have a positive impact on clients need to be followed up if they are to become a part of clients' New way of being.

By observing discrepancies, mixed messages, conflict, and incongruity in the client's statements and behavior, we can identify instances of immobility. These inconsistencies are usually an important part of the client's problems, difficulties, and concerns. The resolution of these discrepancies is central to the helping process.

Confrontation is a therapeutic intervention that seems to cut across all theories. Confrontation, similar to the concept of Piagetian perturbation, requires clients to examine their relationship to the world. Through feeding back, summarizing, and paraphrasing discrepancies and conflict in the client's statements and behavior, you will encourage the clients to look at themselves and to disequilibrate or decenter from an unsatisfactory past, and to move toward change and developmental movement.

The Confrontation Impact Scale (CIS) is a practical measure for assessing, through client language and behavior in the interview, the impact of your interventions. With practice, you will be able to classify client responses to your interventions, questions, and confrontations and you will be able to determine whether your intervention was heard and assimilated by the client. This feedback will help you to plan your interventions in the session to facilitate client growth. Furthermore, this scale can be used as a measure of progress of client cognitions, emotions, and behaviors.

Kübler-Ross's five stages of death and dying were presented to expand and clarify the ideas of this chapter. Her work provides a rich and practical base that may help in transferring the ideas presented in this chapter to other settings.

Change may be viewed as either a loss or an opportunity for development. You may expect many of your clients to experience real feelings of loss as they are perturbed and move toward new ways of thinking, feeling, and behaving. They will sometimes resist and sabotage their own best efforts toward change. Your personal support and warmth throughout the change process are particularly important.

Challenges: Confrontation is a powerful therapeutic and counseling skill that should be used carefully and must be based on a thorough understanding of theory and practice. Skills necessary for the effective use of confrontation include paraphrasing, reflection of feeling, and summarization. Some of the most effective confrontations use the client's language and perceptions as a base. Other confrontation skills include interpretation, reframing, and questioning. The Confrontation Impact Scale is useful for analyzing the effectiveness of interventions.

Research issues:

- Examine your own interviewing practice. Generate a transcript of one of your own sessions. Classify on the CIS how the client responds to your interventions. Have another person do the same classifications. Compute your interrater agreement. Now, look more broadly at how the client or family conceptualized the problem at the first part of the interview. Can you find measurable evidence that your clients moved from denial or partial understanding of an issue to higher levels of understanding as measured by the CIS?

- The specific components of the confrontation techniques and the Confrontation Impact Scale can be applied to Kohlberg-type moral dilemmas (see Chapter 2). A useful and potentially significant exercise would be to combine moral reasoning with developmental assessment and treatment strategies. Can the results of moral development perturbations, using the Kohlberg system, be reliably assessed following the methods presented in this chapter?

- In addition, clients' reactions to general issues of loss and death and dying may be evaluated empirically by adapting the CIS to the work of Kübler-Ross.

THEORY INTO PRACTICE: DEVELOPING YOUR PORTFOLIO OF COMPETENCE

Self-Assessment Exercises

Exercise 1. What has been your reaction to loss or failure?

Kübler-Ross's five stages of death and dying were used to draw a parallel to similar stages we all work through when we face losses and defeats in life. Recall a loss or defeat you have experienced: failure in school or on the job, the breakup of a significant relationship, not making a team, or moving to a new home or school. You may wish to explore more powerful losses and sadness such as those related to the death of a loved one, having an alcoholic family member, or suffering a physical disability. Or you may want to interview a friend or family member who has experienced a loss.

See if you can identify in yourself or the other person the specific stages of loss described by Kübler-Ross. Cite specific examples for the most relevant stages. Also, did you find yourself moving through stages in a linear stepwise direction or did you find that you moved through the issues of the stages in a more random, nonlinear fashion, perhaps even recycling through the stages at times?

Denial

_____

_____

Anger

_____

_____

Bargaining

_____

_____

Depression

_____

_____

Acceptance

_____

_____

Identifying and Classifying Confrontation and Related Strategies

Exercise 2. The primary circular reaction

The primary circular reaction is a key theoretical concept. This concept can be confusing unless you restate the main ideas of the process in your own language and apply the concept to your own practice of counseling and therapy. Briefly outline the key points of the primary circular reaction below and then, in a longer paper, describe how these central ideas may be utilized in your own helping sessions.

_____

_____

_____

_____

_____

Exercise 3. Confrontation practice exercises

Six basic types of discrepancies, mixed messages, or conflicts have been identified in this chapter and are listed below. Think back on your own personal life experience or observations in counseling and therapy. Provide an example of each type of incongruity in the space provided. When have you, a friend, or a client demonstrated the several types of mixed messages, incongruity, or discrepancy?

After each example, write a confrontation statement that a counselor or therapist might use to clarify the discrepancy. The confrontation statement has two parts: (1) feeding back the essence of the discrepancy, using the client's main words, and (2) asking the client how he or she synthesizes the discrepancy (for example, "How do you put that together?" or "What sense do you make of that?")

1. Between two verbal statements (any of the four DCT levels):

   _____

   _____

   Confrontation statement:

   _____

   _____

2. Between statements and actions outside the interview (formal/concrete or concrete/concrete):

   _____

   _____

   Confrontation statement:

   _____

   _____

3. Between statements and nonverbal behavior in the interview (between any of the four DCT styles and sensorimotor behavior):

   _____

   _____

Confrontation statement:

_____

_____

4. Between two nonverbal behaviors (sensorimotor):

_____

_____

Confrontation statement:

_____

_____

5. Between two or more people (any developmental level):

_____

_____

Confrontation statement:

_____

_____

6. Between any of the above and the context (dialectic/systemic):

_____

_____

Confrontation statement:

_____

_____

Exercise 4. The Confrontation Impact Scale

Imagine what a client might say at each of the five levels of the Confrontation Impact Scale to two of your confrontation statements from the preceding section. Write statements that represent each level of the CIS.

Confrontation statement 1:

Level 1: Denial

_____

_____

Level 2: Partial examination

_____

_____

Level 3: Full examination but no change

_____

_____

Level 4: Creation of new dimensions

_____

_____

Level 5: Development of new, larger, more inclusive constructs, patterns, or behaviors (creation of the New)

_____

_____

Confrontation statement 2:

Level 1: Denial

_____

_____

Level 2: Partial examination

_____

_____

Level 3: Full examination but no change

_____

_____

Level 4: Creation of new dimensions

_____

_____

Level 5: Development of new, larger, more inclusive constructs, patterns, or behaviors (creation of the New)

_____

_____

Toward Multicultural Competence

Exercise 5. Anticipating the relationship between DCT and racial/cultural identity

Chapter 8 focuses on multicultural development, with special attention to five stages of cultural identity. Key terms of the Racial/Cultural Identity Model (Atkinson, Morten, & Sue, 1998) are presented below. For each term, write you own brief definition and then indicate how these concepts relate to the four major styles of DCT and to the stages of death and dying. Once you have made this early attempt, please turn to page 249 and compare what you have developed with what is presented there. How to confront issues of self as a multicultural being will be addressed more fully in Chapter 8, which addresses multicultural counseling and therapy.

Stage 1—Preencounter _____

_____

Stage 2—Encounter _____

_____

Stage 3—Immersion/emersion _____

_____

Stage 4—Internalization _____

_____

Additional observations _____

_____

Interviewing Practice Exercise

Exercise 6. Practice using the CIS in a role-played session

Follow usual ethical procedures.

Step 1: Divide Into Practice Groups

Step 2: Select a Group Leader

Step 3: Assign Roles for the Practice Session

- *Role-played client.* The role-played client will talk freely about the topic but be somewhat resistant.
- *Interviewer.* The interviewer will attempt to identify key client discrepancies and then confront these discrepancies. Simultaneously, the interviewer will attempt to observe the level of response to confrontation of the client. Does the client deny (level 1), show partial understanding (level 2), demonstrate understanding but no change (level 3), or perhaps generate new ideas (levels 4 and 5)?
- *Observer 1.* The first observer will write down each interviewer statement. It is possible to reconstruct a total session using only brief notes. The observer will make a special effort to note confrontation statements.
- *Observer 2.* The second observer will complete the feedback sheet provided and will make a special effort to note client responses on the Confrontation Impact Scale.

Step 4: Plan the Session

- The interviewer and client need first to agree on the topic. Useful topics for this session include working through the breakup of a long-term relationship (either now or in the past) or role-playing a friend or family member who experienced such a breakup. The topics of procrastination or a past or present interpersonal conflict are also good.

- The client may think through how he or she wishes to talk about the agreed-on topic throughout the session.
- The two observers will examine the feedback form.

Step 5: Conduct a 15-Minute Interviewing Session
Again it is helpful to videotape or audiotape practice sessions.

Step 6: Provide Immediate Feedback and Complete Notes (5 Minutes)
Allow the client and interviewer time to provide immediate personal reactions to the practice session. At this point, the observers should let the participants take control. Use this time to complete your classification and notes.

Step 7: Review Practice Session and Provide Feedback (15 to 30 Minutes)
The interviewer should ask for feedback rather than getting it without having asked. The observers can share their observations from the feedback form and from their observations of the session. Avoid judgmental feedback.

Generalization: Taking Confrontation Skills Home

Exercise 7. Observation and actions that can enable you to test the concepts of this chapter in the real world

Observing incongruities. Look for and report incongruities you observe in yourself and others over a one-week period of time. Classify the discrepancies into the five types suggested in this chapter. What other categories beyond these five do you observe?

Testing out confrontation. Gently and supportively try confrontations with people with whom you come into contact. Be nonjudgmental and use their key words as you paraphrase and summarize for them what you have observed. Use confrontation skills with sensitivity and care.

Observing developmental movement on the CIS. Observe how people you encounter in your day-to-day life are at different levels on the Confrontation Impact Scale. You can make this assessment in two ways: First, you can classify their reactions to comments using the scale. However, there are lifestyle issues involved as well. Some people go through life functioning at levels 1 and 2, denying all or part of the reality that surrounds them. Second, you can write down evidence of your observations of individual responses and of general lifestyle issues.

Attending a meeting. Using the suggestions from activity 1, visit an open meeting of a community governance group, a PTA, or a business organization. Record your observations of discrepancies and reactions to confrontation. Look especially for positive examples of groups that enable members to achieve new discoveries representative of levels 4 and 5 of the Confrontation Impact Scale. What are these groups doing right?

With permission of the family, observe a family meal using the suggestions from activity 1. What aspects of family life lead to growth and development? At what general level is this family functioning?

Examining your own style in the session. Using an audiotape or videotape of one of your own interviews with an individual or family, list discrepancies and incongruities you observe. You may have confronted the client or clients at some point or you may have used a major intervention. At what level on the Confrontation Impact Scale did the family or individual respond to your efforts? Provide specific evidence supporting your conclusion.

An even more important test is to identify the creation of the New in your clients. What specific acts of creation leading to new points of view, new behavior, or even multiperspective seeing can you document in your own work?

Apply the techniques of this chapter carefully with a client or family in counseling or therapy each day. As you learn the value of the conceptual and practical developmental model, you may find yourself using the concepts in regular interviewing practice.

Portfolio Reflections

Exercise 8. Your reflections on developmental change processes

What stood out for you from this chapter? What sense do you make of what you have read and experienced? What are your key points from this chapter? Write your answers here and add them to your Portfolio Folder in your computer.

_____

_____

_____

_____

_____

_____

REFERENCES

Atkinson, D., Morten, G., & Sue, D. W. (1998). *Counseling American minorities: A cross-cultural perspective* (5th ed.). Dubuque, IA: Wm. C. Brown.

Bolman, L., & Deal, T. (1990). *Artistry, choice, and leadership.* San Francisco: Jossey-Bass.

Bolman, L., & Deal, T. (2000). *Escape from cluelessness: A guide for the organizationally challenged.* New York: AMACOM.

de Waal, E. (1997). *Living with contradiction: An introduction to Benedictine spirituality.* Harrisburg, PA: Morehouse.

Figley, R., Bride, B. E., & Mazza, N. (Eds.). (1997). *Helping traumatized families.* San Francisco: Jossey-Bass.

Hill, C., & O'Brien, K. (1999). *Helping skills.* Washington, DC: American Psychological Association.

Ivey, A. (1973). Media therapy: Educational change planning for psychiatric patients. *Journal of Counseling Psychology, 20,* 338–343.

Ivey, A. (1993). *Developmental strategies for helpers.* North Amherst, MA: Microtraining Associates.

Ivey, A. (2000). *Developmental therapy: Theory into practice.* North Amherst, MA: Microtraining Associates. (Original work published 1986)

Ivey, A., D'Andrea, M., Ivey, M., & Simek-Morgan, L. (2002). *Theories of counseling and psychotherapy: A multicultural perspective* (5th ed.). Boston: Allyn & Bacon.

Ivey, A., & Ivey, M. (2003). *Intentional interviewing and counseling: Facilitating development in a multicultural society.* Pacific Grove, CA: Brooks/Cole.

Kübler-Ross, E. (1997). *On death and dying.* New York: Scribner. (Original work published 1969)

Linkletter, A. (1957). *Kids say the darndest things!* Englewood Cliffs, NJ: Prentice-Hall.

Merton, T. (1999). *The seven storey mountain* (50th anniversary edition). Philadelphia: Harvest Books.

Miller, M. (1997). Counselor intentionality: Implications for the training of beginning counselors. *Counseling and Values, 41,* 194–203.

Minuchin, S., Wai-Yung, L., & Simon, M. (1996). *Mastering family therapy.* New York: Wiley.

Piaget, J. (1963). *The origins of intelligence in children.* New York: Norton. (Original work published 1952)

Piaget, J. (1965). *The moral judgment of the child.* New York: Free Press.

Piaget, J. (1972). *The child's conception of physical causality.* Totowa, NJ: Littlefield, Adams.

Schmidt, J. J. (1994). *Counselor intentionality and effective helping.* Greensboro, NC: ERIC/CASS.

Sharpley, C., & Sagris, I. (1995). Does eye contact increase counselor-client rapport? *Counseling Psychology Quarterly, 8,* 144–145.

Tillich, P. (1964). The importance of New being for Christian theology. In J. Campbell (Ed.), *Man and transformation.* Princeton, NJ: Princeton University Press.

Answers to CIS Classification Exercises (pp. 182–183)

Example 1: 1, 2, 3, 4, 5
Example 2: 3, 2, 5, 4, 1
Example 3: 1, 3, 2, 4, 5

CHAPTER 7
Developing Treatment Plans
DCT and Theories of Counseling and Psychotherapy

CENTRAL PRACTICE OBJECTIVE

Mastery and practice of concepts in this chapter will enable you to shift your counseling style to meet the developmental needs of varying clients. You will be able to work with multiple theories of counseling and therapy and integrate DCT developmental concepts into your treatment plans.

This chapter shows how to use developmental counseling and therapy (DCT) in treatment planning. Multiple strategies from differing theoretical orientations may be systematically combined and used with a single client or family. A network treatment model is presented for helping clients who utilize one or more of the four major cognitive/emotional styles. You will find specific ideas for matching strategies of counseling and therapy theory with the needs of the client.

We as individuals exist in a community within a multicultural frame—a network of interactions. DCT is an integrative metatheory of counseling and psychotherapy. It brings its own strategies, but it also recognizes and recommends full utilization of traditional theories—first force psychodynamic, second force cognitive-behavioral, and third force existential-humanistic. In addition, the newer fourth force multicultural counseling and therapy (MCT) is central to effective practice.

Knowledge of and skill in the concepts of this chapter can enable you to:

1. Identify how the integrative wellness approach of DCT relates to the four major theoretical and practical approaches to counseling and therapy.
2. Outline flexible treatment plans that bring together diverse theories and strategies for the approach that best matches the client's cognitive/emotional needs.
3. Be specific about integrative treatment planning through review of a case of child abuse. A step-by-step treatment-planning model is presented.
4. Understand and use style-shift counseling theory as part of regular practice. The general goal is to match your cognitive/emotional style to the client and shift your style and therapeutic strategies to meet changing client needs.

INTRODUCTION: ECLECTICISM AND INTEGRATIVE THEORY

You encounter multiple theoretical orientations to counseling and therapy in any serious study of the field. While some programs have a commitment to a single school (e.g., cognitive-behavioral, psychodynamic), most prefer to provide the student with a broad coverage of the field. This continues as you enter professional life with multiple possibilities for continuing education, the demands of professional journals, and the divergence of theoretical and practice differences among your colleagues. Each theory and strategy may have much to commend it, but clearly no one person can master such a vast body of theory, research, and clinical experience.

Out of such profusion you will need to define your own theoretical orientation and approach to counseling and therapy. Eclecticism, selecting aspects of varying theories, is one method that many use. As most theories and strategies have some demonstrated value, eclecticism makes considerable sense and helps you to define your own unique approach and theoretical integration. As you use your personal eclectic approach more and more, it will become more systematic and predictable. And the more you use this approach, the more it becomes a theory of helping in its own right.

This chapter seeks to facilitate your integration of a diversity of theories in your practice of counseling and psychotherapy. And we hope that it expands your interest in and willingness to explore some approaches that you have not considered before because you are not completely comfortable with the framework they come from. In this chapter you will see how DCT organizes existing theories and strategies. You'll find that some strategies are particularly strong in facilitating sensorimotor development whereas others lend themselves to expanding concrete action, to using formal reflection, or to building awareness of systems that affect clients. Many theories of helping are multilevel in the DCT sense, but very few cover all the cognitive/emotional styles in depth.

As you develop your own eclectic and integrative theory of counseling and psychotherapy, we encourage you to include strategies that can reach all four cognitive/emotional styles. This will likely require you to use strategies from theories that are not central to your thinking. However, developmental counseling and therapy can provide a theoretical framework into which you can incorporate your choices. An important goal for you in this chapter is to ensure that you develop a theoretical orientation that will help your clients grow cognitively and emotionally in the broadest fashion possible.

DCT AND THE FOUR MAJOR THEORETICAL FORCES OF COUNSELING AND THERAPY

Developmental counseling and therapy, as a metatheory, can support and integrate alternative approaches to human change—even though at times varying theories may appear contradictory. You will find that developmental sequences such as those described in the preceding two chapters are useful tools to help us work within multiple theoretical approaches. Out of this eclectic/metatheoretical approach more comprehensive and systematic client treatment plans become possible.

Theoretical Strategies for Varying Cognitive/Emotional Styles

Different theories tend to place varying emphasis on the four cognitive/emotional styles. Fritz Perls, with his Gestalt therapy, was one of the first to emphasize here and now strategies oriented toward sensorimotor body awareness. Behavioral psychology and behavior modification most often focus on concrete and observable aspects of therapy. Rogers's person-centered counseling and psychodynamic approaches have, for the most part, focused on formal-operational aspects of human change. Feminist therapy and multicultural counseling and therapy often emphasize dialectic/systemic issues in treatment—how is the person affected by the system and context? These last two approaches often complement individual therapy with direct action in the community. They might encourage a rape survivor to join a campus community effort to make the campus safer.

There is value and truth in all theories and strategies. Your task is to select the appropriate ones to help your particular client. For example, if you are working from a cognitive perspective and your client needs more help in understanding patterns of cognition, you may first try an automatic thoughts inventory with your client. However, the client may not respond and you may then try another strategy that might bring about much the same result—for example, an REBT "ABCDEF" analysis, as described by Albert Ellis. On the other hand, you might gain the needed information through a storytelling, narrative approach. There are multiple strategies available. Start with the client's style and change your strategy to meet her or his needs if the first approach does not produce results.

Box 7-1 offers several strategies for each DCT cognitive/emotional style. This is not a comprehensive list and you may wish to add below the box some that you favor. Match the items in this list with the predominant cognitive/emotional style you believe would work best with that strategy, keeping in mind that many strategies will be effective with more than one style.

Box 7-1   Illustrative Strategies Corresponding to Each DCT Style[1]

Predominantly Sensorimotor/Elemental Strategies	Bodywork—acupuncture, massage, yoga Catharsis Exercise—walking, jogging, swimming Focusing on emotions in the here and now Gestalt here and now activities Guided imagery Medication Meditation Psychodynamic free association Relaxation training
Predominantly Concrete/Situational Strategies	Assertiveness training Behavioral counts and charts Brief therapy Cognitive automatic thoughts chart Crisis intervention Decision and problem-solving counseling Desensitization and establishment of anxiety hierarchies Narratives and storytelling Psychoeducational skills training Reality therapy REBT "ABCDEF" analysis Thought stopping
Predominantly Formal/Reflective Strategies	Adlerian therapy—early collections (Chapter 10) Bibliotherapy Cognitive therapy Dream analysis Logotherapy Narratives, reflecting on stories Person-centered therapy Psychodynamic therapies Rational emotive behavior therapy Reflection on narratives

[1]Please note the word "predominantly." While one dimension may be most prominent in a strategy, many are multidimensional and may affect more than one cognitive/emotional style. In addition, a sensorimotor strategy such as imagery is often followed in therapy by concrete discussion of the story associated with the image, then formal reflection on the image and the story. In some cases, counselors will also encourage clients to examine the systems and contextual issues related to the image.

(continued)

Box 7-1	*(continued)*
Predominantly Dialectic/Systemic Strategies	Advocacy for social justice Community or neighborhood action Community genogram Family dream analysis Family genogram or chart Multicultural counseling and therapy
Theories and Strategies Applied Across All Four Styles	Consciousness-raising groups Developmental counseling and therapy Feminist therapy Multicultural counseling and therapy Self-help groups (AA, ACOA, eating disorders) Trauma therapy *if* it also takes a look at systemic effects on the person

Theory or Strategy	Predominant Cognitive/Emotional Style

Major Theories and DCT

Albert Ellis (1999), perhaps the major figure in the cognitive-behavioral tradition, summarizes the essentials of how DCT relates to rational emotive behavior therapy (REBT) and, by implication, many other theories as well. First, he stresses that emotion (the E of REBT) represents the sensorimotor cognitive/emotional style. The concrete behavioral self (B of REBT) is addressed through drawing out the linear and specific reasoning of the client. R, rational reflection on these discoveries, is essential for cognitive change—formal-operational thinking is central to the REBT approach. However, moving to dialectic/systemic issues, Ellis comments (1999, p. 2):

> (DCT) . . . can be defined as . . . one of the ways individuals or collective systems process information. When using this information, individuals and families can look at the ways they have been affected by and also influence the wider sociocultural contexts in which they reside. Additionally, viewing the world from this vantage point helps individuals and families reflect on and challenge the rules and assumptions they have come to believe as they interact, over time, in different contexts.

To be sure, REBT has not emphasized dialectic/systemic counseling as much as it is heavily encouraged in DCT and SCDT *(systemic cognitive developmental therapy)*. Quite possibly, it—and most other popular therapies—is relatively lax in this respect. The unique aspect . . . is the way they stress this fourth process; and REBT had better consider emphasizing it more than it sometimes has done in the past and learn from DCT and SCDT.

It is nonetheless accurate, as Rigazio-DiGilio, Ivey, and Locke (1997, p. 241) note: "Theories of counseling and practice that perpetuate the notion of individual and family dysfunction without giving equal attention to societal dysfunction and to the dysfunctional interactions that can occur between individuals, families, and societies (e.g., intentional and unintentional power differentials) may unwittingly reinforce the oppressive paradigm." *All systems of counseling had better give serious thought to this hypothesis—as, in fact, few of them have to date.*

In summary, Ellis points out that REBT uses the first three of the four DCT styles and that he is reconsidering the importance of the fourth—dialectic/systemic thought and action. Ellis's words are important as they illustrate how traditionally important theoretical systems relate to the integrative approach of DCT.

DCT integrative metatheory focuses on the underlying structural dimensions of all counseling and therapy: information processing and cognitive/emotional style. You will find that most psychodynamic, cognitive-behavioral, and existential/humanistic therapies use two or more of three styles (sensorimotor, concrete, and formal), but their strategies and ways for reaching these client styles vary. On the other hand, feminist and multicultural counseling and therapy (MCT) are examples of major theoretical systems that give prime attention to dialectic/systemic issues. Like developmental counseling and therapy, feminist therapy and MCT also seek to integrate traditional first, second, and third force psychology into broadly based treatment plans.

Cognitive therapy also covers the first three styles very well, although strategies from this approach give less attention to sensorimotor dimensions (Beck, 1976, 1995). Cognitive therapists often start with the client's concrete story and may then ask clients for a sensorimotor image of the story. Of course, they do not use the word "sensorimotor" and do not use this area often for therapeutic intervention. However, these images often serve as the emotional foundation for cognitive therapy. The automatic thoughts log helps clients see the concretes of their situation. Needless to say, much of cognitive therapy is oriented toward reflection on thoughts and feelings. But cognitive therapy gives little or no attention to dialectic/systemic issues.

Carl Rogers (1963) more than anyone else brought the importance of the relationship to the counseling and therapy field. The basic mode of operation tends to be style 3—formal-operational/reflective. Witness the term *reflection of feeling*, very different from Gestalt therapy's sensorimotor emphasis on feeling in the here and now. Nonetheless, Rogers's emphasis on immediacy and here and now interaction often leads to deep sensorimotor experiencing. Perhaps the difference between successful and less successful person-centered therapists relates to their ability to bring out the basics of experienced emotion. And you can't have emotion without direct experience, an important aspect of Rogers's theory and practice.

Rogers brought clarity and understanding to empathy—seeing the world from the other person's frame of reference. DCT adds to empathic understanding by pointing out that just understanding a person's mode of being may not be enough. A more complete empathic understanding may be communicated through words that match the client's cognitive/emotional style. Thus, a client with a concrete style will benefit from the concrete expression of empathy whereas the more abstract client may find a formal-operational reflection of feeling quite satisfactory. *Being with the client also requires matching cognitive/emotional style.*

Psychodynamic thought includes Adler, Freud, Jung, and many others. Traditional analytic therapy tends to be primarily formal-operational and reflective—and perhaps that is one of the reasons it is so time-consuming. More modern approaches such as that of the Afrocentric psychodynamic theorist Bruce Taub-Bynum (1992, 1999) seek to include all four styles with a strong emphasis on an affective sensorimotor base. Taub-Bynum speaks of the way family systems and cultural issues relate to our experience. Concrete, linear discussion, although not stressed, remains part of the process.

The philosophy and values underlying Adlerian Individual Psychology are consistent with DCT (see Chapters 2 and 10). While many practitioners cover all four dimensions by incorporating similar methods, in our experience, DCT can extend the impact of Adlerian interventions. However, few Adlerians have been trained in DCT, which, as noted by Ellis, is a new theory that *should* be embraced by other theoretical perspectives and practitioners. Sensorimotor, concrete, formal, and dialectic styles are found in the practices associated with lifestyle assessment and interpretation of early recollections (Eckstein & Kern, 2002; Clark, 2002), and marriage and family counseling (Sweeney, 1998), and to some extent also in parent and teacher counseling/consultation (Dreikurs & Soltz, 1964/1999; Dreikurs, Grunwald, & Pepper, 1982; McKay, McKay, Eckstein, & Maybell, 2001). Furthermore, both Adler and Dreikurs (Dreikurs & Stolz, 1964/1999) were forerunners in promoting personal responsibility and an end to oppression through social equality.

Multicultural counseling and therapy (MCT) brings with it an array of possible interventions, many of them emphasizing dialectic/systemic strategies. Among the many cognitive/emotional possibilities within MCT are Japanese Naikan therapy with its strong sensorimotor and reflective orientation, consciousness-raising and feminist theories with their emphasis on self-in-systems, cultural identity theory (formal/dialectic/systemic), meditation (deeply sensorimotor), Native American network therapy with its emphasis on multiple systems and styles, and traditional healing practices drawn from African, Asian, Latina/o, and Native American cultures. See Ivey, D'Andrea, Ivey, and Simek-Morgan (2002) for further practical specifics of both theory and practice of MCT.

DCT, Health, and Wellness

Health issues are beginning to figure in counseling and psychotherapy, and work within the sensorimotor style is now recognized as a basic part of treatment. The American Psychological Association presented a special series on health and one of the lead articles was entitled "If You Do Just One Thing, Make It Exercise" (DeAngelis, 2002). Psychologists have found that patients with major depression who exercised were 50% less likely to become depressed six months later than a comparison group (both groups were on medication in the early phases of the study). Over 30 years ago, Ivey (1973) observed that relaxation training with psychiatric inpatients was a valuable part of treatment with the clinically depressed. The importance of sensorimotor work with depression has stood the test of time. In effect, help your client get moving—walking, swimming, exercising in the gym. It is much more difficult to be depressed if your body is moving and you are taking in more oxygen. Box 7-1 has a number of strategies that can be included in a body and physical health–oriented treatment plan. Meditation can be as important as medication in some instances.

Dr. Kenneth Minaker, chief of the Geriatric Medicine Unit of Massachusetts General Hospital, has reviewed the literature (2003) on what is required to reach older age in good health. The list in Box 7-2 is based on *personal choice,* those issues the patient or client can control. Genetics, of course, is influential in aging, but we can do more than we realize. The "secrets" of old age may be more available than generally thought. And each item in the research summary has counseling and therapy implications. One might even wonder whether it is ethical and appropriate not to include physical health issues in any serious longer-term therapy.

Box 7-2   Ten Personal Choice Issues That Contribute to Aging Successfully and Healthfully

Research reveals that the following list is central to a successful and healthy old age (Minaker, 2003).

1. Sleeping 7–8 hours per night (too much or too little is found to be less healthy)
2. Weight control
3. Exercise
4. Limited alcohol
5. Non-smoking
6. Eating breakfast
7. Seldom snacking
8. More education
9. Social connectedness
10. Optimism/happiness

Anger management can be an important health resource (e.g., Deffenbacher, in press; Ivey et al., 2002; Smith, 2003). Those who are angry are more likely to have heart attacks, and hot temper can predict heart disease. The cognitive-behavioral strategies listed in Box 7-1 help clients who are dealing with a wide variety of health issues. Your work with the health issues listed by Minaker (2003) will often employ concrete and behavioral strategies—systematic weight control, smoking cessation, and moderation with alcohol.

An article entitled "Angry Thoughts, at Risk Hearts" speaks to both concrete and formal-operational issues (Smith, 2003). It points out that busy, hard-driving,

"Type A" clients who have heart disease must make major cognitive/emotional change if they are to survive. Person-centered counseling or psychodynamic therapy can offer support and may enable the client to see her or his issues from a new perspective. As noted in Box 7-2, social support and family systems are important to health when we consider dialectic/systemic issues. As just one example, Thompson, Kaslow, Short, and Wyckoff (2002) found that abused and suicidal African American women who received social support from family and friends had more self-efficacy and were at less risk in the future. Again, think of the self-in-relation, the person-in-community.

Box 7-2 points to the importance of a multistyle approach to physical care of the body; obviously, this broad approach needs to become more important in therapeutic literature and practice. Sensorimotor, concrete, formal, and dialectic/systemic work is needed to enable a client to develop a better lifestyle that, in turn, will lead to better mental health.

DCT Theoretical Integration: Case Example

The DCT integrative multistyle approach is illustrated by the case of Michael.

> Michael, a Vietnam veteran, is an example of a client with a concrete style who is a trauma survivor. Michael came to therapy complaining of flashbacks to battle scenes—flashbacks so vivid they seemed real. He described them as if he were in the middle of a movie. Sensorimotor night sweats and random images playing out in his mind accompanied these concrete experiences.
>
> Part of his therapy was involved with discussing concrete, linear stories from the Vietnam war and then thinking about them using formal/reflective thought. Reflective cognitive therapy (Beck/Ellis) was added at times, with sensorimotor imaging strategies. Sensorimotor relaxation training and meditation helped calm Michael's stormy flashbacks. Concrete assertiveness training assists in helping Michael take action at work and in the family to follow up on these new learnings.
>
> Therapy was not complete, however, until the dialectic/systemic orientation came into play. . . . His reactions to war were not just his responsibility, but also related to larger systemic issues such as the unpopularity of that war. . . . Michael was encouraged to join a group of Vietnam veterans who shared their experiences. As Michael came to see his personal issues in a social context, he responded more effectively to traditional techniques such as cognitive therapy, imagery, and assertiveness training. Integrative therapy without providing a social context would have been incomplete for Michael. (Ivey et al., 2002, pp. 378, 380)

Comprehensive treatment planning begins with offering some help in each style area, much as was done for Michael. You are not expected to be expert in all strategies and all theories, but you must have some skill in each of the four style dimensions. Sometimes your favored intervention is not well received by your client. In this case, you might, for example, move from concrete narrative storytelling to an automatic thoughts log, role-playing (with both a concrete and sensorimotor dimension), or some other strategy. *There are many ways to address the client with a concrete style.* Similarly, it is wise to have several ways in which you can enable clients to examine their issues within all styles.

Network Therapy

Carolyn Attneave, the pioneer and founder of Native American psychology, conceptualized network therapy in 1969 (Attneave, 1969, 1982; Speck & Attneave, 1973). Proponents of network therapy claim that individuals and their families cannot be satisfactorily treated in one-on-one counseling or in family sessions. For significant change to occur, they believe that broader social support systems need to be developed in the extended family, the community, and, if possible, in the broader society (Galanter, 1999; Galanter & Brook, 2001; Speck, 1998). Multiple theories and strategies need to be considered.

Many aspects of Native American culture and family life have useful implications for a more integrated practice of counseling and therapy. LaFromboise and Low (1989, p. 121) comment on some of these aspects:

> Traditionally, Indian people live in relational networks that serve to support and nurture strong bonds of mutual assistance and affection. Many tribes still engage in a traditional system of collective interdependence, with family members responsible not only to one another but also to the clan and tribe to which they belong. The Lakota Sioux use the term *tiospaye* to describe a traditional, community way of life in which an individual's well-being remains the responsibility of the extended family. . . . When problems arise among Indian youth, they become problems of the community as well. The family, kin, and friends join together to observe the youth's behavior, draw the youth out of isolation, and integrate that person back into the activities of the group.

Traditional Western therapy too often tries to change individuals and families in isolation. Newer, more ecologically oriented ways of helping employ case management techniques, with the full awareness that an entire community network of extended family and professional helpers may be required to bring about significant and lasting change. This, of course, represents the dialectic/systemic portion of the DCT framework.

For example, in working with an alcoholic woman and her family, network therapists would bring together the woman, the immediate family, the extended family (parents, grandparents, siblings, in-laws), and the woman's employer and colleagues. Beyond that, key individuals such as the owner of the local bar, the police, neighbors, social service workers, individual and family therapists, and the parish priest might be brought in for a session of two hours or longer. Here we see the full dialectic/system network of possible individuals brought together to help solve difficulties.

The network therapist would review the family problem and essentially facilitate a community meeting about how the problem of alcoholism might be solved. As might be anticipated, the bar owner might receive community pressure to stop serving the woman, the social service agency might provide child-care services previously denied, and the extended family might be encouraged to institute stronger controls for the children. The decisional process in network therapy is not hierarchical or theory directed; rather, it is generated from group consensus.

The process of network therapy often reveals that the "problem" of alcoholism resides not in the family alone but also in a community that allows and supports alcoholic behavior. In network therapy, more than just the individual are required to change behavior, unlike the case in traditional Western psychotherapy.

DCT suggests that interdependence—an ever-changing balance between individual and system—may be a more realistic therapeutic goal than individualism—the person-in-relation, the self-in-community. Such an orientation does not denigrate the importance of the individual but rather provides a framework for viewing the person in relationship with the world. The individual actually becomes *more special* because her or his total situation is now part of therapy. We lose the specialness if we fail to see the broader context in which people live.

A CASE OF CHILD ABUSE: DCT AND NETWORK THERAPY

How would DCT's emphasis on cognitive/emotional style be integrated with network therapy in a practical fashion? Let us take a complex and difficult case of child abuse and examine how this might be done. As you read this section, remember that child abuse and neglect are important problems for which there is no one, easy answer. DCT and network therapy offer us an opportunity to work with clients comprehensively if we are to produce significant change.

Presenting Problem. Anthony Marciano was an 8-year-old third-grade student at the time of his second referral to the school guidance office by his teacher who complained of Anthony's fighting on the playground and restlessness and daydreaming in the classroom. Anthony's test scores showed he had average ability, but he was slightly behind classmates in achievement. He lived near the school with his single-parent mother and 13-year-old brother.

Anthony's parents, both of fourth-generation Italian background, had been divorced several years prior to this referral. His father had moved to a nearby town, and his mother was currently working in a local department store. Her manfriend, employed as a mechanic, had moved in with the family about a year ago.

Past History of Counseling. Anthony first came to the school counselor's attention in kindergarten. He was extremely restless, and his teacher thought he might be hyperactive (*DSM-IV-R* attention deficit disorder). Before accepting the teacher's assessment, the counselor visited the classroom. Classroom observations confirmed the teacher's general impressions. Anthony was in and out of his seat, constantly interrupting the teacher or others in the class; at times, however, he could sustain attention well.

Before undertaking counseling or referral, the counselor asked Anthony's mother to come in after school and discuss the situation. After a brief presentation, the young mother broke into tears and talked about going through a difficult divorce. With the mother's agreement, the counselor's interventions at that time focused on a classroom behavioral management program that included rewards and attention for appropriate behavior. Anthony's mother was referred to a community mental health counselor for assistance in working through her issues, since there was not a family therapist in practice in the community at that time. In addition, his mother joined a parent education program. Neither Anthony's father nor his mother's manfriend would participate in the child's treatment plan.

Individual counseling was attempted, but Anthony was not a talkative child, and individual work proved slow and difficult. Some access to feelings was obtained while Anthony played games, manipulated an easy puzzle, or did artwork. Anthony responded especially well to bibliotherapy, in which the counselor's reading stories about divorce was coupled with artwork for Anthony (see Myers, 1998). Psychoeducational classroom activities, educational games, and structured problem solving were increased, partially in an effort to assist Anthony in his peer relations. In addition, the counselor arranged a weekly "divorce group" in which Anthony and other children of divorce shared their experiences in a structured way. Although Anthony didn't say much, he did pay attention to the others' comments.

It is unfortunate that family therapy was not available in the community. A family therapist could have explored to learn whether Anthony's difficulties stemmed from the divorce or problems in his present interaction with his mother. It would have been desirable for Anthony's mother and father to meet with a family therapist to help them work jointly for Anthony's benefit. This would have enabled the therapist to observe the system of interactions within the family. Also, it might have been beneficial to have a therapist work with the mother and her two children. But, no family therapist was available in the community at the time of the first contact; also many families will still refuse to enter treatment. In many situations, you may find yourself as the only resource available for help.

From a DCT frame of reference, sensorimotor and concrete treatment techniques provided Anthony with sufficient support to produce some improvement in his behavior problems. Consultation with the teacher, psychoeducational classroom interventions, and the referral of Anthony's mother to therapy represent dialectic/systemic interventions. The "necessary and sufficient" conditions for therapeutic change of warmth, positive regard, and authenticity—the core conditions Rogers (1963) identified—are important beginning points. A combined network and DCT approach to treatment recognizes that multifaceted interventions are necessary if change is to be instituted and maintained.

This first round of treatment enabled Anthony to negotiate the next two years of elementary school relatively effectively. He achieved at grade style and, in general, seemed an average student with a good peer support group. However, problems resurfaced in the third grade. At this time, a network/DCT approach was used in formulating a treatment plan for Anthony.

As Anthony entered this second treatment phase, it was clear that special attention must be given to many factors if solutions to his fighting, restlessness, and academic achievement issues were to be found. Single intervention programs are likely to fail with children.

Generating a DCT/network treatment plan involves several steps and examples of this approach are presented in detail.

Step 1: Establishing a positive base for treatment

Drawing from wellness concepts, the counselor first considered Anthony's strengths. She knew from experience that it would be difficult for him to talk about his problems. As she prepared for the first session, she identified Anthony's positives: he is lively and energetic; he has a lovely, engaging smile; he has been able to sustain friendships, although his friends also are sometimes likely to get into trouble in school. Anthony had had problems earlier, during the family divorce, but seemed to bounce back until this latest outbreak. His mother tends to be cooperative. Anthony seems to respond positively to attention, but if he doesn't get it, he will use any way he can to gain what he wants. Base a treatment plan on wellness.

Another important positive base for treatment was awareness of community resources that could be used to help Anthony and his family. The personal strengths and knowledge of the counselor also can serve as a positive resource for the client. Never forget yourself as a positive client resource for wellness.

Step 2: Examining key relationship issues that might affect the counselor or therapist

"How clients treat you [and others] is how they were treated." Anthony's personality style is typical of many boys who are impulsive and attention demanding. This behavior contrasts with the more reflective, sometimes passive personality styles of many counselors and therapists.

The counselor knew that working with Anthony was not going to be easy, even given the positives. She was aware of a tightening in her stomach as she thought through the case. She allowed herself to first magnify the tightness, and then she "went with the feeling." She remembered a scene from her own childhood when an energetic boy who looked a little like Anthony used to chase and throw sticks at her. She sighed and said to herself, "Anthony is not James, who made me so angry and frightened in the past. I'd better not confuse the two." Until she had looked at her own past feelings toward acting-out, impulsive boys, her counseling interventions with this type of client had not been effective. She found it easier to relate to active boys now that she had examined her own feelings. This allowed her to establish better and more consistent relationships.

Many therapists and counselors are not comfortable with the acting-out individual, be it child, adolescent, or adult. If you are one of these, it may be beneficial for you to work through your own feelings and developmental history surrounding these issues using the self-examination techniques suggested in Box 7-3, Discovering Your Developmental Blind Spots.

Drawing on knowledge of her feelings about Anthony's behavior, the counselor asked herself, "How does Anthony's relating to me and to others somehow reflect what has happened to him in the past?" The logical first assumption is that Anthony was parented aggressively and impulsively. For example, he might have been in a family that rewarded acting-out behavior, or the father (or mother) might have modeled impulsiveness. Emotional or physical abuse is not uncommon in the families of acting-out children.

There can be alternative explanations, of course. A busy single parent may not have a lot of time to be with a child. Impulsive, attention-seeking behavior may be the only way such a child can obtain parental involvement. Or the acting-out child may have come from a highly controlled home environment. His impulsiveness is, in this case, a reaction to rigidity. In all of the above situations, the acting-out or impulsive child has had the true self held back or crushed by the family. Lacking a sense of self, acting-out children often infringe on and violate other people's boundaries.

Box 7-3 Discovering Your Developmental Blind Spots

How clients relate to us in the here and now of the interview is a major clue to their past developmental history and how they were treated. In turn, the way you treat clients is often a reflection of how you were treated yourself. Rapport, relationship, and empathy are central to DCT practice.

The following self-study exercise can enable you to start the process of discovering your developmental blind spots. These areas may interfere with your empathic relationship with clients as well as in effective treatment planning.

1. Think of a specific person (or an actual client) who may represent special difficulty for you from the past. Get the person and the specific situation with that person clearly in your mind.
2. *Sensorimotor body feelings.* Focus on your thoughts and feelings around this person. Relax and seek to find a clear visual image and/or hear the actual words said in your mind. Out of images and sounds, note the feelings that *are occurring here and now* in your body. Locate a specific part of your body where those kinesthetic feelings are located. You will be surprised how readily your body reacts to these sensorimotor images from the past.
3. *Positive body feelings.* It is wise to repeat the above from a positive standpoint. Does either that person or that client have some positive assets and strengths? (If not, select someone who does give you positive "vibes.") Again locate the positive feeling in your body.
4. *Concrete narrative.* Return to the negative feelings in your body. Stay with them, perhaps even magnify the actual feelings in your body through close attention. Now, describe in linear form the actual situation where this happened in your own words. What were you thinking? What happened before? During the critical event? After? If you wish, repeat this with the positive body feelings.
5. *Formal reflection.* Can you identify other situations, stories, or people like this that affect you? Is there some pattern of your reaction to these people. Reflect on your own feelings when you encounter people and/or situations like this and how you respond. Again, repeat the positive situation, if you wish.
6. *Dialectic/systemic reflection and action.* Where did your thoughts and feelings come from? Particularly, where did they develop in your family and in relation to key people? Are there specific family rules or patterns you recall? What was your family attitude toward these people and situations? What are some strengths in your developmental history that might enable you to encounter them more successfully in the future? How can you actually *use* this information in your own interviewing practice?

This exercise is designed to help you become aware of body feelings that you are likely to have in the counseling and therapy session. You'll find that each client you work with brings out certain feelings in your body. This physical awareness can be a useful tool to avoid countertransference and issues that come up with difficult clients. You can, even in the middle of a session, note the specific feelings in your body and then understand from whence they came.

What have you learned from this exercise that you will take out and actually use in the session?

Working on the theory that Anthony's behavior was most likely a natural response to the need for attention led the counselor to assume the need for a relationship that provided nonjudgmental, firm controls and clear boundaries. Such definition leads the child to individuation, autonomy, and separation. But there must be warmth and support for the child's true self to emerge. Achieving individuation and autonomy can best be done from a firm base of attachment and connection.

In the preceding paragraph, the focus is on helping Anthony become both more autonomous and more relational—an interdependent goal. Each culture has its own approach for balancing separation and attachment tasks, and thus the "correct distance" in the counseling relationship should adjust according to the cultural background of counselor and client.

Step 3: Identifying DCT treatment options using multiple theories

A child may be in tears in the early part of the interview, be happily talking about baseball five minutes later, be groaning about a teacher next, and then worrying about divorce. This random mix of sensorimotor, concrete, and formal styles is common for most children (and adults). Unless you have a map of this complex territory in your mind, you may lose your direction and lose the child.

Anthony as a third grader would be expected to be very concrete. Although it would be desirable to help Anthony see other frames of reference (formal operations), it is likely that a more structured, almost sensorimotor style might be required at first. Later, the counselor could shift counseling style as Anthony showed increasing cognitive-developmental growth. Late concrete causal reasoning might be all that could be expected—for example, "Anthony, *if* you continue that type of behavior, *then* the consequences will be . . ."

Box 7-4 presents assessment and treatment options for children based on the DCT framework. (Note that the constructs of network and systemic action begin to appear most clearly in the dialectic/systemic style.) The counselor planned two sessions that focused solely on rapport building and getting to know Anthony more personally. The first two sessions focused on game playing, with little emphasis on the problem. During the first two sessions, the counselor planned to point out to Anthony his positive strengths and assets. In the third or fourth session, she planned to work through some of Anthony's issues using DCT questioning strategies adapted for children. In the meantime, consultation with the teacher about Anthony's classroom behavior was conducted and a behavioral contract was organized for discussion with Anthony's mother.

Clients may talk about their problems and developmental concerns from four perspectives, but younger children will generally discuss their problems at the sensorimotor or concrete style. Some fifth and sixth graders may operate at the formal style. Relatively few individuals (children or adults) will talk about their issues at the post-formal dialectic/systemic style. Many clients, both children and adults, will discuss their issues at two or more styles. The task of the counselor is to assess the child's cognitive-developmental style(s) on the particular problem being examined. Then the counselor can institute developmentally appropriate interventions that can change as the child develops.

Box 7-4   Four Styles of Developmental Assessment and Associated Child Treatment Strategies

---

Sensorimotor
(What are the elements
of experience?)

Assessment: The child presents concerns in a random fashion, changing the topic frequently, and may exhibit magical or irrational thinking. The child's behavior will tend to follow the same pattern—namely, short attention span and frequent body movement.

Treatment: The counselor needs to provide a firm structure for exploration but must simultaneously listen to random elements of conversation. Listening at this point will help the counselor better identify the problem. Listening skills, closed questions to provide structure, and frequent paraphrasing and summarization are useful. Direction should be provided as needed. Treatments may involve play therapy and games, use of an exercise room, relaxation training and breathing instruction, behavioral structuring of the classroom, and time-outs. Medication is extremely common now for children despite its frequently controversial nature.

Concrete Operations
(What are the
situational descriptors?)

Assessment: Most children talk in very concrete terms. They may either say very little in response to questions (early concrete), or they may talk endlessly about the little details of their experience (middle concrete). Late concrete thinking occurs when children can exhibit if/then causal thinking. The parallel between the counseling term "concreteness" and concrete operations should be apparent.

Treatment: With the quiet child, well-placed closed questions are necessary to elicit concrete data. With the more verbal child, asking the question "Could you give me a specific example?" is the classic concrete opening. The counselor acts more as a coach, alternating between direct action and structuring and careful listening. The child needs help in organizing thought and behavioral patterns. Behavioral techniques, communication skills training, assertiveness training, and problem-solving counseling aimed at specific, single issues are particularly helpful. When dealing with problems in causal thinking, Adlerian logical consequences approach and Glasser's reality therapy may be useful. Classroom and group programs aimed at concrete concepts (friendship groups, divorce groups, social skills groups) are especially helpful.

Formal Operations
(What patterns of
thought and action
may be discerned?)

Assessment: Particularly in the fifth or sixth grade, children start to be able to discuss their concerns from a formal-operational frame of reference. They can talk about themselves and their feelings—sometimes even from the perspectives of others. ("I think it was Jane's fault, but Jane thinks it was mine." Or, later, "I guess I need to think about my friend's feelings.") The child who recognizes commonalities in repeating behaviors or thoughts is moving toward formal thinking. This type of thinking can appear as early as the third grade—usually only on selected topics.

Treatment: In helping the child describe self or situations, we may ask the question "Is that a pattern?" or "Does that happen in other situations?" If the child can see the underlying structural repetition, he or she is showing signs of formal thinking. The elementary counselor often has difficulty here since the treatment requires the counselor to operate more as a consultant, thus giving the child more power. Too many teachers and counselors stay at only the concrete style with children. If they are to develop more complex formal thinking patterns, children must be challenged and encouraged to examine themselves. Formal-operational theories of the self and the

(continued)

Box 7-4 *(continued)*	

	pattern mode of thinking abound, and a Rogerian or cognitive-behavioral style may be used if the child responds. A variety of self-oriented programs, such as self-esteem workshops, me-kits, and friendship groups, can help facilitate the examination of self and perspective taking. Finally, decisional counseling aimed at working with broader patterns of behavior and thought may be useful.
Dialectic/Systemic (How did that develop in a system? How is all this integrated?)	*Assessment:* Most children and adults do not ordinarily make sense of their worlds from this frame of reference. With children, dialectic/systemic thinking will manifest itself most clearly when, for example, a young woman (usually in the upper grades) starts talking seriously about sexism or when a minority student recognizes that personal difficulties may be caused by a racist system. Here, the child is operating on systems of knowledge and is learning how he or she is affected by the environment. The locus of awareness changes from the child or teacher to larger systemic concerns. As counselors, we must be aware that families and classrooms are two important systems affecting the child and give them more attention.
	Treatment: Case management techniques undergird the dialectic approach. Coordinating individual, group, family, school, and community interventions is key. Systems thinking is manifested in family sessions and in classroom consultation. We also use systems orientations to help children deal individually or in groups with issues of racism, sexism, and ableism. When we conduct a case conference with our colleagues and the family, we are utilizing our dialectic/systemic skills. Family counseling, referral of other family members for therapy, and coordination of cases with social services exemplify systemic action. In addition, community developmental activities may be essential. For example, if the community has a serious employment problem or serious problems with racism or other forms of discrimination, the task of the counselor may be to facilitate community action programs.

Step 4: Generating a client-counselor contract for the treatment plan

The counselor who works with children has a particular responsibility to share treatment plans with parents and involve them in the process. Box 7-5 lists some of the services of school counselors. This list should be available to all parents and can sometimes be used for planning and developing a specific client-counselor contract.

Increasingly, therapists and counselors are providing clients with statements about their rights and the skills the therapist has to offer and generating written contracts with the client, as noted in the introductory chapter, Before You Start. The information in Box 7-5 can supplement data on client rights.

The counselor called Anthony's mother and discussed the child's issues with her. The mother's response to the problem was at the formal-operational style, which indicated that she could participate in and support the counseling process (that is, she was able to reflect on Anthony's problem). Some families respond in concrete style and will be able to respond to only one or two specific problems. Occasionally, counselors will encounter adults in the family who are at an embedded sensorimotor

Box 7-5 Counseling Services Offered by School Counselors

The following activities are offered by the school guidance office and are presented to parents so that they are informed as to the process of counseling and its possible goals. The school counselor, Jane Smith, offers the following services. In consultation with Ms. Smith, parents are encouraged to select counseling programs they believe will meet their child's needs.

As you begin, you may first want to list in this space the goals you have for your child and the specific things you might want the school to do. Also, what do you think your child wants?

_____

_____

_____

_____

_____

Following are some services offered in this school. You may wish to check those of special interest to you for your child.

____ 1. Behavioral classroom consultation. Many children benefit from a more structured approach to the educational process. In consultation with the teacher and through observation of your child, it is possible to set up reward systems in the classroom. These programs are most effective if they are coordinated with parents in the home and if the specific program is negotiated with each parent.

____ 2. Skills training. Counseling is an educational process, and it is possible to teach your child, individually or in groups, certain basic skills such as:

____ Relaxation skills   ____ Friendship skills

____ Communication skills   ____ Social skills

____ Problem-solving skills   ____ Stress management skills

____ Conflict resolution skills

____ Other specific skills _____

_____

____ 3. Group counseling. Younger children often benefit from sharing ideas and experiences with one another. Specific topic groups are offered, which include:

____ Friendship groups

____ Groups for children experiencing divorce or family change

____ Anger management

____ Moving groups (for children about to move to another geographical area)

____ Self-esteem groups (to help children learn to appreciate themselves)

____ Other special topic groups: _____

_____

(continued)

Box 7-5   *(continued)*

___ 4. Individual counseling. Individual one-on-one counseling is a less specific activity but may involve one or more of the following, with the resulting specific goals:

___ Problem assessment. Often a child's issues are a mystery to the parents and the school. Exploring current situations may often uncover easy solutions or lead to referral to someone else. The interviews are nonstructured.

___ Developmental counseling. Over a period of several interviews, specific questions are asked that encourage the child to look at an issue from a variety of perspectives. For example, if a child has a problem on the playground, the counselor may seek to explore the actual happenings on the playground, how the child describes the situations, whether or not there are identifiable patterns in the child's behavior and thinking, and how that behavior might have developed. Specific questions are asked and may be reviewed by the parent before counseling begins.

___ Exploration of self. This is usually for the verbal child. The counselor listens to the child's conceptions of self and others. The aim is to develop a better sense of self and to encourage individual decision making.

___ Play and activities counseling. Games are played with children in most individual counseling sessions. These range from checkers and similar games to counseling games oriented to feelings and problem solving. Interspersed in the counseling process may be questions and counseling techniques oriented to more fully understanding the child's thinking process and the problem. At times, play and activities counseling may be the only approach used.

___ Supportive counseling. A child may have experienced a crisis at home, such as divorce or death, or be in a transition stage. During such times, checking in with the counselor weekly or biweekly can be helpful.

___ 5. Consultation, referral, and parent involvement.

___ Parent consultation. The school guidance office is often the place to start if you sense your child is having difficulty in school or is not achieving at his or her full potential. We believe it is essential that you be kept informed and that we obtain your input for the benefit of your child.

___ Parent education and counseling. Individual or group sessions are offered in parenting skills and child management. At times, family meetings are held, with all family members present to explore ways we can work together to facilitate your child's social and academic development.

___ Community referral. The counselor maintains a complete file of available financial, employment, medical, social work, and psychiatric support services for the child and for family members who may be interested in assistance for themselves.

___ Referral to individual educational planning (IEP) team. The counselor is often the first step in referral of a child with academic and social difficulties to the IEP. The IEP can arrange special services for your child, including special teacher support, therapeutic teaching, medical and psychiatric support, and other services.

___ Other services: _____

style and are unable even to understand or name the problem. Clearly, the client-counselor contract must change as cognitive-developmental style changes.

Anthony's mother was given the list of services offered by the counselor. In a mutual process, the counselor and Anthony's mother discussed a behavioral management program in the classroom, Anthony's participation in a self-esteem group, and his involvement in exploratory assessment and developmental counseling so that a more complete understanding of his issues could be gained. The counseling contract was brief, as follows:

> Specific goals for Anthony's counseling during the three weeks are to (1) improve classroom and playground behavior, (2) openly explore reasons that Anthony's behavior has changed for the worse, and (3) share these goals of counseling with Anthony and involve him in the planning process as much as possible.
>
> Attached is a list of checked methods that the counselor will employ to reach these goals. (List is attached to contract.)

Step 5: Proceeding with individual treatment

The first two interviews went as planned and expected. Anthony accepted the general goals of counseling. He was glad to play games and get out of the classroom but was not open to talking about himself or his issues. The counselor rewarded his standard social behavior with smiles, warmth, and approval. Rapport seemed to be developing. The third interview continued the same approach. In the interview Anthony was quiet and noncommunicative. When asked if something was bothering him or if he wanted to talk, he asked to play a game. The counselor suggested a board game dealing with feelings. Anthony played listlessly. When the counselor asked him what he liked best about school this year, like most children he said, "Recess," but he seemed sad.

During the next week, Anthony got into trouble several times for fighting on the playground and was especially rebellious in the classroom. After one particular fight, the teacher sent him to the counselor.

The counselor took a nonjudgmental approach and asked Anthony to tell her what had happened that day on the playground. Anthony at first talked in the random, angry fashion typical in such situations: "It wasn't my fault. He hit me first." Listening and paraphrasing eventually elicited a more linear concrete picture of the fight. With encouragement, Anthony slowly presented a detailed concrete-operational description of his last fight.

Important in this process was the counselor's willingness to listen to a child whose primary mode of functioning is detailed concrete-operational. As is true of most concrete children, Anthony often wandered to other topics, mostly using concrete description but also adding elements of sensorimotor and random meaning making. Throughout this discussion, it was important that the counselor maintain a focus on the primary topic of fighting but also be willing to help the child develop an adequate foundation of trust. Skilled paraphrasing, reflection of feeling, and summarizing are critical interviewing skills for building a sensorimotor and concrete base of understanding.

As the counselor listened, the value of the base of trust established in the first three sessions was apparent. The counselor focused the interview on sensorimotor functioning but with a new framework—the DCT systematic questioning process. The key five minutes of that session are summarized in brief form below:

Counselor: What did you see just before you hit him? Can you see him now?

Anthony: I see his red ugly face. He is panting and shouting.

Counselor: What are you feeling right now in your body?

Anthony: My stomach feels queasy, like I want to throw up.

Counselor: Where have you had the same feeling before?

Anthony: When Don (manfriend living with mother) came in drunk last week and threw the dog against the wall and then he hit me.

This questioning sequence that led to the discovery of abuse contained the following elements: (1) accepting and listening to the random events leading to the argument and fight on the playground; (2) organizing these events in a concrete linear sequence; (3) returning to the sensorimotor style, with an emphasis on what is seen, heard, and felt coupled with a free-association exercise based on the expectation that the same feeling occurred in some other situation. Here the counselor expects a pattern but introduces conditions so that the child can bring out the information. Basing counseling on a solid sensorimotor and concrete foundation is particularly important as we seek to understand the complexities of childhood cognitions. (Exactly the same sequence of counselor actions is also extremely effective with adolescents and adults in helping them discover developmental roots of present disturbance.)

Many children who are acting out or impulsive are reacting to a current problem or stage in their developmental history. Children like Anthony cannot express fear, frustration, or anger at absent parents or their abusers. Their tendency is to strike out at others. Similarly, abusive individuals themselves usually have a developmental history of significant trauma and, through their abusive behavior, enact their own problematic developmental history.

After uncovering the basis of Anthony's problem, the therapeutic task is to draw out more of the sensorimotor feelings and linear concretes of the situation and then search for formal patterns of repeating events—both the repetition of the trauma in the home and the repetition of the anger not expressed to the manfriend can be misdirected to others on the playground. This type of work takes time and is not ordinarily completed by school counselors; referral to others is required, and the counselor's role with the child becomes that of developmental case manager (coordinating various treatment services) while continuing to provide supportive counseling, group work, and classroom consultation.

Step 6: Expanding individual treatment through network involvement

On discovering the abuse, the counselor notified the Division of Social Services, the mandated state requirement, and also contacted the mother. She came in wearing makeup over what appeared to be a black eye. She appeared to be slow moving and depressed but was able to focus on her son. The counselor reviewed her sessions with Anthony and the discovery of abuse. The mother broke into tears, saying, "He hit me too, but now he's gone." In some sense, this case is easier than many abusive situations. In this case, the family did not hide the abuse but was willing and able to examine it. In some situations, the mother might have defended her manfriend and withdrawn Anthony from counseling, forcing the school to take stronger action.

In cases of abuse, systems and network interventions are critical. Individual counseling for Anthony may be beneficial, but unless the situation changes at home and support is provided in the classroom, the chances that Anthony will resume normal development are greatly impaired. In this case, youth services were called in, and a child therapist was found for Anthony. Anthony's mother was referred for individual counseling at a community mental health center. Unless key family members are able to manage their lives, work with the child is likely to be fruitless. Discussion with Anthony's brother revealed that he, too, had experienced abuse from the manfriend. Individual counseling for him was also arranged. We now have several agencies involved. You will find through experience that the problem does not go away and many times the child and family will need your help again. State referrals don't always work. You also need to be prepared to help arrange broad treatment plans yourself.

At this point, a family meeting was arranged. When working with a multiproblem family or an individual from a multiproblem family, there is always the possibility that treatments for different members can conflict. Thus, a family network meeting can be helpful in coordinating treatment and ensuring that all involved are aware of individual and family goals. "No secrets" is one motto of such meetings. Rather than hide problems and issues, open discussion of difficulties with key parties is important. Out of such meetings come commitments on the part of all. All family members, including children, are part of the planning process.

At this family meeting, the school counselor, a consulting family-oriented psychiatrist, and a representative from youth services met with Anthony, his mother, and his brother. If it had been possible, Anthony's father and the manfriend also would have been there. More information came out in this session, and it was agreed that individual work for all three was desired, plus a series of family sessions. The mother asked that special attention be given to Anthony's academic difficulties and his present lack of friends. The mother also requested some counseling to help her work through these difficult issues.

Consultation with Anthony's teacher was important in this case. The teacher needed guidance in dealing with Anthony at this difficult time, particularly since the teacher herself was facing divorce. The school counselor had to counsel the teacher in addition to developing class management programs. A "big brother" from the high school peer counseling program volunteered to meet with Anthony twice weekly after school.

Anthony's mother worked with a community therapist who provided concrete behavioral interventions and specific homework assignments, and through this, her parenting skills improved. With the therapist's guidance, the mother not only began to understand how the family system was affecting the children but also to see her pattern of selecting men who might eventually abuse her. With this discovery, she was able to break the relationship with the abusive male. Later she was able to trace back her pattern of interactions with men to examples from her own family of origin.

As sometimes happens, Anthony did not relate well with the therapist at the community mental health center and soon refused to return. Since the mother's relationship with the abusive manfriend had terminated, the school counselor took Anthony as a longer-term client. The treatment consisted of weekly counseling and involving Anthony in a self-esteem group. Needless to say, an 8-year-old boy is not expected to put together how the patterns of neglect and abuse result in his acting-out behavior. But the concept of repeating patterns is useful to the counselor in conceptualizing events and planning counseling interventions.

Through further individual therapy, Anthony's mother became more assertive and supported the counseling interventions in the home. She came to four group psychoeducational programs on parenting skills taught by the counselor. With support from the counselor, the teacher became more able to plan for this sometimes-difficult child in the classroom.

Counseling and therapy are too often defined as individual or family centered. In complex cases such as Anthony's, individual change is virtually impossible unless the full network of services is utilized effectively. The school counselor in this case can be considered a developmental case manager who orchestrated the many parts of the network necessary for a satisfactory result that will last over time.

Not every community provides a complete network of services. There are not enough guidance counselors in elementary schools throughout the country and fewer family therapists. Schools generally do not want to provide "therapy," despite the fact that the school setting could be organized to provide a more therapeutic and supportive atmosphere. At present, the tendency remains to blame the individual (or family) for problems. However, as suggested by this case, a network approach to human development is and will continue to be cost-effective, in both financial and emotional terms.

APPLYING THE DCT AND NETWORK TREATMENT MODELS WITH ADOLESCENTS

With children, the network model proposed here seems especially fitting: One cannot expect children to change unless their environment changes as well. For adolescents and adults, the network model, with its emphasis on balancing individual and environmental interventions, might seem to some less appropriate. This sense of "lack of fit" most likely results from the individualistic emphasis of North American culture in which the responsibility for change is placed on the individual adolescent or adult. In truth, children and early adolescents are more clearly selves-in-relation than adults. However, the network/DCT model is equally useful for adults.

LaFromboise and Low (1989, p. 131) describe how they used their systemic network approach with a drug-abusing Native American adolescent.

Mark, a 16-year-old Indian male of average intelligence, has been "acting out" for more than a year. Often truant, Mark has fallen behind in his academic work. He uses drugs and alcohol, has had several violent encounters with fellow students, and has been in minor trouble with local authorities. Mark has lived with his maternal aunt and uncle on the reservation for the last ten years. His mother is a chronic alcoholic, and Mark rarely sees her. The identity of Mark's father is unknown. Recently, Mark's uncle lost his job and began to disappear for days on end. A school counselor, who has become increasingly concerned about apparent depression, has referred Mark.

Getting Mark to therapy first required the support of his family to ensure that he would come. Mark's therapist emphasized the development of rapport and of defining the problem as Mark saw it. A critical cultural and individual issue in this case was negative stereotypes about Native Americans' problems with drinking. Early intervention strategies focused on challenging irrational beliefs, behavior change, and social validation. The school problem was approached through consultation with Mark's teachers, who were asked to use more small group work as opposed to the traditional lecture format. Mark was encouraged to participate in social gatherings, such as basketball tournaments, rodeos, powwows, and feasts, to help him reaffirm his Native American identity.

LaFromboise and Low suggest engaging key family members in therapy, which may require the participation of community leaders in a network meeting at the first stage. Particularly important in this session is the Native American belief that any individual's behavior reflects on the total community. Interventions with clients such as Mark and his family need to focus on cooperation, connectedness, and interdependence. The goal of such therapy is not individualistic self-actualization but the interdependent actualization of the individual in a family and community context.

Interdependence (self-in-relation) provides a goal for more ecologically oriented counseling and psychotherapy. The network model can be described as a case management approach. Counseling and therapy theory and training often focus on the myth of a skilled therapist sitting in his or her office, stimulating change in clients by brilliant conversation. Although this may be the case for a few lucky therapists, most professional helpers soon realize that their efforts are likely to be ineffective unless coupled with family, school, work, and community interventions. Furthermore, it usually takes more than one counselor or therapist when dealing with serious problems. Treatment teams and community networks of helping professionals are becoming more the norm.

Let us now follow up these ideas with a concrete case example.

AN ADULT CASE EXAMPLE USING STYLE-SHIFT COUNSELING

In this section we first explore style-shift counseling as an additional strategy that you can use in working with clients. We then take a sample style-shift case and apply network and DCT methods in developing a specific treatment plan. However, the treatment plan in this case will be primarily your responsibility.

Defining Style-Shift Counseling

Style-shift is the term Anderson (1987a, 1987b, 1998) employs in his developmental approach to the interviewing and treatment processes. The tenets of style-shift counseling and therapy parallel those of DCT and involve a five-step process:

1. Assess the general developmental style of the client.
2. Choose a helping style that matches that style.
3. Identify developmental tasks of the client and intervene.
   (Clients may be at multiple developmental styles on varying developmental tasks.)
4. Evaluate and plan alternative actions.
5. Shift style if needed and as client develops.

Anderson's (1987b) Style-Shift Indicator is a learning instrument developed to provide an introduction to developmental assessment and treatment planning. Eight cases are presented in the instrument, and the tasks are to (1) identify the developmental style of the client and (2) rank order four treatment alternatives in order of preference. From rankings of clients, it is possible to obtain counselor and therapist scores on preferred helping styles and effectiveness of style matching.

A case from the Style-Shift Indicator follows (Anderson, 1987b, p. 8). You will be asked in the next section to help develop a comprehensive treatment plan for Jorge.

Jorge, age 25, out of work

Jorge has been a good, steady worker with a local construction company since he failed grade 10 and quit school. Due to lack of work, he was laid off from his job. Jorge was quite persistent at first in looking for another job. However, as the weeks went by he began to spend more and more time at home. Lately, his drinking has increased, and he spends a lot of late nights out, then comes home to watch the late shows.

You are a career counselor at a local community agency, and Jorge comes to you seeking help because he knows he is not going anywhere with his life and says he wants to go to work soon. Jorge is getting discouraged with his prospects and realizes that his life is going nowhere fast. He has no real plan for the future, is tired of construction work, and can't seem to think clearly about the future. He seems to value a "macho" approach to life, keeping emotional distance between himself and others.

Given this description, at what cognitive-developmental style is Jorge? Rank order your responses by writing 1 (for first), 2, 3, and 4 next to the styles.

___ Sensorimotor	___ Formal
___ Concrete	___ Dialectic/systemic

From the data provided, Jorge appears to use primarily a concrete style. A major question, of course, is the alcohol issue. If it is a serious problem that interferes with his functioning and if he is denying that fact, Jorge would be considered to be at the sensorimotor style. Distinctions between the formal and dialectic/systemic styles are more difficult. In the dialectic/systemic form of therapy, there is often mutuality between the client and counselor. Jorge might be more likely to think in this style than in the formal style. He does not appear to be reflective or interested in looking at himself and his life patterns (although he may be formal on some life developmental tasks). The Style-Shift Indicator suggests a 2-1-4-3 ranking for Jorge. (Using rankings for several cases, it is possible to determine a counselor trainee's assessment capacities and preferred treatment style [Anderson, 1987].)

The Style-Shift Indicator provides four treatment options for Jorge, as follows. Which treatment would you use first? Second? Third? Fourth?

A. Respond to Jorge's feelings of poor self-worth; assist him to focus on how these feelings arose from deeper problems and help him see how they affect his ability to do career planning or to find a job now. Help Jorge clarify some of his values and priorities in life and encourage him to set his own goals so he can reach his desired position. Help him to look at self-defeating, repeating patterns in his lifestyle.

B. Call a friend who has a construction company and needs casual labor. This friend has a reputation for taking on somewhat immature young men and helping them develop into responsible, skilled workers. Your friend has training sessions in the evenings to facilitate personal and work development. Follow up to ensure that Jorge engages effectively in this plan.

C. After developing a relationship with him to earn his trust, tentatively confront him with his unproductive and self-destructive (drinking) behavior in a respectful way and see how much of this he wants to share with you. Assist him in evaluating his own behavior and work toward a specific job search. Include role-playing so that he knows how to present himself favorably in a job interview.

D. Discuss openly his strengths and weaknesses. Explore options available to him that will make use of his strong points. Try to keep a mutual relationship with him, providing information and sharing your experience with him. Be creative in generating ideas mutually to deal with the future rather than trying to influence or help him directly.

Which of the above four treatments would you select as your preferred mode of action? Which would be your second choice? Third choice? What would be your least preferred treatment? List your choices in the spaces provided below.

First _____   Second _____

Third _____   Fourth _____

The style-shift evaluation of the case is as follows:

Having identified Jorge as primarily concrete in his thinking, the Style-Shift Indicator suggests that the coaching, concrete-operational approach is the place to start. Jorge has several developmental tasks; the most obvious of these is the matter of jobs, and the most important may be the drinking issue. He may have other family problems, interpersonal skill deficits, and so on. The DCT and style-shift models suggest joining the client's concrete frame of reference (option C above) and using coaching techniques to assist him in becoming more rational, conscious, and consequential in his thinking. Concrete behavioral treatment alternatives could be used to help him try new behavioral patterns.

A second choice might be the environmental structuring approach that a sensorimotor diagnosis would suggest (option B). Here you take greater responsibility for the client. It also assumes that alcohol is the central issue. If, for example, you could respectfully influence Jorge to enter an alcohol treatment center and receive career and life planning, then you, as part of his environment, could be catalytic in "bumping" him into a new environment where he will more likely receive a concentrated and controlled therapeutic impact to counteract his quite well-established, self-defeating behavior patterns. At the sensorimotor style, counselors provide more direct influence in their client's lives.

A third choice could be the mutual, creative dialogue of option D. This might work out to an extent if Jorge perceived you as "cool," somehow like him, and a fellow struggler who has made it in a number of ways. However, Jorge's creative powers have not been realized yet. He is stressed; he needs to dry out from a possibly debilitating dependence on alcohol and begin to have a dream for his future before he can do a lot of brainstorming and mutual problem solving.

The least preferred choice might be the formal-operational approach (option A) of attempting to help Jorge examine, explore, and understand himself and the alternatives he has. This sounds ideal, but the information we have about Jorge indicates that he is not only developmentally unready for the depth of this style but is perhaps unwilling to engage in the emotional intensity of it as well.

If we counsel Jorge in a concrete coaching style and things go well, we can shift our style to a more formal-operational self-examination approach as his developmental maturity increases. If his drinking becomes worse, we may want to shift our style to a more influential sensorimotor approach. Furthermore, on the many developmental tasks of the young adult, we can anticipate that Jorge may operate at different cognitive styles on each task. Flexibility and adaptability are watchwords of Anderson's style-shift theory. Supporting the entire framework is a mutual, systemic approach in which client and counselor work together, looking at the family and environment as well as just the individual.

Developing a Case Treatment Plan

The case of Jorge provides you with a framework for generating a network treatment plan. Although the entry point for counseling probably should be at Jorge's concrete style, full treatment will require action at multiple cognitive-developmental styles. It may be helpful at this point to generate your own approach to a client such as Jorge, using the steps of the DCT treatment plan framework.

1. *Establish a positive base for treatment.* What strengths can you identify in Jorge that may be helpful in designing a successful treatment plan? Given the brevity of the case presentation, you will have to improvise on positives you might expect. You may find it helpful to think of a person you have known who is somewhat similar to Jorge and use that person's qualities to "flesh out" your description.

_____

_____

_____

What positive strengths and resources can you identify in the environment and in important support systems such as family, friends, work, and community?

_____

_____

_____

2. *Examine key relationship issues that might affect you as the counselor or therapist.* First, what are you own general feelings about a client such as Jorge? What has your personal experience been with such individuals? What feelings do you experience in your body? What images come to mind from your own developmental history? How would these events and patterns affect the here and now of your relationship with a person such as Jorge?

_____

_____

_____

Given this knowledge, what type of relationship do you think you could offer Jorge? What balance of attachment and separation, autonomy and relationship do you think is most appropriate?

_____

_____

_____

3. *Identify treatment options you would consider.* What key developmental tasks do you believe Jorge faces? You may also find it helpful to review Erikson's life-stage and family life-cycle theories. List at least three key developmental tasks and the treatment options you might consider. Include the possibility of varying types of network interventions.

Developmental task 1: _____

_____

_____

Developmental task 2: _____

_____

_____

Developmental task 3: _____

_____

_____

Develop an ideal network treatment program that includes not only individual counseling and therapy but also family therapy and involvement of the employer, community and self-help groups, and other key individuals or groups. How would you coordinate these interventions?

_____

_____

_____

What cultural, ethnic, racial, or religious group did you think Jorge was a member of? Identify that group and then examine your treatment plan to see if it coordinates with Jorge's cultural heritage. Then imagine that Jorge comes from another racial background. What impact does this change have on your treatment plan?

_____

_____

_____

4. *Generate a client-counselor contract for a treatment plan.* On a separate piece of paper, write your own statement for a therapist-client contract in which you outline your knowledge, skills, and competencies. (See the sample informed consent form in Before You Start.)

In addition, imagine you have worked with Jorge for one or two sessions. List below specific goals for counseling and clear statements of what successful treatment would consist of. (Use language Jorge would understand.)

_____

_____

_____

Treatment plans, of necessity, must relate to your own knowledge and competencies. One of the values of the above exercise is that the counselor gains a sense of humility by acknowledging the very human limitations we all share. We must first identify what we can do and then contrast it with a more ideal treatment plan. Then, rather than just depending on our own inevitably limited skills, we can refer the client for assistance on some issues, working with other helpers and community members in a mutual way. Using a network framework for therapy requires willingness to examine oneself, admit frailties, and work with colleagues in a mutual, non-hierarchical manner. Also required is the ability to reflect on one's own skills, beliefs, and attitudes—something that not all counselors and therapists, even those who have had lengthy training, are capable of doing.

SUMMARY

DCT is both a theory within itself and an integrative metatheory—a theory about other theories. The essence of the metatheory is that all counseling and therapy strategies can be organized into sensorimotor, concrete, formal, and dialectic/systemic categories.

Clients can expand their cognitive/developmental style(s) through work within any specific theory so long as that theory reasonably matches their basic style. Also, clients who might be resistant to a Gestalt therapy sensorimotor strategy (e.g., the empty chair) may find a cognitive-behavioral strategy (e.g., relaxation training) acceptable. Thus, using varying theoretical approaches, you can integrate seemingly disparate techniques in a positive fashion.

Most theoretical strategies cover the concrete and formal styles quite well with a lighter emphasis on the sensorimotor area. The dialectic/systemic and multicultural frame is important in DCT. Albert Ellis, the prominent cognitive-behavioral theorist, has stressed this uniqueness and raised the possibility that other theories had better take serious note of this hypothesis although "few of them have to date." At the same time, we should note that DCT relies extensively on feminist theory and multicultural counseling and therapy as key related approaches.

Native American network therapy facilitates understanding of the importance of dialectic/systemic issues in the helping process. In working with children, particularly, it is vital that broader family and contextual issues be constantly considered as part of the treatment plan.

Six steps for conceptualizing a DCT treatment plan were presented: (1) establishing a positive base for treatment; (2) examining key relationship issues that might affect the counselor or therapist; (3) identifying DCT treatment options using multiple theories within the four cognitive/emotional styles; (4) generating a client-counselor contract for the treatment plan; (5) proceeding flexibly with individual treatment; and (6) expanding individual treatment through network involvement.

Style-shift counseling consists of five key elements: (1) assess the general developmental style of the client; (2) choose a helping style that matches that style; (3) identify developmental tasks of the client and intervene (clients may be at multiple developmental styles on varying developmental tasks); (4) evaluate and plan alternative actions; (5) shift style if needed and as client develops.

Challenges: Although there is much to recommend a broadly based network approach, at times the client may feel he or she is confronting a small army of professionals. In such situations, the individual or the family may be overwhelmed by numbers and may not feel comfortable participating actively in the therapy process. Awed by professionals, clients quietly do what they are told or quickly leave therapy. In some cultures, this might appear to be culturally appropriate. However, regardless of culture, a reasonable balance of individual initiative and environmental constraint needs to be achieved. DCT proponents would argue that the concept of interdependence of individuals and their environments might serve as a useful basis for achieving this balance.

Research issues: Given the complexity of the network approach, traditional empirical research methods are not easily identified. However, an individual case study plan can be used in which measures of certain key data are made before, during, and after therapy. The case study approach is especially useful when specific goals for behavior and attitudinal change are contracted for early in the process. The measures can then be adjusted to fit the individual or family.

For example, for Mark, the Native American Indian adolescent discussed in this chapter, measures might be made of number of days absent from school, time between violent incidents, number of conflicts with the law, self-concept, and cultural identity. Mark should be actively involved in decisions about criteria for evaluation of interventions. For Mark's family, the return of his uncle to work and informal observations of community members could be the data measured.

Action research data such as these examples can become part of the treatment process, serving as objective indicators of client progress. Some treatment clinics require some form of action research as part of the treatment process. Clients can share in the process and be made constantly aware of their progress toward goals. The action research plan can be part of the treatment contract, thus making counselors and therapists more accountable.

As psychologists, social workers, and counselors in private practice or working in community agencies and schools, we have a responsibility to be accountable for our work. Integrating some way to systematically assess our interventions with individuals, family, or communities is a professional responsibility too many of us neglect.

Paraphrasing Kurt Lewin, we should have no therapeutic or counseling action without some form of research, and research should not exist independent of action in the real world. "No action without research, no research without action."

THEORY INTO PRACTICE: DEVELOPING YOUR PORTFOLIO OF COMPETENCE

Self-Assessment Exercise

Exercise 1. Assessing your skills in multiple theories and strategies

Review Box 7-1, which lists an array of theories and strategies. In addition, you are probably aware of others not listed there. Write below the strategies you would like to have available for your own practice. Circle those you already feel comfortable using and consider the rest as a plan of study for the future.

What sensorimotor strategies appeal to you?

_____

_____

What concrete strategies?

_____

_____

What formal strategies?

_____

_____

What dialectic/systemic strategies?

_____

_____

Identification and Classification Exercise

Exercise 2. Generating network treatment plans

Using the case of Jorge, generate a treatment plan using multiple cognitive/emotional strategies.

What sensorimotor strategies might you use?

_____

_____

What concrete strategies?

_____

_____

What formal strategies?

_____

_____

What dialectic/systemic strategies?

_____

_____

How would you integrate style-shift practice into your use of these varying methods?

_____

_____

Multicultural Competence Exercise

Exercise 3. Cultural identity development and the treatment plan

Jorge could be of a different racial, religious, ethnic, gender, age, or sexual orientation from yours. He could have a physical or intellectual handicap. Furthermore, he might be at any of the five styles of minority identity development. Each situation changes the nature of the network you must consider. How would the counseling approach change with any of these factors? What impact would they have on the contracting process?

_____

_____

_____

_____

_____

Interviewing Practice Exercises (Small Group)

Exercise 4. Sharing treatment plans

In a small group, share treatment plans for a client such as Jorge. Note similarities and differences of your plans. How do the skills, knowledge, cultural background, and beliefs of each individual in the group, including yourself, affect the treatment plan? In answering this last question, you may each want to share your responses to question 2 on page 230 in which you talked about your own developmental history and attitudes toward individuals such as Jorge. How does your own life developmental history affect your approach to the interview and to treatment planning?

_____

_____

_____

_____

Exercise 5. Generating specific goals in client-therapist contracts

Again, in a small group, have one person role-play Jorge. In consultation with him, generate a written contract for methods and goals of counseling. It is useful in this exercise if the person role-playing Jorge first does the exercise as a formal-operational 25-year-old; second, as a more concrete-style individual. How does the language change in the two situations?

_____

_____

_____

_____

Generalization: Taking Network Skills Home

Exercise 6. Moving toward your own interviews

For a single client or family, go through the specific steps of the treatment plan in consultation with a colleague or supervisor. What did you learn about yourself and your relationship with that client? How did you respond to the network concept of treatment? What specific agencies or people can you count on as resources for helping clients?

Test your treatment plan with your client and involve the client in determining specific goals for counseling and therapy. How do you use (or not use) network concepts of treatment?

_____

_____

_____

_____

Portfolio Reflections

Exercise 7. Your reflections on the integrative metatheory of DCT as it relates to broadly based network treatment plans

What stood out for you from this chapter? What sense did you make of what you read and experienced? What are your key points from this chapter? Write your thoughts here and add them to your Portfolio Folder.

_____

_____

_____

_____

_____

_____

_____

_____

REFERENCES

Anderson, T. (1987a). *Style-shift counseling and developmental therapy with the style-shift indicator.* North Amherst, MA: Microtraining Associates.

Anderson, T. (1987b). *Style-shift indicator.* North Amherst, MA: Microtraining Associates.

Anderson, T. (1998). *Tranforming leadership.* Boca Raton, FL: CRC Press.

Attneave, C. (1969). Therapy in tribal settings and urban network interventions. *Family Process, 8,* 192–210.

Attneave, C. (1982). American Indian and Alaska Native families: Emigrants in their own homeland. In M. McGoldrick, J. Pearce, & J. Giordano (Eds.), *Ethnicity and family therapy.* New York: Guilford.

Beck, A. (1976). *Cognitive therapy and the emotional disorders.* New York: International Universities Press.

Beck, J. (1995). *Cognitive therapy.* New York: Guilford.

Clark, A. J. (2002). *Early recollections: Theory and practice in counseling and psychotherapy.* New York: Brunner-Routledge.

DeAngelis, T. (2002, July/August). If you do just one thing, exercise. *Monitor on Psychology,* 49–51.

Deffenbacher, J. (in press). Psychosocial interventions: Anger disorders. In E. Coccaro (Ed.), *Aggression, assessment, and treatment.* New York: Marcel Dekker.

Dreikurs, R., Grunwald, B. B., & Pepper, F. C. (1982). *Maintaining sanity in the classroom* (2nd ed.). New York: HarperCollins.

Dreikurs, R., & Soltz, V. (1999). *Children: The challenge.* New York: Plume. (Original work published 1964)

Eckstein, D., & Kern, R. (2002). *Psychological finger prints: Life style assessments and interventions.* Dubuque, IA: Kendall/Hunt.

Ellis, A. (1999, March). *A continuation of the dialogue on counseling in the postmodern era.* Presentation to the American Counseling Association Convention, San Diego.

Galanter, M. (1999). Network therapy. In P. J. Ott & R. E. Tarter (Eds.), *Sourcebook on substance abuse: Etiology, epidemiology, assessment, and treatment* (pp. 264–271). Needham Heights, MA: Allyn & Bacon.

Galanter, M., & Brook, D. (2001). Network therapy for addiction: Bringing family and peer support into office practice. *International Journal of Group Psychotherapy, 15*(1), 101–122.

Ivey, A. (1973). Media therapy: Educational change planning for psychiatric patients. *Journal of Counseling Psychology, 20,* 338–343.

Ivey, A., D'Andrea, M., Ivey, M., & Simek-Morgan, L. (2002). *Counseling and psychotherapy: A multicultural perspective.* Boston: Allyn & Bacon.

LaFromboise, T., & Lowe, K. (1989). Psychological interventions with American Indian adolescents. In J. Gibbs & L. Hwang (Eds.), *Children of color.* San Francisco: Jossey-Bass.

McKay, G. D., McKay, J. L., Eckstein, D., & Maybell, S. A. (2001). *Raising respectful kids in a rude world.* Roseville, CA: Prima.

Minaker, K. (2003, March). *Myths and realities of aging.* Presentation at the Sarasota Massachusetts General Hospital Meeting, Sarasota, FL.

Myers, J. E. (1998). Bibliotherapy and DCT: Co-constructing the therapeutic metaphor. *Journal of Counseling and Development, 76*(3), 243–250.

Rigazio-DiGilio, S., Ivey, A., & Locke, D. (1997). Continuing the postmodern dialogue: Enhancing and contextualizing multiple voices. *Journal of Mental Health Counseling, 19,* 233–255.

Rogers, C. (1963). *On becoming a person.* Boston: Houghton Mifflin.

Smith, D. (2003, March). Angry thoughts, at risk hearts. *Monitor on Psychology,* 46–47.

Speck, R. (1998). Network therapy. *Marriage and Family Review, 27*(1), 51–69.

Speck, R., & Attneave, C. (1973). *Family process.* New York: Pantheon.

Sweeney, T. J. (1998). *Adlerian counseling: A practitioner's approach* (3rd ed.). Englewood Cliffs, NJ: Prentice Hall.

Taub-Bynum, B. (1992). *Family dreams: The intricate web.* Ithaca, NY: Haworth.

Taub-Bynum, B. (1999). *The Afrocentric unconscious.* New York: Teachers College Press.

Thompson, M., Kaslow, N., Short, L., & Wyckoff, S. (2002). The mediating roles of perceived social support and resources in the self-efficacy–suicide attempts of relation among African American abused women. *Journal of Consulting and Clinical Psychology, 70,* 942–949.

SECTION III

Multiple Applications of DCT for Counseling and Psychotherapy Practice

Developmental counseling and therapy, with its wellness orientation, offers many possibilities for direct action. In this section, you will see how DCT is applied and coordinated with multicultural counseling and therapy. This is followed by a chapter that shows how to use DCT to engage and treat clients who have been diagnosed through the American Psychiatric Association's *Diagnostic and Statistical Manual of Mental Disorders*. In addition, you will find new information on Adlerian theory and how to use DCT with families and with early recollections and bibliotherapy. The use of DCT with issues of spirituality is the subject of the concluding applications chapter.

The final chapter of this book will enable you to examine your progress through this book and assess your ability to take theory into your own practice of counseling and psychotherapy.

Chapter 8. Multicultural Counseling and Therapy. Despite the positive intentions of both individual and systemic therapeutic theories, it is possible that the Black identity movement, the women's movement, and gay liberation have done more for the mental health of oppressed individuals and groups than have all of the counseling and therapy theories combined. These movements have helped us all become aware of the critical role that societal and cultural factors play in individual and family development.

This chapter will show you how to use cultural identity theory in the interview. These ideas can help your clients learn more about themselves as multicultural beings and enable them to see the cultural context of their issues and problems. Oppression is a major issue in multicultural counseling and therapy. Psychotherapy as liberation provides a clear theoretical framework accompanied by practical interventions to liberate your clients from oppressive thinking and may enable them to act to change the systems that brought about their distress.

Chapter 9. Reframing the *Diagnostic and Statistical Manual of Mental Disorders*: Positive Strategies From Developmental Counseling and Therapy. Traditionally, mental health care has focused more on individual problems and less on society's responsibility for those problems. Thus, responsibility for the illness and for change is placed on the individual. The field of social work, however, has continued to emphasize that the individual lives in a social context and that change in the environment is of equal or more importance than change in the individual. The mental health of individuals living in oppressive situations may be better addressed by making changes in society. This chapter will enable you to reframe severe distress as a logical biological and psychological response to environmental conditions. You will be able to develop comprehensive treatment plans, using multiple theoretical orientations and strategies, to work with issues such as depression, personality style ("disorder"), and post-traumatic stress.

Chapter 10. Early Recollections: Using DCT With Early Memories to Facilitate Second-Order Change. This chapter builds on the Adlerian and wellness theory presented in Chapter 2. You will find that clients can better understand their present circumstances after connecting their early life experiences with the attitudes, emotions, and behaviors associated with their presenting issues for counseling. This offers them alternatives to a better future through the positive uses of early recollections, current developmental issues, and new rules, choices, and behaviors. DCT provides specific strategies that can enable an in-depth analysis and discovery of what one's developmental past means for the future. You will learn to use early recollections in your practice as a way to understand and mobilize a client's wellness strengths. You will then be shown how to use early recollections as a way to help clients understand the past as a source of present rules, self-talk, emotional responses, and choices. Used in conjunction with DCT, early recollections help clients move toward the future by creating new expectations and solutions to previously unsatisfactory outcomes through new perspectives, choices, and results.

Chapter 11. Using Developmental Counseling and Therapy With Families. As people-in-relation, we learn our concepts of self and of culture through our families of origin. This chapter focuses on the family life cycle and the manner in which family members relate to one another as they move through stages and phases from birth through old age. This chapter will enable you to understand and work with families at various stages of the life cycle and apply DCT questioning strategies to facilitate couple and family development.

Chapter 12. Bibliotherapy, Metaphors, and Narratives. Drawing out client narratives and life stories is central to DCT. The use of media (art, articles, books, television, movies) is explored as a way to help clients understand and rewrite their stories. Metaphor is presented as a creative process and as a way to help clients understand and reframe their stories. Mastery of the concepts of this chapter will enable you to bring more creative and artistic processes into the counseling and psychotherapy interview. You will be able to use DCT facilitative strategies to encourage clients to become more fully creative themselves.

Chapter 13. Spirituality, Wellness, and Development: Applying DCT to Core Values in Clients' Lives. Spirituality is first presented as a cultural phenomenon through contrasting the Judeo-Christian creation narrative with that of Aboriginal Australians. Discernment of life's meaning and goals through DCT questioning strategies is central to the chapter. A holistic lifespan view of spiritual development is presented and specifics for introducing spiritual issues into the counseling process are considered. Mastery of the concepts of this chapter will enable you to conceptualize the place of spiritual and religious issues in the interview. You will be able to use DCT discernment processes to help clients find and make meaning in their lives and help them examine their faith development; in addition, you will be able to use spiritually oriented strategies in the here and now of the therapeutic session.

Chapter 14. Epilogue: Your Future Development. The concluding chapter focuses on you and your personal understanding and integration of the developmental, wellness, and lifespan models. You will be challenged to examine yourself and your mastery and competence in the practice of developmentally oriented counseling and psychotherapy.

CHAPTER 8
Multicultural Counseling and Therapy

Mastery and practice of concepts in this chapter will enable you to assess and to facilitate clients' expansion of cultural identity and multicultural consciousness. You will also be able to use the specific steps of psychotherapy of liberation to help clients discover, name, reflect, and act on issues related to multi-cultures and to oppression.

Multicultural counseling and therapy (MCT) has been termed the fourth force of counseling and psychotherapy theory, a major addition to the traditional three theoretical forces of psychodynamic, cognitive-behavioral, and existential-humanistic. MCT is not in opposition to traditional theory; rather, it brings three major ideas to the counseling and therapy process:

1. MCT is a metatheory, a theory about theory. With MCT, culture is the underlying defining issue in counseling and therapy. It provides a different way to examine traditional theory and to bring it into greater accord with a broader contextual view of the process of helping. A therapist using MCT is working with a client in a social context rather than with an autonomous "self."
2. MCT uses all major theories and strategies, but seeks culturally appropriate use of these theories and may, at times, supplement traditional theory with multicultural strategies.
3. MCT also brings new theory and strategies to the therapeutic encounter, thus increasing alternatives for action.

This chapter, however, is not a comprehensive summary of MCT. The focus here is on how the theory relates to the evolution of consciousness, that major dimension of both Platonic thought and DCT. Some sources for a more complete view of multicultural counseling and therapy are Ponterotto, Casas, Suzuki, and Alexander (2001) and Sue, Ivey, and Pedersen (1996).

Knowledge of and skill in the concepts of this chapter can enable you to:

1. Examine culture and multicultures as core constructs underlying all counseling and therapy.
2. Consider yourself as a multicultural being with special attention to issues of privilege, power, and oppression.
3. Understand some central concepts of cultural identity theory and their relationship to DCT.
4. Utilize specific skills and strategies to facilitate client liberation of consciousness.

INTRODUCTION: DEFINING CULTURE AND MULTICULTURALISM

Both counselor and client identities are formed and embedded in multiple levels of experience (individual, group, and universal) and contexts (individual, family, and cultural milieu). The totality of interrelationship of experiences and contexts must be the focus of treatment. (Sue et al., 1996, p. 15)

As we begin to explore multicultural counseling and therapy, it is important to define culture and multicultures more precisely. The word *culture* in this book is in-

---

This chapter is based on material presented in Allen E. Ivey and Mary Bradford Ivey, "Developmental Counseling and Therapy and Multicultural Counseling and Therapy: Metatheory, Contextual Consciousness, and Action," in Don C. Locke, Jane E. Myers, and Edwin L. Herr (Eds.), *The Handbook of Counseling*, pp. 219–236. Copyright © 2000 by Sage Publications. Reprinted by permission of Sage Publications.

terpreted broadly. Culture can be associated with a racial group (African American, Asian) or an ethnic group (Polish, French, Cuban, Mexican) as well as with gender, religion, economic status, nationality, physical capacity or handicap, or sexual orientation. These larger categories also have subcategories. For instance, African American culture in the United States can be further subdivided into Caribbean, Mississippi, Harlem, or African culture.

There may be even more variability in individuals than in cultures. Class and economic differences, religion, and family experiences contribute to each individual's unique personal history—a distinctive personal culture. It is dangerous to use multicultural approaches to stereotype individuals. Justice must serve both the community and the individual.

Thus, culture consists of two sometimes conflicting components: Each group has a distinctly different culture, and each individual has a distinctive personal culture. If we become accustomed to thinking in a cultural framework, we may fail to see the unique individual before us. If we focus too much on the individual, we may fail to see how this individual is affected by cultural history.

Culture, then, is both an abstraction and a concrete particular. In its abstract form, culture cannot be seen, heard, or felt. It is a way of being—the norms and customs of a group. Culture becomes a concrete particular in the specific individual and his or her family. But no one individual or single family totally represents the culture.

YOU AS A MULTICULTURAL BEING

Multiculture is a way to talk of the many cultures within each of us. We are not solely ethnic/racial beings. We also are men and women; we have a sexual orientation, and religious and spiritual beliefs. Gender, sexuality, and spiritual orientations are all the basis of cultural groups. The RESPECTFUL cube is shown in Figure 8-1. Here you see that any one individual participates in multiple cultural groups. At one point, ethnic/racial issues may be most important, but at another point, one's physical ability or economic class may be the central issue related to the counseling and therapy process. All White people or People of Color are more than just their race: We are all multicultural beings and all of us are deeply affected by our multicultural status.

For the practice of counseling and therapy, especially from a DCT perspective, we need to be aware of culture and multicultures and their many and changing manifestations. The sensorimotor and concrete experience of each individual is deeply affected by abstract formal and dialectic/systemic dimensions. Each individual, family, and culture represents a different way of being.

Figure 8-1 also speaks to the locus within which culture exists and is meaningful. Not only do individuals have multicultures, but also so do their families, their groups, and communities. The individual may or may not be in synchrony with the culture of the family (e.g., the adolescent who is gay in a heterosexually oriented family). Similarly, one may be Jewish in a predominantly Christian community. Older persons may find themselves surrounded by a culture oriented to youth. The locus within the multicultural cube helps remind us even more that client context is vital to our understanding of any one individual.

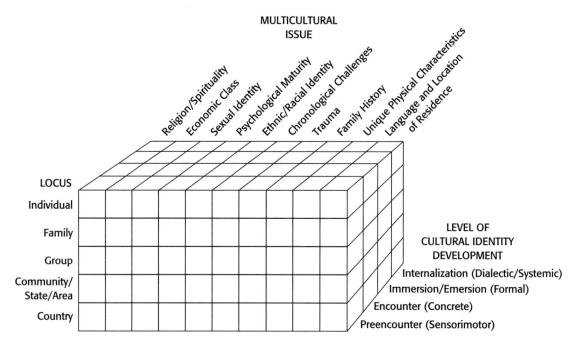

Figure 8-1   The RESPECTFUL Cube. (Reprinted by permission of Allen E. Ivey, 1992, 2004. See Ivey, D'Andrea, Ivey, & Simek-Morgan, 2002.)

The cultural identity portions of the cube are discussed in more detail later in this chapter. The degree to which an individual is aware of culture and multicultures varies. Cultural identity development—becoming aware of one's multicultural being (racial, gender, sexual orientation, etc.)—is a major goal of multicultural counseling and therapy. This chapter offers ideas for assessing a person's cultural identity level while simultaneously suggesting specific ways to facilitate growth of contextual and multicultural awareness.

Privilege and power issues are also found in the RESPECTFUL cube. The work of McIntosh (1989) has been central in this area; she coined the term "White privilege," indicating that in North America, it is European Americans who have the vast majority of power. Along with that power over others come privileges, such as not worrying about how others will respond to the color of one's skin, finding bank loans more easily, and being in the company of people "like oneself" most of the time. This privilege and power brings a basic comfort level that may be described simply as an easier lifestyle. (You can visit http://www.utoronto.ca/acc/events/peggy1.htm for the full text of this influential paper.) According to the 2000 census, the White majority no longer exists in the state of California. Thus, in this microcosm of what will later be representative of the United States as a whole, new definitions of privilege and power are emerging and merit further study. Cultures and multicultures are constantly in flux in our global society, and lifelong study of changing cultural issues and definitions is essential for all persons in helping professions.

Each area of the cube raises issues of power and privilege. Male privilege is obvious to women whereas gays and lesbians see clearly that heterosexual culture has the advantage of privilege, power, and—of course—law. Those who survive the trauma of cancer learn that power rests in hands other than theirs, although it obviously helps if one has a privileged economic status. In another example, Christians in predominantly Christian countries can be sure their major holy days are considered in establishing school holidays and retail closings, whereas Buddhists, Jews, and Muslims see their holidays given less attention. Similarly, when Christians are nondominant—as in portions of Africa, the Middle East, and Asia—they will be aware of their pronounced lack of power and privilege.

Out of privilege and power often comes oppression. Locke (1992) has defined some key terms related to cultural oppression:

> *Prejudice* is defined as judging before fully examining the object of evaluation. *Racial prejudice* refers to making a judgment based on racial/ethnic/cultural group membership before getting to know the person being judged. *Racism* combines prejudice with power—power to do something based on prejudiced beliefs.

Expanding on Locke, oppression is another word for sexism, heterosexism, anti-Semitism, or any other form of systemic prejudice plus power. Reflect on the place of older people in society. Because of cultural beliefs, vast numbers of these individuals experience oppressive events simply because of their chronological age. Virtually all of us will experience this prejudice and oppression at some point in our lives; and as we grow older this prejudice will express the arbitrary criterion of youth as a more privileged status. On the other hand, if we choose to develop positive attitudes toward older persons and persons of all ages, we can help change societal attitudes as we ourselves experience the universal processes of aging.

Power and privilege, then, are not just issues affecting People of Color. You will find that your clients vary widely in their access to privilege and power and that multiculturally sensitive counseling and therapy requires you to be alert to the ways oppression related to these factors may appear in and affect the lives of your clients.

As a first step in this direction, review the RESPECTFUL cube and indicate which areas you are in that give you more or less privilege and power. Check the items below where you believe that you are in the more privileged group. Privilege, in truth does not mean that one is "better than another"; rather, it means that one has more access to power and resources.

____ R Religion

____ E Economic status

____ S Sexual identity

____ P Psychological maturity (cognitive/developmental style)

____ E Ethnic/racial identity

____ C Chronological challenges (age)

____ T Trauma

____ F Family history

____ U Unique physical characteristics

____ L Language and location of residence

This brief exercise can be thought provoking, particularly as you think of personal experiences of prejudice and power in relation to your own developmental past and present. Please note your reflections and observations in regard to the RESPECTFUL cube in the exercise at the end of this chapter.

When we review the three dimensions of the multicultural cube, it becomes apparent that almost all counseling and therapy sessions in some way touch on multicultural issues. And any time we start viewing the individual as a self-in-relation or person-in-context, we are considering contextual multicultural issues. In short, the MCT view is that *virtually all counseling and psychotherapy are multicultural.*

CULTURAL IDENTITY DEVELOPMENT AND THE EVOLUTION OF CONSCIOUSNESS

Cultural identity development is a major determinant of counselor and client attitudes toward the self, others of the same group, and the dominant group. These attitudes, which may be manifested in affective and behavioral dimensions, are strongly influenced not only by cultural variables, but also by the dynamics of dominant-subordinate relationships among culturally different groups. The level or stage of racial/cultural identity development will both influence how clients and counselors define the problem and dictate what they believe to be appropriate counseling/therapy goals and processes. (Sue et al., 1996, p. 17)

Cognitive/emotional development is a major goal of much of counseling and it is perhaps even more central to DCT and MCT. Both theories recognize that people over time develop increased awareness of self and others, self and context, and the role of cultural factors in their lives. As DCT and MCT are both integrative theories, each embraces others within its framework and includes many interlacing concepts.

Plato's Allegory of the Cave, presented briefly in Chapter 1 and again in more detail in Chapter 4, perhaps should be reviewed and read again at this point. The journey toward multicultural consciousness and cultural identity is much like the experience of the individual moving from the cave to the light. Steele (2003, p. 16) comments, "We are like Plato's cave dwellers, staring robotically at the wall marked "oppression," when in fact our true problem is something outside the cave. . . . This new 21st-century racial problem might be called the problem of emergence." The person who is not aware of how culture affects the nature of personal being has not been shown the light of culture/environment context. For people to be truly unique, autonomous, and free, they must become aware of their multicultural roots, which so deeply affect anyone's humanity.

The MCT developmental framework rests in cultural identity theory (Cross, 1971, 1991, 1995; Cross & Vandiver, 2001; Fischer & Moradi, 2001; Helms, 1985, 1990, 2003; Thomas, 1971). Cross and Thomas independently generated cultural identity theory as they observed cognitive/emotional development among African Americans who experienced the Black identity movement of the 1960s. During this time, *Black awareness* developed and matured. Cross and Thomas noted that when African Americans moved from denial and naiveté about the color of their skin to

Black pride, a major change in consciousness occurred. Much like Plato's cave dwellers, they became aware of the light—the racist surroundings that had limited their awareness of their own dignity.

Women, gays and lesbians, persons with disabilities, and many other groups have experienced expansion of their consciousness just as African Americans did earlier. Each of these groups has moved from denial of their worth as human beings to a state of pride. This evolution of consciousness has resulted in major changes in society over the last 50 years and a vast improvement in opportunity and mental health for many. But we must remain aware that social justice and full equality still have not been reached.

The most influential model of cultural or racial identity was developed by Cross (1971) and is summarized below:

- *Preencounter.* The individual (or group) may be locked into a White perspective and may devalue and/or deny the vitality and importance of an African American worldview. The goal of some African Americans who take this perspective may be to be as "White" as possible.
- *Encounter.* The African American meets the realities of racism in an often emotionally jarring experience. This perturbs one's consciousness and often leads to significant change.
- *Immersion/emersion.* Discovering what it means to be African American and to value Blackness becomes important; often, one simultaneously denigrates Whites. Emotions can run strong with pride in one's culture and anger at others. This is often a stage of action for African American rights.
- *Internalization.* An internalized reflective sense of self-confidence develops and emotional experience is more calm and secure. This is often characterized by "psychological openness, ideological flexibility, and a general decline in strong anti-White feelings" (Parham, White, & Ajamu, 1999, p. 49). However, the strength of commitment to the African American world may even be stronger. In addition, Cross (1995) suggests a fifth style, very similar to internalization with the addition of a commitment to action and social change.

Cross and Vandiver (2001) have added important new dimensions of complexity to the basic four-stage cultural identity model. Preencounter individuals, for example, can represent three types. The first preencounter African American individual thinks of herself or himself solely as an "American" with little or no attention to Black culture and may even actively support White interpretations of Blackness. Individuals of another type may be more aware of the issues, but may compartmentalize and think of themselves as "better than" other African Americans. The third preencounter group may engage in self-hatred and self-blame. At the immersion/emersion level, one may find African Americans who are angry and mistrustful of all things White as well as African Americans who ignore White society as much as possible and base their lives totally in a Black cultural framework. The "internalization nationalist" focuses on African American issues and the surrounding world and may be a realistic advocate for change while the "internalization biculturalist" seeks the strengths of both African American and White cultures. Cross and Vandiver describe the "internalization multiculturalist" who moves within multiple areas as focusing on oppression wherever it is found and regardless of to whom it may be directed.

For purposes of this book, we remain focused on the four major types of cultural identity consciousness that have direct parallels to developmental counseling and therapy's four cognitive/emotional styles. Nonetheless, regardless of the race, ethnicity, gender, sexual orientation, spirituality, or other multicultural factor, expect variations in the individual's approach to each cultural identity level.

Cultural identity is often described sequentially, but Parham (in Parham et al., 1999) also sees cultural identity holistically and speaks of recycling. Individuals may achieve internalization, for example, on certain concepts, but then they may encounter a new form of racism. They then find that while they may be thinking primarily from an internalization frame of reference, the new experience helps them realize that parts of them are still using the encounter style. Life is a constant state of development and change. There is no one "right" or final stage or style. Cross (1995) makes the same point when he comments that each style or stage has value in certain situations. There is danger in thinking of one way of being as "best" at all times.

Parham has made two additional important contributions to cultural identity theory. He points out that for a child or adolescent who is "exposed to and indoctrinated with parental and societal messages that are very pro-Black in orientation . . . the personal identity and reference group orientation initially developed by that youngster might be pro-Black as well" (Parham et al., 1999, p. 50). In short, from Parham's frame of reference, a circle rather than a linear chart might be a more useful way to present identity development.

Parham's third point is that "identity resolution can occur in at least three ways: stagnation (failure to move beyond one's initial identity state), stagewise linear progression (movement from one identity stage to another in a sequential linear fashion), and recycling (movement back through the styles once a cycle has been completed)" (Parham et al., 1999, p. 53).

Cultural identity theory, then, is moving toward a broad developmental framework that allows it to be related to traditional lifespan ego development theory (e.g., Erikson, 1950/1963). However, developing a perspective of one's being not in isolation from others and one's culture, but rather as self-in-context, person-in-community, and/or being-in-relation (to others) will result in a far more culturally centered view of development than presently exists. Cultural identity theory, in short, suggests specific ideas for updating and modernizing traditional theory.

A large number of theorists and researchers have validated the sequential stages of cultural identity development in many cultural settings and extended them to other groups. Important among these have been Atkinson, Morten, and Sue (1993; general theory of cultural identity development), Hardiman (1995; White identity development), and Helms (1990; African American and White identity development). While the language varies, the general sequence identified by Cross holds for these theorists. Cultural identity theory need not apply only to racial and ethnic issues; rather, it is a broad-based approach that has significant importance for the counseling and therapy process.

DCT and cultural identity theory are compared in Table 8-1. Despite some similarities, they are not the same. DCT involves *developmental styles* and validates the importance of all styles. More styles and style flexibility are the goals. Cultural identity theory also recognizes the value of all stages or levels, particularly depending

Table 8-1 Two Models of Holistic Consciousness Compared

Cultural Identity Theory	DCT
Preencounter	Sensorimotor
Encounter (with elements of immersion)	Concrete
Immersion/Emersion	Formal
Internalization	Dialectic/Systemic

on the situations in which individuals live or find themselves. Both theories encourage awareness of self-in-system, and development of dialectic/systemic intelligence. They emphasize the importance of direct action to attack social oppression that may exist within the social context.

Cultural identity theory is centered on expanding awareness of one's racial/ethnic identity. Increasingly we are finding identity theories focused on other multicultural issues. Cass (1979, 1984, 1990) has been influential in applying cultural identity theory to gay issues. Marszalek and Cashwell (1998) and Marszalek, Cashwell, Dunn, and Heard (in press) have presented a DCT-based theory of gay and lesbian identity development. Ivey, D'Andrea, Ivey, and Simek-Morgan (2002) suggest that many groups (e.g., women, cancer survivors, persons with disabilities, Vietnam veterans) go through parallel issues of identity as they discover the power of context in their individual lives.

The cultural identity movement will continue to grow in influence and can be expected to change with further research and as new populations deal with privilege and power. For example, Degges-White, Rice, and Myers (2000) used a sample of adult lesbians in a qualitative study of Cass's sexual minority identity development theory and found that definitions of the integrative or dialectic/systemic aspects of development were no longer valid; rather, a new stage appears to be evolving, the nature of which remains unclear. Important in this change, perhaps, is that societal awareness and acceptance of alternative lifestyles have increased over time. Simultaneously, the challenges to gay and lesbian individuals from some portions of society have become more intense. As culture changes, we can expect further issues in the developmental process to appear among many groups. Important among these will be increasing awareness that we all have many multicultural identities, rather than just one. The RESPECTFUL cube should be considered a useful beginning.

DCT: MULTIPLE NARRATIVES OF CONSCIOUSNESS

Ivey and Payton (1994) have related cultural identity to early Platonic roots:

> Meaning-making has been identified as a central aspect in the development of a cultural identity. . . . The essence of this framework is Plato's observation in *The Republic* that the transition to enlightenment involves four levels of consciousness and that each level builds on previous perceptions of reality, preparing the way for the next higher level. Ivey points out that the progressions of

knowledge portrayed in the "Allegory of the Cave" may be construed as a useful framework for the generation of cultural consciousness.

In connecting Plato to cultural consciousness, it may be helpful to recall that the prisoners in the Cave thought that the flickering shadows in front of them [were] "reality." As one prisoner was removed from his chains and taken out of the cave, he would eventually realize that what he saw in the cave was not reality, but only a perspective. However, as Plato soberly notes . . . if the former prisoner were returned to his fellows with news of the new truth, "they would kill him." The birth of consciousness is lonely and often fraught with real pain.

Cultural identity theory moves people from the cave of naive consciousness about self to awareness of self in relation to system. The parallels to the Platonic journey are not perfect, but do suggest that coming to a new view of reality may involve some difficulty. As Cornford notes, "One moral of the allegory is drawn from the distress caused by too sudden passage from dark to light" (1941/1981, p. 227).

Developmental counseling and therapy emerged from a reference point different from that of MCT's cultural identity theory, but the two have considerable congruence around the concept of consciousness development. DCT offers a different but complementary theoretical base plus narrative specifics leading toward action to enhance identity development.

Whereas cultural identity theories tend to focus on specific groups, DCT takes a narrative approach to the evolution of consciousness. Individuals (and families and groups) have life stories that they tell about themselves, guiding the way they think and behave.

Specifically, DCT theory asserts that clients come to counseling with varying levels of consciousness or meaning-making systems that they use to understand their world. These consciousness orientations lead to different stages or styles of thinking and behaving. The task of the counselor is to assess and understand the cognitive/emotional stages clients use to make sense of what they are experiencing. Then the counselor joins the client where the individual is in her or his cognitive/emotional understanding and assists expansion of development both vertically and horizontally. No one type of consciousness is best, although more styles and stages permit more possibilities for thought and action.

The parallels between the orientations of Cross's cultural identity development and DCT meaning making can be seen in Table 8-1, Two Models of Holistic Consciousness Compared. The holistic model notes that development can occur within multiple states/stages or levels/orientations/styles simultaneously. We should recall that individuals or groups could be expected to move at any time from one consciousness model to another. Types of thought, feeling, and action vary within each consciousness model.

Comparisons between DCT and cultural identity theory are interesting and useful. For example, preencounter and sensorimotor thought and emotion can be limited and constraining when a client is dealing with a complex issue. At the same time, preencounter and sensorimotor experience can be more open to here and now experience and thus provide an opportunity for the client to grow and change. Parham points out that many individuals may be caught in denial and stagnation and use preencounter cognitions to prevent change. Yet the concrete and specific encounter with a racist incident can perturb individuals and help them move out of sensorimotor magical thinking patterns, characteristic of the preencounter stage.

Encounter is so important to the change process that Cross and others usually present it as a separate stage. In DCT this process would be termed *late sensorimotor* and be considered necessary for a full concrete consciousness.

Immersion/emersion concepts relate to concrete and formal consciousness. The most likely result of consciousness during the encounter stage is concrete and specific awareness of racism and prejudice, accompanied by anger—and often concrete and specific action to fight the situation. At a later time, during this stage, the reflective consciousness becomes prominent. The ability to reflect is essential if one is to operate at the internalization or dialectic/systemic level.

The formal/reflective consciousness—thinking about thinking—is characteristic of DCT clients who think about self. It is also typical of reflective individuals in cultural identity theory who think about cultural identity. As clients think about cultural identity, they have moved back and taken a new perspective on themselves as cultural beings.

A requirement of internalization is systemic thinking and the ability to take multiple perspectives. Thinking of the self-in-relation or person-as-community requires dialectic/systemic thought. Developmentally, some African American or other minority individuals may actually be operating at this frequently more sophisticated level and they may be fully aware of how oppression operates in a systemic sense. Many who see themselves as oppressed or treated unfairly may be especially able to think at this level. But, as Parham notes, they may not yet be able to see the perspective of the dominant group, whom they often regard as oppressors.

Thus, linear models of consciousness development do not really describe the complexity; a holistic model may be more realistic than linear stage frameworks. Developmentally, some young African American, Asian American, or Native American youth may experience post-formal thought and dialectic/systemic awareness much earlier than their majority-culture peers as a result of life experiences, which include personal experience with prejudice.

Both the DCT model and Parham's addition to cultural identity theory suggest that "higher is not necessarily better." There is value in the embeddedness of preencounter and sensorimotor approaches to reality. The ability of an individual at the encounter or concrete stage to act on the world and tell clear stories is important. No one can deny that the formal reflective consciousness of immersion/emersion is important. And from both the counseling/therapeutic model of DCT and the multicultural framework, it is patently clear that the ability to take multiple perspectives on reality is important. Consciousness may at times work in a linear fashion, but ultimately it is holistic and moving, perhaps ultimately existential and spiritual in nature. Is not our consciousness our spirit?

THE LIBERATION OF CONSCIOUSNESS

The effectiveness of MCT is most likely enhanced when the counselor uses modalities and defines goals consistent with the life experience and cultural values of the client. No single approach is equally effective across all populations and life situations. The ultimate goal of multicultural counselor/therapist training is to expand the repertoire of helping responses available to the professional regardless of theoretical orientation. (Sue et al., 1996, p. 19)

This assumption of MCT is a culturally appropriate restatement of traditional counseling theory and practice—*join the client where he or she is.* Counselors and therapists are, for the most part, deeply committed to empathy and understanding the client's frame of reference. What has been missing in traditional empathic, relationship, and therapeutic alliance writing is cultural context and awareness of the self-in-relation.

DCT is committed to a co-constructed counseling and therapy process with an emphasis on an equal relationship between counselor and client, therapist and patient. This commitment includes awareness of the social context of both counselor/therapist and the *client consultant.* The term *client consultant* emphasizes that the client can and often does have a significant impact on the helper.

Joining clients where they are involves diagnosing stages and levels of consciousness development, respecting that person where he or she *is,* and facilitating expansion of consciousness in consultation with the client.

The first task of a therapist focused on consciousness is to assess the client's stage and style of meaning making. This will show most clearly in the person's verbal behavior in the interview, but it also may be manifested in behavior in her or his daily life. Both cultural identity theory and DCT suggest ways to assess the client's consciousness development.

Liberation of Consciousness as a Theory and Practice

The liberation of consciousness is a basic goal of MCT theory. Whereas self-actualization, discovery of the role of the past in the present, or behavior change have been traditional goals of Western psychotherapy and counseling, MCT emphasizes the importance of expanding personal, family, group, and organizational consciousness of the place of self-in-relation, family-in-relation, and organization-in-relation. This results in therapy that is not only ultimately contextual in orientation, but that also draws on traditional methods of healing from many cultures. (Sue et al., 1996, p. 22)

Liberation of consciousness is a goal of both MCT and DCT. We seek to encourage clients to find new ways of examining their lives and eventually of acting on these insights.

Paulo Freire's *Pedagogy of the Oppressed* (1970) is valuable in showing ways to liberate consciousness. In a liberation orientation, the word *level* is preferred over *style* in the belief that the more complete versions of consciousness do require one to become more cognitively complex. In this case, "higher is generally considered better." Nonetheless, presenting oneself as being at a different level of consciousness than where one "really is" can be wise. For example, it would not always be wise for an oppressed group of peasants in South America to challenge the plantation owner openly. An individual migrant worker in South Florida, California, or Texas should also be careful in expressing her or his beliefs about unionization.

Freire discusses some specifics of consciousness raising in Chapter 3 of his book. He tells of meeting with a group of peasants over a campfire. The shared objective would be literacy training in which the peasants were to select and name the words they wished to learn to read. Freire worked out of their life experience, so reading education would naturally focus on the life of the peasant. In this way, he was as much a learner as were his "students."

Freire and his students would identify objects in their natural environment and daily life. He stressed the importance of *codification* in which themes of the culture were identified. He used visual, tactile, and auditory channels as the peasants identified things in their environment. Counselors and therapists using the developmental counseling and therapy model would recognize this as sensorimotor questioning ("What are you seeing? Hearing? Feeling?") in which direct experience is accessed as most fundamental. Neurolinguistic programming (Andreas & Faulkner, 1996) uses this type of questioning to help the client colleague anchor present and past life experiences. However, note that Freire was using specifics of neurolinguistic programming long before this psychotherapeutic mode became popular. Freire was key to the inclusion of these concepts in the methodology of developmental counseling and therapy, particularly as related to contextual issues.

Freire followed codification of experience with naming. His groups would describe the events of their lives and name what they saw, heard, and felt. The named words of lived experience would serve as the foundation of their reading. In psychotherapeutic terms, we want to know the nature of direct experience and how the client names this experience.

It is here that cultural identity theory can be helpful in understanding what Freire was doing. The peasants and Freire were operating in a state of naiveté and were passively accepting conditions of life on a plantation (see Table 8-2). In Platonic terms, they were "imagining" life rather than truly experiencing it. The act of naming experiences enabled the peasants first to know what was happening and later to reflect on their condition.

For a concrete example, Freire might ask the peasants to describe what they saw, heard, and felt during a typical day. Important would be specific sensorimotor images of events. Then, he might ask them to describe the daily life of the plantation owner as they saw, heard, and felt it, thus helping them identify contradictions and make them concrete. The words used in these descriptions would be the foundation for literacy training. The concrete *names* they used to describe their own lives and that of the plantation owner often brought them to new and complex forms of cognition and emotion about their previously lived experience, cognitions and feelings that had been impossible before. In short, the act of naming and identifying contradictions is fundamental to cognitive, emotional, and behavioral growth.

In the above example, the names given to life experiences are primarily those of the client colleague. The names are not taken from a previously agreed-on theory developed by remote experts. The names also help the leader or counselor identify new ways to conceptualize experience.

To bring and extend these concepts to cultural identity theory and counseling practice, the task for varying cultural groups is first to identify experience as lived (what they see, hear, and feel), then to name the experience and sometimes to act on it as a result of naming. As part of this type of examination, clients naturally reflect

Table 8-2   Cognitive/Emotional Developmental Change: Five Theoretical Perspectives

Cultural Identity Theory	DCT	Plato	Freire	Actions Needed to Produce Change to the Next Level/Stage
Preencounter (Naiveté with acceptance of status quo)	Sensorimotor	Imagining	Magical consciousness (conforming)*	Ask clients to describe life experiences through stories of oppression.
Encounter (Naming and resistance with anger a common emotion)	Concrete/situational	Belief	Beginning of critical consciousness (reforming)	Name and confront contractions between self and contextual systems.
Immersion/emersion (Redefinition and reflection)	Formal/reflective	Thinking	Reflective consciousness sees patterns of oppression	Support pattern recognition and self-in-system reflections.
Internalization (Multiperspective integration)	Dialectic/systemic	Dialectic	Critical consciousness (transforming), conscientizacào	Continue emphasis on dialogic thought and co-investigation of reality. Joint action to transform reality.

*Conforming, reforming, and transforming are terms coined by Alschuler (1986) that are helpful in defining the changes that occur with critical consciousness.

and redefine the meaning of their experience. These therapeutic and educational processes relate cultural identity theory, the Platonic epistemology, and Freire's original thought. These comparable dimensions are outlined in Table 8-2.

Table 8-2 points out that specific actions can be employed within each level of consciousness to facilitate movement to the next level. Freire used many techniques similar to those used daily in counseling and psychotherapy, but his goal was achieving equality and action in the system, not leading individuals to conform to the status quo. Institutional or environmental change as a result of naming was also often engaged in by joint action of the leader and the group.

As one current example, DCT and the liberation model have been used in a Native American context (Cameron, Chavez, King, & turtle-song, 2001). The authors present a case example of their treatment method with a student who commented, "People sometimes stare at me, but they're looking at the Indian, not me." DCT questioning sequences helped the student to discover strengths in himself and the culture—and to become more aware of how issues of prejudice and racism were impacting him. The liberation model was considered most successful when the client decided to join in critical action against oppression in the community. But perhaps most important here is that the authors took the basic model and reframed it to address issues within the Native American Indian culture.

The goal of *conscientizacào* is critical consciousness—the client colleague who experiences self, perhaps for the first time, and then begins to see how self was constructed in a sociocultural relationship. Freire and the cultural identity theorists provide a diagnostic frame that can serve as a place to design helping interventions and assess their effectiveness. And moving beyond awareness, there is a call to action—almost a demand that one *act* on issues of oppression and unfairness that brought about the oppressive thought patterns. Many of these interventions will follow a social justice model and require direct action in the community (Arredondo & Perez, 2003; Helms, 2003).

Skills and Strategies for Liberation of Consciousness

"Psychotherapy as liberation" is a specific attempt to apply the concepts of Freire to the counseling and therapy progress (Ivey, 1995). The goal is to help clients see their issues in social context. Client narratives are particularly useful for assessment. This section presents specific questions designed to achieve the critical consciousness described above in relation to Paulo Freire.

Questions such as the following typically stimulate sufficient information:

- Could you tell me a story that occurs to you when you think about yourself (as African American, Korean American, Mexican American, Jewish American, Polish American, woman, gay male, person-with-AIDS, etc.)?
- Could you tell me about a situation in which you may have experienced or seen prejudice (racism, sexism, heterosexism, ableism, etc.)?
- What does it mean to you to be (insert term here)?

DCT has generated a set of questions designed to extend narratives at each stage of consciousness. Specific applications of these questions for each level of *cultural* identity theory might be as follows.

Expansion of Preencounter or Sensorimotor Consciousness

These questions are designed to encourage experiencing what it is like to be at a specific consciousness level or orientation. They can help those at the preencounter level expand their awareness of where they are (and thus perhaps prepare them to move on to other levels of consciousness). They are also useful for people at immersion/emersion states who may not be fully in touch with their emotions and here and now experience.

The focus in the following questions is on here and now sensory experience related to the story. The client might be asked to generate an image of the general situation just described.

- Could you think of one visual image that occurs to you as most important in that story? (Or auditory, kinesthetic, or other depending on preferred sensory modality of the client or group.)

Visual perceptions
- What are you seeing?
- Describe in detail the scene where it happened.

Auditory perceptions
- What are you hearing?
- How are people sounding?
- Describe the sound in detail.

Kinesthetic perceptions
- What are you feeling in your body at this moment?
- Where is that feeling in your body?
- What are you feeling as this is going on?

Encouraging Movement to Another Consciousness Level

In-depth generation of sensorimotor experience in itself may bring about the spontaneous emergence of a new way of thinking about old ways of being. Oppression in all its forms affects the body and is ultimately a sensorimotor experience. Often, just getting fully in touch with that experience is enough to jar consciousness.

Helping move to new states of consciousness is often facilitated by supportive but challenging perturbation. Pointing out discrepancies and incongruities in the story or situation, particularly when the story is supported by emotionally based here and now experience, is often helpful in moving consciousness.

Essential to the following types of supportive confrontations is first hearing the client carefully and listening to her or his situation and unique perceptions and feelings. In presenting what you have heard, seen, or felt yourself, use the client's key words so that it is she or he who develops the resolution, not you. Hearing the client's story and narrative accurately and fully is vital in multiculturally oriented therapy, just as in any other model (Semmier & Williams, 2000).

The story is summarized with accurate paraphrasing and reflection of feeling. Important keywords of the client or group are used.

- On one hand, I hear that you said . . . , but on the other hand, they said . . .
- I hear you saying you felt . . . , but then . . .
- Could you point out to me the contradictions in the story and how you felt about it? (This type of lead may encourage more self-discovery.)

Similar questions can help people at other levels of consciousness consider alternative perspectives. For example, the person at the immersion/emersion stage of consciousness might benefit by returning to the emotional dimensions of preencounter or by being challenged to move toward more reflective consciousness at the later stages of immersion/emersion. The person whose consciousness is at the internalization level can profit by experiencing other, more direct ways of being.

Expanding Immersion/Emersion, Concrete, and Formal Consciousness

The goals at the early stages of immersion relate most closely to DCT's concrete orientation to consciousness whereas later, formal/reflection questions may be useful. Note that these questions are useful in consciousness-raising groups and may help individuals relate their experience to others in the group.

Concrete examples useful for the earlier stages of immersion/emersion:

- Could you share a story of what happened? I'd like to hear it from beginning to end.
- What happened first, and then what happened; what was the consequence?
- What did he/she say? What did you say? Then what was said?
- What did you feel?
- What do you think the other(s) felt?

- Reflect feelings—"You felt XXX because XXX."
- Particularly helpful in moving to reflective thought is summarizing two or more individual or group stories (which will often contain similar key words) and then asking the individual or group how the stories are similar.

Formal reflective examples to facilitate later stages of the immersion/emersion stage:

- How is your story similar to stories you have told me in the past?
- How is your story similar to (and different from) stories of other members of the group?
- How are your feelings similar?
- Is that a pattern (in the individual or the group)?
- What does this story say about you as a person?
- What do these stories say about us all (identity group—for example, a women's or gay liberation session)?

Expanding Internalization and Dialectic/Systemic Consciousness

Useful in moving to internalization and dialectic/systemic thought are questions that focus on the relationship of the individual to the social context. Critical here is encouraging people to see themselves and their group in relation to broader systemic issues, often through multiperspective thought. This level of consciousness can become heavily embedded in intellectual thought and abstraction. Thus, focusing on action and generalizing learning to the real world through concrete action may be essential. This is also an important place to identify client metaphors (see bibliotherapy chapter) and underscore client strengths for coping with life challenges.

It is often useful to summarize major portions of an individual or group conversation. This is followed by asking people to reflect on the conversation and asking them questions such as these:

- How do you put together/organize all that you have told me (or the group)? What one thing stands out for you?

Often this question or a variation will result in a broadened point of view toward the issue discussed.

Other questions:

- How many different ways could you describe the situation? How would it look from another perspective different from your own (different ethnic group, sexual orientation, etc.)?
- How would external conditions (e.g., trauma, racism, sexism, heterosexism) affect what is occurring with you (or the group)?
- What rule(s) were you operating under in this situation? What rule(s) are in the other person's mind?
- Where did those rules come from (family, culture, etc.)?
- Can you see some flaws in your own reasoning that the others might think of? What do you see as flaws in the others' reasoning?
- Do your feelings and emotions change as you look at the situation from a new perspective?

Internalization and dialectic/systemic consciousness may lead some clients to become enmeshed in thought and fail to act. "Some Blacks fail to sustain a long-term interest in Black affairs. Others devote an extended period of time, if not a life-time, to finding ways to translate their personal sense of Blackness in a plan of action or general sense of commitment" (Cross, 1995, p. 121). Both MCT and DCT would agree that thought without action is empty.

Below are some potentially useful questions to encourage following up on these issues:

- We've heard the "what" and the "why." Now what are you/we going to do about it?
- What one thing might you want to do tomorrow/next week to act on what you've learned and said?
- How can we take these thoughts into action?
- How might we behave differently?
- Let us develop an individual/group action plan.
- This is what I am going to do about it! (In some cases—for example, a school-teacher oppressing a student or a manager harassing a woman—the client may not have sufficient power and the therapist is then faced with the decision of how to act in the client's best interests. Needless to say, this is not a traditional view of the helping relationship.)

It is important for the counselor or group leader to note that these are all concrete action plans and may also be typical of what we might expect to find in the often highly motivated early stages of the concrete immersion/emersion consciousness. At this point we move consciously into social action promoting change in the systems that often are at the root of client problems. Increasingly, issues of social justice are coming to the fore in the counseling and therapy fields (Ivey & Collins, 2003; Vera & Speight, 2003). It is important to extend this idea beyond racism to other areas of oppression. For example, Mothers Against Drunk Driving (MADD) is a personal and group statement about the effect of alcohol abuse in our society. Women who march for their rights are directly attacking what many describe as an oppressive rape culture. Cancer survivors often meet in groups and take action to work with insensitive physicians or to support others in the struggle against the dis-ease. The search for gay rights is a clear indication of taking internalization consciousness into action against heterosexism and oppression.

Action against the oppressive conditions of life can lead toward better mental health and increased holistic wellness. Passively sitting and discussing oppression is not enough. Action seeking to address oppressive external conditions is essential.

The Value of Each Level of Consciousness

Each style, stage, level, or orientation to consciousness has its value. The ability to experience life directly, associated with the sensorimotor and preencounter style, can be useful in both survival and heightened awareness of what is happening. We need concrete narratives to describe our experience and we need to reflect on the meaning of the narratives. Finally, dialectic/systemic internalization thought tends to help us see problems and issues in social context and, if balanced with action, can lead to significant change. So-called higher stages are not necessarily better. More useful is the ability to work with multiple levels of consciousness. Both Thomas Parham and William Cross endorse the wisdom of all states of being and they also imply "more is better." The ability to take multiple positions seems to offer the most intentionality and perhaps the most flexibility to deal with the ultimate complexity and pervasiveness of oppressive experience.

SUMMARY

The multicultural counseling and therapy metatheoretical framework places cultural issues at the core of all helping theories while simultaneously endorsing traditional theories, assuming that they are adapted to meet individual and group needs. MCT is not an either-or absolutist frame of reference. Rather, it builds on traditional approaches, adding new dimensions to enrich the uniqueness of each person. If we fail to see the context in which the individual develops, we miss the richness that each individual has to offer.

We are all cultural beings participating in many multicultural dimensions. The RESPECTFUL multicultural cube was presented to remind us that vital to our being are many identities ranging from religion and spirituality to ethnic/racial identity to language and location issues. Privilege and power (and sometimes oppression) can occur in the dominant group in each multiculture.

Cultural identity theory points out that awareness of oneself as a cultural being is a developmental issue in which a person moves from lack of awareness to multiperspective understanding. William Cross's theory was presented with its focus on ethnic/racial issues. However, the cultural identity model can be used to describe the growth process of any multicultural group.

Evolution of consciousness is a broad goal, not only for cultural identity, but also for all clients, almost regardless of the issue on which they are working. Parallels were presented between and among DCT, cultural identity theory, the work of Paulo Freire, and the writing of Plato. All are concerned with multiple narratives of consciousness in which clients learn to examine their issues from many perspectives. An important part of the wellness perspective is becoming aware of self-in-context and self-in-relation in most concerns presented by clients.

Paulo Freire's concept of education as liberation strategies provides both a value structure and a methodology for helping clients discover how they are selves-in-systems. The Brazilian educator's methods have had a powerful impact in Latin America and can be adapted for facilitating client awareness in the counseling and therapy field.

Skills and strategies adapted from DCT provide specifics for implementing a counseling and psychotherapy of liberation in the here and now of the interview. The chapter closed with many suggestions for how the interviewer could take the ideas of this chapter into direct and immediate practice.

Challenges: The concepts of multiculturalism are not easily accepted by all, although more and more people are becoming aware of the necessity to build increased understanding. The state of California by 2005 will have more residents that are People of Color than of White European background, with other Southwestern states soon to follow. By mid-century, the United States will be a true multicultural nation with no one group in the majority. These facts are perhaps the best argument to those who are resistant to multicultural issues.

Research issues: The research on cultural identity theory has become extensive. See Cross and Vandiver (2001) and Fischer and Morardi (2001) for useful presentations. One important study of ethnic/racial identity is by Utsey, Chae, Brown, and Kelly (2002), who examined stress and quality of life. Studying three ethnic groups (African American, Asian American, and Latina/o), these researchers found that African Americans had the greatest amount of race-related stress. The African Americans also had a higher level of racial identity, perhaps because of being forced to develop this awareness through living in a racist society. In addition, on quality-of-life issues, African Americans reported having poorer health, less satisfaction with relationships and social networks, and less satisfaction with lifestyle than other groups. All of these issues can appear in the counseling or therapy office and we may expect that many Asian Americans and Latina/o clients will present with parallel difficulties. Nonetheless, in a society that pays particular attention to color, we can anticipate continued challenges for African Americans.

THEORY INTO PRACTICE: DEVELOPING YOUR PORTFOLIO OF COMPETENCE

Self-Assessment Exercises

Exercise 1. Your RESPECTFUL awareness of your own multicultural self

At the beginning of this chapter, you were asked to place yourself in the multicultural cube as you might experience power and dominance, either as a person of privilege or a person who deals with privileged others. We'd like you to return to the RESPECTFUL cube and use the four-level cultural identity theory model to rate your level of awareness in each category. For example, how aware are you of yourself as a spiritual being, the importance of your language, or your racial/ethnic heritage?

Based on your own subjective impressions, where do you see yourself in terms of your awareness of the importance of your multicultural identities? Please revisit Table 8-1 to help you make your decisions. Circle 1 for preencounter, 2 for encounter, 3 for immersion/emersion, and 4 for internalization. (Note: It may help if you think first of the general effect of the category and then about its effect on you. You may find, for example, that you never thought of it before, which is a clear indication of level 1 preencounter. In another example, many people never think of their economic status, but it deeply affects who they are and their opportunity.)

1 2 3 4 R Religion

1 2 3 4 E Economic status

1 2 3 4 S Sexual identity

1 2 3 4 P Psychological maturity (cognitive/developmental style)

1 2 3 4 E Ethnic/racial identity

1 2 3 4 C Chronological challenges (age)

1 2 3 4 T Trauma

1 2 3 4 F Family history

1 2 3 4 U Unique physical characteristics

1 2 3 4 L Language and location of residence

Exercise 2. Your personal reflections on multicultural identity

As you think of the above indicators of your personal awareness plus your earlier ratings on power and privilege, what implications do you find for your own self-awareness and for the counseling and therapy process?

_____

_____

_____

_____

_____

_____

Exercise 3. Using DCT strategies to explore personal thoughts about oppression

It is helpful to become aware of your own experiences with discrimination. Most of us, whether we are in a majority or a minority, have experienced discrimination of some type. This discrimination may have manifested as actual racism, jokes about your ethnic heritage, not being allowed to do something because of your sex, religious bigotry, not having enough money to do something necessary for you or your family. If you are gay or lesbian or have close friends who are, you undoubtedly know the personal pain that comes from discrimination. Other topics can help you get in touch with your own history of discrimination. For example, many athletes find themselves stereotyped as "dumb jocks." Good students are seen as "nerds." You're considered "out of it" if you don't wear the right clothes. Perhaps you were teased unmercifully as a child. Or you may be the child of alcoholic parents. Individuals who won't go along with the prevailing majority often suffer forms of discrimination not unlike racism and sexism. Being different is often a route to being oppressed.

Review the discussion above and select a discriminatory issue that is relevant to you. The exercise will be more profitable if you can identify a specific issue you have experienced personally, but you may wish to work through the exercise focusing on a friend or family member. What area of multicultural awareness did you select, and why is it important to you personally?

_____

_____

_____

_____

Give a specific instance when you or a friend suffered from some type of discrimination? Get a visual image of that situation. What do you see? Hear? Feel? Can you locate a specific feeling in your body? Where in your body? Focus particularly on your emotions and kinesthetic feelings. Can you recreate the past situation in the present?

_____

_____

_____

_____

Describe the concrete events surrounding the situation. What happened before? What happened afterward? Who was there? How did they act? What did they say and do? How did you feel before the event, and how did you feel afterward?

_____

_____

_____

_____

Did things similar to that event happen in other situations? Was it a pattern? How did that pattern affect you and your sense of self? How did you feel about other people, perhaps in your family, who suffered from the same pattern of discrimination?

_____

_____

_____

_____

Look back at your responses above. What sense do you make of the incident now? Note particularly your responses using the sensorimotor and concrete-operational styles. At what level of multicultural identity theory were you operating? Given what you have observed, what are you going to do?

_____

_____

_____

_____

The following exercise is more difficult. Select one of the suggested areas of discrimination above with which you are less familiar. It is important to choose a topic you know is difficult for you to understand and encounter. What topic did you select? Why?

_____

_____

_____

_____

_____

Imagine that you are an individual of that cultural group. Generate a visual image of a type of discrimination you might encounter. What would you see, hear, and feel? Where was the feeling located in your body?

_____

_____

_____

_____

_____

What sense would you make out of this discriminatory situation? What would it mean to you if you experienced that event?

_____

_____

_____

_____

_____

Imagine a series of concrete events, such as the one above, that repeat again and again. What would life be like? What would it mean to you if you experienced repeated discrimination? What would it mean to your family?

_____

_____

_____

_____

_____

How do you integrate this brief exercise with the previous exercise in which you examined your own personal experience with discrimination? What was similar? What was different?

_____

_____

_____

_____

_____

Identifying and Classifying Cultural Identity and Fostering White Awareness

Exercise 4. Classifying cultural identity stages

Each of the following clients represents a different cultural identity level. While we all must recall that many clients will present different cultural identity levels in the interview, we still should be able to classify the *predominant cultural identity level* at that time. Refer to page 252 for definitions of the four stages.

Rate each of these from 1 through 4:

1 2 3 4   1. (Cambodian) The United States is best. I just want to be an American like everyone else.

1 2 3 4   2. (Cambodian) I've been ripped off. America doesn't care about me. White people are just plain racist and Blacks aren't much better.

1 2 3 4   3. (Cambodian) I need to get back to my roots and think about my homeland. It's too much hassle dealing with this culture. I need time to think.

1 2 3 4   4. (Cambodian) As I look at it now, the United States does have much to offer, although I know I must fight racism. I'm glad I took time to recapture my Cambodian identity.

1 2 3 4   5. (woman) I've just come back from the picket line. The affirmative action program at the plant just isn't working. I'm going to do something about it. It really makes me angry.

1 2 3 4   6. (woman) I don't see why people are picketing the plant. I'm doing fine. Sure, I work hard as a secretary and I'd like more pay, but I sure don't want to handle lumber in the yard.

1 2 3 4   7. (woman) I'm tired of the hassle. I'm supporting the strike, but I need time to think for a while. I just want to be with women and think it through. Men just seem irrelevant to me.

1 2 3 4   8. (woman) Well, I'm going to work on the picket line, but I also know that we've got to work with those men in the plant who understand our point of view. We've got to work together to change a lot of people's minds.

1 2 3 4   9. (blind) I've learned a lot about life by listening and touching. I know I've missed a lot in terms of seeing. I've been angry at the discrimination I've faced, but I'm

excited to see all the improvements for us that have come in recent years. It's been worth it.

1 2 3 4   10. (Chinese) I'm fed up with this university. Everywhere I turn, I find more and more racism. The history texts distort my background; the housing office ignores the discrimination. We've got to get organized.

1 2 3 4   11. (Jewish) There's no discrimination in this country. I've gotten along fine. I do have to watch things a bit, but things are OK.

1 2 3 4   12. (Nigerian international student) Discrimination is certainly an issue for me in this country. But I've learned to sit back and live and play with other Nigerians. We have our own agenda anyway.

1 2 3 4   13. (lesbian teen) What is "wrong" with me? I find that I'm attracted to women and men don't interest me. I feel so alone.

1 2 3 4   14. (lesbian, two years later) I understand now. I'm glad I came out, but I am really angry at the way I was treated

1 2 3 4   15. (Muslim) I can understand the discrimination that occurs toward our people, but I'm glad for the understanding and support that I get from some of my Christian and Jewish friends. Nonetheless, I have decided that I am going to act more carefully in the future to protect my family. It is a difficult balance I face.

1 2 3 4   16. (cancer trauma survivor) I shouldn't have ignored that lump in my breast. I'm going to go out and educate others and help them understand the disease more fully. We have to act to take care of ourselves.

1 2 3 4   17. (counseling student) People are people. Why all this fuss about racism and sexism? We're all struggling.

1 2 3 4   18 . (counseling student) I now see what I've been missing. It really ticks me off. The therapy theory course doesn't mention issues of racial or sexual discrimination. I'm going to see that something is done about it.

1 2 3 4   19. (counseling student) I can certainly understand why people get upset about racism, but as I think about it, there isn't a lot I can do. I need to go off and think about it some more.

1 2 3 4   20. (counseling student) Developing full multicultural understanding may take some time. My own goal is to work more on where I come from ethnically. As I understand my background, I should be better able to understand others. At the same time, I can't let that be enough. I'll take some action as well.

Exercise 5. Fostering White awareness: The frontier of multicultural training

In U.S., Canadian, and European society, the dominant White Euro-American cultural group is in particular need of self-awareness. Efforts at multicultural awareness will be fruitless unless Whites begin to examine and know themselves.

Cultural identity theory provides a four-stage model for evaluating racial consciousness of White counselor trainees (Ponterotto, 1988). The framework can also be applied to White identity development in general. Four stages of thinking and behavior of counselors in training are identified: (1) preexposure, (2) exposure,

(3) zealotry or defensiveness, and (4) integration. These stages are roughly comparable to the four styles of DCT.

Where are you personally in terms of your awareness of White culture? If you
are of White European ancestry, classify yourself as a counselor, according to the suggestions of Ponterotto. If you are non-White, identify one or two White people you
may work with and classify them. Each person will require differing types of counseling when issues that relate to racial awareness come up.

_____

_____

_____

_____

Interviewing Practice Exercises

Exercise 6. Practice in a role-played session using multicultural awareness questions

The format for this exercise is similar to that of other role-plays, the exception being
that the client is asked to play her or his real self and to honestly explore how he or
she has personally experienced issues of prejudice and racism. The specific questions
used in Exercise 3 of this chapter can serve as the framework for the practice session.
Follow usual ethical guidelines with your group.

Step 1: Divide Into Practice Groups

Step 2: Select a Group Leader

Step 3: Assign Roles for the Practice Session

■   *Role-played client.* The role-played client will explore one or more personal
multicultures, as in the RESPECTFUL cube, when he or she experienced discrimination and/or prejudice. The client should share only what he or she feels comfortable sharing.

■   *Interviewer.* The interviewer will ask the specific DCT/Freire four-style questions, as outlined in this chapter (pages 257–260). The questions are adapted to
meet the specific needs of this client. The interviewer will not be intrusive and will
especially try to understand the client's frame of reference.

■   *Observers 1 and 2.* The observers will observe the session but will not take notes.
They will be available after the role-play for discussion and mutual support.

Step 4: Plan the Session
The interviewer and client need first to agree on the specific topic to be reviewed.

Step 5: Conduct a 15-Minute Interviewing Session
You will find it helpful to videotape or audiotape practice sessions.

Step 6: Provide Immediate Feedback (15 to 20 Minutes)
Allow the client and interviewer time to provide immediate personal reactions to the
practice session. After this has been done, the observers and the role-played client
can focus on the thoughts and feelings of all members of the group. An open sharing of issues may be beneficial. Avoid judgmental feedback.

Step 7: Generate a Fantasy About Another Cultural Group (20 Minutes)
In the groups, generate a fantasy about how a member of an oppressed multicultural group might experience the same DCT four-style questions. Do this as a group rather than an individual discussion.

Exercise 7. Counseling and psychotherapy as liberation

Before starting this exercise, please review the specific questions based on Paulo Freire's thought on page 257. Your task in this session is to explore the specifics of the systematic questioning procedure in a practice session. For this practice session, we strongly recommend that you have the actual questions before you and that you share them with the client. Work through them carefully together.

Step 1: Divide Into Practice Groups

Step 2: Select a Group Leader

Step 3: Assign Roles for the Practice Session

■   *Role-played client.* The role-played client will talk freely about a topic of discrimination or oppression, perhaps selected from the topics presented in Exercise 3.

■   *Interviewer.* The interviewer will share the questions to be asked of the client and work with the client carefully through each style. Be sure to use reflective listening to encourage openness and depth of expression.

■   Due to the length of the session, it will not ordinarily be possible to have observers. If possible, audiotape or videotape the session and, following ethical procedures with appropriate permissions, have classmates review the session and provide feedback. Ideally, your client will be present during the feedback session.

Step 4: Conduct an Hour or More Interviewing Session
Again it is helpful to videotape or audiotape practice sessions.

Step 5: Review Practice Session and Provide Feedback
The interviewer should ask for feedback rather than getting it without having asked. The observers and the client can share their observations of the session. Avoid judgmental feedback.

Generalization: Taking Multicultural Concepts Home

Exercise 8. Observe individuals in daily life

Listen to friends and colleagues when they talk about various groups and note these individuals' levels of consciousness. You may ask close friends or family, in a non-judgmental fashion, "How do you see or think about (the particular group)?" Note their responses and then assess their level or levels of consciousness. Many, perhaps most, people you listen to will be at preencounter (sensorimotor) consciousness. You may wish to perturb or confront them gently with new or additional data.

Exercise 9. The interview

The basic helping model to apply in your sessions, either with individuals or families, is as follows: (1) Join the client's construction of the problem where the client is. How does the individual or family understand the problem? (It is useful to follow the classification systems of cultural identity theory, which will help you understand the level of consciousness.) (2) Perturb the client's current level of thinking by using confrontation skills that focus on discrepancies between the individual and the environment. (3) Help the client struggle with that understanding and realize that anger (common in stage 2) may result from your confrontation. Understand and join the client struggling to incorporate this new perspective.

To consolidate this new level of understanding, expand awareness through sensorimotor, concrete, formal, and dialectic/systemic interventions. An angry client or family may need relaxation training to temper high emotion, or concrete skills training for specifics on coping with the environment, or a formal understanding of patterns that they can expect to repeat in the society.

Portfolio Reflections

Exercise 10. Your reflections on multicultural issues and counseling and therapy as liberation

What stood out for you from this chapter? What sense did you make of what you have read and experienced? What are your key points from this chapter? Write your thoughts here and add them to your Portfolio Folder in your computer.

_____

_____

_____

_____

_____

_____

REFERENCES

Alschuler, A. (1986). Creating a world where it is easier to love: Counseling applications of Paulo Freire's theory. *Journal of Counseling and Development, 64,* 492–496.

Andreas, S., & Faulkner, C. (Eds.). (1996). *NLP: The new technology.* New York: Quill.

Arredondo, P., & Perez, P. (2003). Expanding multicultural competencies through social justice leadership. *The Counseling Psychologist, 31,* 282–289.

Atkinson, D., Morten, G., & Sue, D. W. (1993). *Counseling American minorities* (3rd ed.). Dubuque, IA: Brown.

Cameron, S., Chavez, C., King, G., & turtle-song, I. (2001, March). *Reframing DCT: A Native American approach.* Presentation to the American Counseling Association Convention, San Antonio.

Cass, V. C. (1979). Homosexual identity formation: A theoretical model. *Journal of Homosexuality, 4,* 219–235.

Cass, V. C. (1984). Homosexual identity formation: Testing a theoretical model. *Journal of Sex Research, 20,* 143–167.

Cass, V. C. (1990). The implications of homosexual identity formation for the Kinsey model and scale of sexual preference. In D. P. McWhirter, S. A. Sanders, & J. M. Reinisch (Eds.),

Homosexuality/heterosexuality: Concepts of sexual orientation (pp. 239–266). New York: Oxford University Press.

Cornford, F. (Ed.). (1981). *The republic of Plato*. London: Oxford University Press. (Original work published 1941)

Cross, W. (1971). The Negro to Black conversion experience. *Black World, 20,* 13–25.

Cross, W. (1991). *Shades of black.* Philadelphia: Temple University Press.

Cross, W. (1995). The psychology of Nigrescence: Revising the Cross model. In J. Ponterotto, J. Casas, L. Suzuki, & C. Alexander (Eds.), *Handbook of multicultural counseling* (pp. 93–122). Thousand Oaks, CA: Sage.

Cross, W., & Vandiver, B. (2001). Nigrescence theory and measurement. In J. Ponterotto, J. Casas, L. Suzuki, & C. Alexander (Eds.), *Handbook of multicultural counseling* (2nd ed., pp. 371–393). Thousand Oaks, CA: Sage.

Degges-White, S., Rice, B., & Myers, J. (2000). Revisiting Cass' theory of sexual identity formation: A study of lesbian development. *Journal of Mental Health Counseling, 22,* 318–333.

Erikson, E. (1963). *Childhood and society* (2nd ed.). New York: Norton. (Original work published 1950)

Fischer, A., & Moradi, B. (2001). Racial and ethnic identity: Recent developments and needed directions. In J. Ponterotto, J. Casas, L. Suzuki, & C. Alexander (Eds.), *Handbook of multicultural counseling* (2nd ed., pp. 341–370). Thousand Oaks, CA: Sage.

Freire, P. (1970). *Pedagogy of the oppressed.* New York: Herder & Herder.

Hardiman, R. (1995). *White identity development: Origins and prospect.* (Videotape). North Amherst, MA: Microtraining Associates.

Helms, J. (1985). Toward a theoretical explanation of the effects of race on counseling: A Black and White model. *The Counseling Psychologist, 12,* 153–165.

Helms, J. (1990). *Black and White racial identity: Theory, research, and practice.* New York: Greenwood.

Helms, J. (2003). A pragmatic view of social justice. *The Counseling Psychologist, 31,* 305–313.

Ivey, A. (1995). Psychotherapy as liberation. In J. Ponterotto, J. M. Casas, L. Suzuki, & C. Alexander (Eds.), *Handbook of multicultural counseling and therapy.* Beverly Hills, CA: Sage.

Ivey, A., & Collins, N. (2003). Social justice: A long-term challenge for counseling psychology. *The Counseling Psychologist, 31,* 290–298.

Ivey, A., D'Andrea, M., Ivey, M., & Simek-Morgan, L. (2002). *Counseling and psychotherapy: A multicultural perspective.* Boston: Allyn & Bacon.

Ivey, A., & Payton, P. (1994). Toward a Cornish identity theory. *Cornish Studies, 2,* 151–163.

Locke, D. (1992). *Increasing multicultural understanding: A comprehensive model.* Beverly Hills, CA: Sage.

Marszalek, J. F., III, & Cashwell, C. S. (1998). The gay and lesbian affirmative development (GLAD) model: Applying Ivey's developmental counseling therapy model to Cass's gay and lesbian identity development model. *Adultspan Journal, 1,* 13–31. (Also published in *The Journal of Adult Development and Aging: Theory and Research* [Online journal], *1*(1), http://www.uncg.edu/ced/jada)

Marszalek, J. F., III, Cashwell, C. S., Dunn, M. S., & Heard, K. (in press). Comparing gay identity development theory to cognitive development: An empirical study. *Journal of Homosexuality.*

McIntosh, P. (1989, July–August). White privilege: Unpacking the invisible knapsack. *Peace and Freedom,* 8–10. (Also see http://www.utoronto.ca/acc/events/peggy1.htm for a complete text of this article.)

Parham, T., White, J., & Ajamu, A. (1999). *The psychology of Blacks: An African centered perspective.* Upper Saddle River, NJ: Prentice Hall.

Ponterotto, J. (1988). An organizational framework for understanding the role of culture in counseling. *Journal of Counseling and Development, 53,* 410–418.

Ponterotto, J., Casas, J., Suzuki, L., & Alexander, C. (Eds.). (2001). *Handbook of multicultural counseling* (2nd ed.). Thousand Oaks, CA: Sage.

Semmier, P., & Williams, C. (2000). Narrative therapy: A storied context for multicultural counseling. *Journal of Multicultural Counseling and Development, 28,* 51–62.

Steele, S. (2003, April 29). The souls of Black folk. *Wall Street Journal,* p. 16.

Sue, D. W., Ivey, A., & Pedersen, P. (1996). *A theory of multicultural counseling and therapy.* Pacific Grove, CA: Brooks/Cole.

Thomas, C. (1971). *Boys no more.* Beverly Hills, CA: Glencoe.

Utsey, S., Chae, M., Brown, C., & Kelly, D. (2002). Effect of ethnic group membership on ethnic identity, race-related stress, and quality of life. *Cultural diversity and ethnic minority psychology, 8,* 366–377.

Vera, E., & Speight, S. (2003). Multicultural competence, social justice, and counseling psychology. *The Counseling Psychologist, 31,* 253–272.

Answers to Exercise 4. Classifying Cultural Identity Stages (pp. 266–267)

1. 1	5. 2	9. 4	13. 1	17. 1
2. 2	6. 1	10. 2	14. 2	18. 2
3. 3	7. 3	11. 1	15. 4	19. 3
4. 4	8. 4	12. 3	16. 4	20. 4

Reframing the *Diagnostic and Statistical Manual of Mental Disorders*

Positive Strategies From Developmental Counseling and Therapy

CENTRAL PRACTICE OBJECTIVE

Mastery and practice of concepts in this chapter will enable you to reframe severe distress as a logical biological and psychological response to environmental conditions. You will be able to develop comprehensive treatment plans, using multiple theoretical orientations and strategies, to work with issues such as depression, personality style ("disorder"), and post-traumatic stress.

In recent years, counselors and therapists have found a marked increase in clients who are experiencing severe distress. You can expect that a portion of your practice, regardless of the setting, will entail working with clients who present really challenging issues. The average American child today reports more anxiety than child psychiatric patients did in the 1950s (Tomsho, 2003). In a study covering 40 years, Twinge (2000) found that neuroticism and anxiety levels in both children and adults had increased almost a full standard deviation. "Correlations with social indices (divorce rates, crime rates) suggest that decreases in social connectedness and increases in environmental dangers may be responsible for the rise in anxiety" (p. 1007). Depression is also increasingly prevalent throughout the world (Muñoz, 2001). Out of a more anxious and tense age comes greater possibility of severe stressors—and thus more clients in deep need of your sensitive care.

Given that severe distress is increasingly common, how can we integrate a positive developmental approach with current models of psychopathology? All of us work at times with children, adolescents, adults, and families in severe distress and most of us would admit that the *Diagnostic and Statistical Manual of Mental Disorders (DSM-IV-TR)* (American Psychiatric Association, 2000) speaks with at least some accuracy about the human condition. *DSM-IV-TR* is an update of *DSM-IV* (American Psychiatric Association, 1994). Virtually all the language in the text revision *(TR)* is the same as that of the earlier version. However, more attention has been given to gender and cultural issues in the newer version than in previous editions, and there is some updating of language and references.

The developmental view of *DSM-IV-TR* embodied in developmental counseling and therapy may be useful in helpful us taking a positive, proactive view as we work with so-called pathology. This chapter suggests that *there is no necessary conflict between a developmental and a pathological view.* We do suggest, however, that a new perspective is needed, a synthesis that retains the integrity of our positive developmental frame and yet provides concrete ways to approach problematic human conditions with specific actions and treatment plans.

Developmental counseling and therapy (DCT) prefers to use the words *severe distress* rather than psychopathology or mental illness. The stressors causing the distress may be biological, interpersonal, or intrapersonal. More broadly, they represent the result of major stressors that occur between the individual and the environment. Severe distress (or "psychopathology") is described as a logical response to often insane environmental conditions. Thus, both the individual and the social context are addressed within DCT treatment planning. This chapter focuses on a practical system for dealing with clients who present with severe distress. You will not find all the answers here, but you will find an integrated philosophy and practice that will enable you to conceptualize and work more effectively with challenging clients who face complex and very difficult situations.

Portions of this chapter are reprinted from Ivey, A., and Ivey, M., "Reframing *DSM-IV*: Positive strategies from developmental counseling and therapy," *Journal of Counseling and Development, 76,* 334–350 (1998). © American Counseling Association. Reprinted with permission. No further reproduction authorized without written permission of the American Counseling Association.

Knowledge of and skill in the concepts of this chapter can enable you to:

1. Challenge traditional views of "disorder" and "mental illness" and view severe emotional and psychological distress from a positive developmental frame of reference.
2. Understand and work with personality "disorder," described in Axis II of *DSM-IV-TR*, from a positive frame of reference. Specifically, you will be able to describe how developmental personality styles are logical responses to developmental history—biological and psychological.
3. Frame the serious "disorders" of Axis I as the failure of Axis II defensive structures.
4. Understand how developmental history, particularly as outlined by John Bowlby's attachment theory, and multicultural issues relate to severe emotional stressors. Important among these stressors is post-traumatic stress.
5. Generate developmentally appropriate treatment plans from a positive DCT and wellness perspective.

INTRODUCTION: DISORDER OR DEVELOPMENTAL ISSUE?

Let us begin by reviewing how *DSM-IV-TR* defines "mental disorder" (American Psychiatric Association, 2000, p. xxxi):

> a clinically significant behavioral or psychological syndrome or pattern that occurs in an individual and that is associated with present distress (e.g., a painful symptom) or disability (i.e., impairment in one or more important areas of functioning) or with a significantly increased risk of suffering, death, pain, or disability, or an important loss of freedom. In addition, this syndrome or pattern must not merely be an expectable and culturally sanctioned response to a particular event, for example, the death of a loved one. Whatever its original cause, it must be currently considered a manifestation of a behavioral, psychological, or biological dysfunction in the individual. . . . Neither deviant behavior (e.g., political, religious, or sexual) nor conflicts that are primarily between the individual and society are mental disorders unless the deviance or conflict is a symptom of a dysfunction of the individual as described above.

DSM-IV-TR provides us with only four lines of text on the topic of treatment (p. xxv), noting that substantial information is required before moving to action based on diagnosis. Koerner, Kohlenberg, and Parker (1996) sharply challenge the idea that diagnosis should be so separate from treatment. The critical test of any diagnostic classification system, they say, is whether it enables more effective intervention. These authors, taking a radical behavioral perspective, comment that diagnostic classification systems should link "problems, outcomes, and the proposed processes of change" (p. 1170). In that view, *DSM-IV-TR* becomes a potential barrier to client growth and change because of its lack of linkages useful for the therapeutic process.

Nonetheless, a number of efforts have been made over the years to suggest specific treatment alternatives for *DSM-IV-TR* issues. Beck, Freeman, and Associates

(1990) provide concrete ideas for linking Axis II diagnoses to treatment, giving some attention to etiology. Another useful approach is that of Jongsma, Peterson, and McInnis (1996), who suggest specific treatment plans for children. The American Psychiatric Association has developed a video series, *Treatment of Psychiatric Disorders,* for continuing education. In one of these segments, Rush (1995) presents materials on etiology and treatment of mood disorders. An earlier work, Masterson's (1981) object relations conception of the borderline and narcissistic individual, has been influential in enabling connections between the past when the condition developed, the present, and specific treatment suggestions. Nonetheless, all of these approaches tend to locate the problem "in the individual" and work from a pathological rather than a developmental frame.

The pathological view of working with severe distress continues to this day. The traditional medical model of repair and restore continues to be the model of choice for most. Muñoz (2001) reviews the literature and argues for a preventive and psychoeducational approach to treatment. He focuses on a public health frame of reference in which wellness and positive mental health are stressed. His conclusions are consistent with Larson's (1999) suggestion that multiple approaches to health care are needed, incorporating both the medical and wellness models in a comprehensive system of health care. Thus, a review of Chapter 2 may be beneficial as you consider, or reconsider, the applications presented here.

An alternative viewpoint is provided by Seem and Hernandez (1997), Paniagua (1998), and Smart and Smart (1997), who remind us that the *DSM-IV-TR* exists in a cultural context—all etiological, diagnostic, and treatment approaches need to be managed with awareness of culture perspectives. They also question the absence of linkage to etiology and treatment within *DSM-IV-TR.* These authors are important in moving the field to a culture-centered frame of reference.

Agreeing with the authors above and the radical behavioral assumption that diagnosis needs to be tied clearly to treatment, developmental counseling and therapy (DCT) adds the importance of a positive developmental approach in conceptualizing client history within a cultural context, understanding client behavior in the here and now of the interview, and utilizing multiple treatment alternatives in a network model of treatment and action (see Ivey, 1991, 2000; Ivey & Ivey, 1993).

This chapter is based on the idea that so-called disorder is a logical response to developmental history and environmental/biological conditions. We need to transcend a somewhat defeatist orientation to severe emotional distress, move beyond our orientation to psychopathology, and replace old systems with a positive developmental view. Those who are acquainted with the developmental and wellness orientations are well prepared to undertake a new approach that will enable us to work more effectively in mental health teams as we face the severe emotional distress of clients. Let us start with an exploration of the meaning of pathology within a developmental orientation.

Transcending Pathology

"According to . . . *DSM-IV-TR,* human life is a form of mental illness" (Davis, 1997, p. 63). Davis notes that bad writing (315.2), coffee nerves (305.90), and jet lag (307.45) are examples of how the field has tended to pathologize even the most normal behavior. Socioeconomic issues are glossed over, indicating, for example, that those who are poor may suffer from a limited vocabulary (expressive language disorder, 315.31). Perhaps most important, Davis comments that seldom does *DSM-IV-TR* touch on the nature of sanity, mental health, and normality. While perhaps over-critical of *DSM-IV-TR*, these comments remind us that diagnostic systems need more balance and attention to the reality of human experience, wellness, and positive psychology.

Seem and Hernandez (1997) sharply criticize *DSM-IV-TR* for insufficient attention to cross-cultural and feminist issues. They describe *DSM-IV-TR* as an exercise in power and dominance, citing Jean Baker Miller (1976): "Once a group is defined as inferior, the superiors tend to label it as defective or substandard in various ways. . . . the actions of the dominant group tend to be destructive of subordinates" (p. 6). Seem and Hernandez conduct a cultural and feminist analysis of *DSM-IV-TR*, ending with an appeal for a more culture-centered and egalitarian approach to diagnosis.

Table 9-1 presents the *Diagnostic and Statistical Manual* system as usually constructed in psychiatry and psychology in contrast with the DCT frame. The contrast between the two is summarized here:

DSM-IV-TR —pathology is most often described as located *"in an individual"* (American Psychiatric Association, 2000, p. xxi, italics ours). Etiology and treatment are not stressed.

DCT—distress (rather than "pathology") is a logical result of biological and developmental insult. The stressor may be located within the individual and/or in broader systemic and historical factors. Treatment plans related to assessment are central.

For example, let us contrast the two models around the construct of depression. Both models would use the behavioral/attitudinal categories of *DSM-IV-TR*, but the

Table 9-1 *DSM-IV-TR:* The Contrast Between Traditional and DCT Meaning-Making Systems

Issue	Traditional Pathological DSM-IV-TR Meaning	Developmental Meaning
Locus of problem	Individual	Individual/family/cultural context
Pathology	Yes	No, logical response to developmental history
Developmental and etiological constructs	Peripheral	Central
Culture	Beginning awareness	Culture-centered
Helper role	Hierarchy, patriarchy	Egalitarian, co-construction
Cause	Linear Biology vs. environment	Multidimensional; considers both biology and environment
Family	Not stressed	Vital for understanding individual development and treatment
Treatment	Not stressed	Central issue

meaning attached would be markedly different. Depression is traditionally seen as something that exists in the individual and as pathological. We would argue that this tends to victimize the client. The developmental model sees depression existing in the interaction among the individual's biological and social history, the family, and the cultural context. Depression is constructed as *a logical response to developmental concerns*, blocks, or difficulties in one or more of these dimensions. Treatment focuses on multiple dimensions so that the client understands distress in social context.

We should recognize that *DSM-IV* has made useful beginnings to include culturally relevant issues, including the following key statement (American Psychiatric Association, 1994, p. xxiv): Clinicians "may incorrectly judge as psychopathological those normal variations in behavior, belief, or experience that are particular to the individual's culture." Paniagua (1998) points out that *DSM-IV* does not make such possible cultural issues central; rather, they remain peripheral. He also notes that the discussion of depression in *DSM-IV* includes cultural issues only in regard to Major Depressive Disorder.

We should not forget that, developmentally, depression may result from external circumstances; for example, in African Americans or women, depression could result from cultural racism or sexism. Carter (2003) identifies constant racial harassment as a traumatic insult to the person. Through repeated instances of microaggressions encountered daily, depression, high blood pressure, and other physical and psychological issues logically follow. Where is the disorder located—in the person or in the environment?

People with disability suffer parallel problems. Allen Ivey's father went through sudden blindness, the loss of sight overnight. Grieving over the loss in the hospital, he was considerably upset and depressed—a reaction that would seem to be a logical and reasonable response to most people. Not grieving the loss of sight would seem truly disturbed. However, the physicians rapidly diagnosed him as experiencing clinical depression and started organizing *DSM-IV* treatment recommendations, failing to provide time for the author's father to even experience and reflect on the trauma.

In the DCT view, the distress of depression is considered one expected result of the interaction of person and environment. This environmental orientation, however, does not rule out biological factors; rather, environment interacts with personal biology. However, *DSM-IV-TR* still locates the depression *in the individual.*

The psychotherapy as liberation concepts presented in the chapter on multicultural issues is important in the reframing of *DSM-IV-TR.* The assignment of names is a process that occurs in an egalitarian setting in which the client becomes an active participant in diagnosis. Labels and their meanings are openly discussed with the individual. Co-construction of diagnosis is essential from a DCT perspective whether you work with severe psychological distress or instances of oppression from a multicultural counseling and therapy frame of reference.

The naming/meaning process within a developmental orientation "provides for the transformation of the person in terms of body and mind; it provides transcendence of the person's relationship with the universe" (Levers & Maki, 1994, p. 83). Within this developmental frame is the possibility for the inclusion of culture-related issues such as race/ethnicity, gender, sexual preference, spirituality, and others as part of the movement toward the future. In the DCT frame, a diagnosis that is not culture-centered with awareness of multiple contextual issues is seen as incomplete at best and potentially dangerous and misleading. The naming process most commonly associated with *DSM-IV-TR* is the placing of an individual in a diagnostic box.

The Importance of Axis II

Clinicians give *DSM-IV-TR*'s Axis I major attention, for here we find the focus on diagnosing severe distress (schizophrenia, depression, panic reactions, etc.). The DCT approach, however, suggests that we start with an examination of Axis II personality style. Axis II provides a framework of basic personality "disorders" with some very negative labels such as "narcissistic," "borderline," or "histrionic." Although the listing of behaviors and styles within *DSM-IV-TR* is useful, DCT assumes that all personality *styles* (not "disorders") represent logical adaptive functioning. For example, all of us need to be cautious in some situations and even mistrustful of others at times. Carried to extreme, of course, caution and mistrust result in what *DSM-IV-TR* terms the paranoid personality "disorder." DCT would point out that behind many, perhaps most, paranoid styles is a documented history of significant persecution. For example, indigenous and minority populations in the Western world have a disproportionate amount of diagnosed paranoia. We would suggest that cautious "paranoid" behavior may be a logical response to external environmental conditions.

Stiver (1991) places a positive meaning on the personality style of dependency, pointing out that so-called dependent individuals have the potential to attach and care. They are deeply aware of the importance of interpersonal relationships. In a Western society that emphasizes separation and autonomy, there is great need to reawaken us to our interdependency with others. This focus on positives within client issues is basic to the DCT frame of reference, so much so that we recommend, *"If you can't find something positive in the client's behavior and history—refer!"*

Kjos (1995) has linked career counseling to Axis II concerns. For example, *workaholics* are constructed within the obsessive-compulsive style. The high standards of perfection required in some jobs can make this style useful. But carried to excess, it can lead to serious problems and poor job performance. Treatment, according to Kjos, needs to focus on client strengths as well as difficulties. Each developmental personality disorder/style has healthy dimensions.

Each personality style has its positive dimensions and they are detailed briefly in Table 9-2. These positive dimensions, coupled with developmental understanding, can lead to new and cooperative treatment plans, even in the difficult area of deeply ingrained personality styles. The positive asset search has been basic in microcounseling's approach to skills training for more than 30 years (Ivey & Gluckstern, 1974; Ivey & Ivey, 2003). From a DCT perspective, much of the success of narrative therapy (White & Epston, 1990) and brief therapy (de Shazer, 1982; Littrell, 1998; O'Hanlon & Weiner-Davis, 1989) rests on the constant search for positives and exceptions to the problem.

In truth, we find relatively few individuals with a single personality style. Rather, most of us are mixes of varying styles. The balanced individual needs to be

Table 9-2 Developmental Personality Styles

Style and Positive Aspect	Behavior/Thoughts in Session	Possible Family History	Predicted Current Relationships	Possible Treatment Approach
Paranoid—it is important to watch out for injustice	Suspicious, takes remarks out of context and interprets them to support own frame of reference	Possible history of persecution, active family rejection	Controlling behavior, anticipates exploitation, quick to anger, may mistrust friends and family	Always be honest, never defensive; structure ahead of time; don't argue, you'll only lose
Schizoid—it is useful to be a loner or independent of others at times	Relationship with therapist fragile, constricted body stance, little emotion shown, problems accepting support	Cold family; received little affection, rewarded for being alone and on own, may be identified patient in otherwise normal family	Loner; few friends, superficial relationships	Be consistent, warm, supportive—no pressure; social skills training may be helpful
Schizotypal—ability to see things differently than others see them	Ideas of reference, social anxiety; odd magical beliefs, odd behavior, limited affect, distant, vague	Chaotic family style; family anxious/ambivalent with mixed messages, combination of intrusion/rejection	Loner; no close friends, perhaps an unusual or "different" peer group	Same as above; behavior may be seen as engulfing; important to maintain verbal tracking on single topic
Antisocial—it is sometimes necessary to be impulsive and take care of our own needs	Acts out; cannot sustain task; involved in crime, drugs, truancy, physical fights; cruel, maltreats family; tries to "con" therapist	Probable abuse as child; avoidant family forced child to take matters into own hands; little affection in home	Abusive, exploitive relationships; fear of abandonment	Be open, honest, and set clear limits; avoid entanglement; expect client to leave treatment if you get close
Borderline—intensity in relationships is desirable at times	Pushes therapist's "buttons" skillfully; impulsive, intense anger or caring, suicidal gestures	Enmeshed family during early childhood; lack of support for individuation; possible sexual abuse	Serial, intense relationships; may have close friends, relationships may move rapidly between extreme closeness and distance	Confront engulfment and support individuation—that is, do opposite of family; group/systems approaches are useful
Histrionic—all could benefit at times from open access to emotions	Seeks reassurance; seductive, concerned with appearance, too much affect, self-centered, vague conversation	Enmeshed, engulfing family, with little support for individuation; possible sexual abuse/seduction; little family expectation for accomplishment; aware of others not of self	Similar to the borderline without the externalized anger; actions directed inward rather than outward	Encourage individuation; use assertiveness, skills training, consciousness raising; examine history of problem; use cognitive-behavioral and systems interventions

(continued)

Table 9-2 *(continued)*

Style and Positive Aspect	Behavior/Thoughts in Session	Possible Family History	Predicted Current Relationships	Possible Treatment Approach
Narcissistic—a strong belief in ourselves is necessary for good mental health	Grandiose, self-important, sees self as unique; sense of entitlement; lacks empathy, oriented toward success and perfection	Received perfect mirroring for accomplishments rather than for self; engulfing family; child enacts family's wishes; anxious/ambivalent caregiver	Focuses on selfish needs, tends to engulf others with needs; is charming to get wishes met, Don Juan type, may be paired with borderline	Interpret behavior; look to past; employ cognitive-behavioral, systems, sensitivity training in a group
Avoidant—it is useful to deny or avoid some things	Avoids people, shy; unwilling to become involved; distant, exaggerates risk	Either engulfing family or avoidant family; enacting what the family modeled	Not many friends; easily becomes dependent on them or therapist	Use many behavioral and cognitive techniques, assertiveness training and relaxation training useful
Dependent—we all need to depend on others	Dependency on therapist even outside of session; indecision, little sense of self	Engulfing, controlling family; not allowed to make decisions; rewarded for inaction, told what to do	Dependent on friends; drives people away with demands	Reward action, support efforts for self, use paradox, assertiveness techniques
Obsessive-compulsive—maintaining order and a system is necessary for job success	Perfectionistic and inflexible; focuses on details, making lists, devoted to work; limited affect, money oriented, indecisive	Overattached family that wanted achievement; oriented to perfection, like narcissist, but keenly aware of others with a limited sense of self	Controlling, limited affect, demands perfection from others, hard worker; cries at sad movies	Reflect and provoke feeling, orient to client's personal needs, support development of self-concept, orient to body awareness
Passive-aggressive—all of us are entitled to procrastinate at times	Procrastination; seems to agree with therapist, then undercuts; seems to accept therapist, then challenges authority	Perhaps controlling family; individual instead moves away from perfectionism and fights back; a more healthy defense needs to be developed	"Couch potato," skilled at getting back at and criticizing others; defends by doing nothing; resents suggestions; not pleasant on the job	Let them learn the consequences of their behavior; do not do things for them, but confront and interpret and pay special attention

dependent on others at some times and suspicious or cautious at other times—and certainly needs a degree of healthy narcissism. In short, DCT suggests that a developmental balance of these styles may represent positive mental health.

Manifesting to an extreme degree one or two personality dimensions rather than a balance of several is a result of developmental history in family and culture, personal physiology, and severe stressors. The individual who forsakes dependency on others for acting-out antisocial behavior has become stuck with a limited range of thought, feeling, and action. And it is important to recall that people who live the antisocial style very often come from a history of severe neglect and abuse.

In short, DCT argues that we all need to seek a balance of defensive styles and recognize that so-called pathology is really our best effort to make meaning and find workable behaviors in a complex and confusing world. A related issue from Axis I is the child or adolescent diagnosed with attention-deficit/hyperactivity "disorder." The medicalized *DSM-IV-TR* approach too often allows us to put the "problem" *in the child* solely. Environmental stressors, family issues, and insensitive teachers become almost irrelevant as we rely on medication as the way to solve behavioral issues. ADHD conceptualized more systemically would likely result in less medication; moreover, it also would require the system to adapt to the uniqueness of the child.

THE DEVELOPMENTAL MEANING OF PERSONALITY STYLES

This section explores how personality styles are learned in family and social context. While biology remains important, the DCT approach suggests that we need to examine developmental history in any consideration of severe distress and trauma. Special attention is given to a positive reframing of strengths within each personality style. A five-stage theoretical framework outlines possible developmental history and events behind each style. From this framework, we can learn how to anticipate developmental history from client behavior in the session, develop appropriate empathic relationships, and begin to generate comprehensive treatment plans.

Given a positive development frame, the therapist seeks to make meaning in and from personality styles (Ivey, 1991; Ivey, D'Andrea, Ivey, & Simek-Morgan, 2002). In particular, the DCT framework suggests the need to seek positive assets and developmental strengths in client meaning making and behavior. For explaining emotional and cognitive development, the work of James Masterson (1981) as he conceptualizes the borderline style has been particularly helpful. Masterson draws from Bowlby's (1969, 1973, 1988) attachment theory and Mahler's (1975) object relations approach. However, Masterson still uses a pathological meaning-making system and gives insufficient attention to sociocultural factors, although his explanation of family issues is highly useful.

We all need basic attachment to our caregivers. From this base of relatively secure attachment, we can later separate into autonomous beings. Masterson talks about the borderline personality as frequently born out of an enmeshed caregiver-child system. Efforts of the child to separate are met inconsistently by the caregiver, who might respond to autonomous efforts of the child one time with fear, the next time with anger, and the next with indifference. Anything the child does is bound to fail. Thus, adolescent or adult borderline behavior is seen as rooted in earlier attachment patterns in the family, particularly, in Masterson's frame, with the mother. What the child needs is a *balance* of separation and attachment tasks. Within the DCT framework, this concept of balance can be extended to cultural variations, as different child-rearing styles tend to lead to varying pictures of the appropriate balance of individuation and connectedness.

While attachment is the foundation for effective separation and individuation, the second task is separation from the caregiver. *Separation difficulties lead to depression, which, in turn, tends to lead to personality "disorder";* this is a brief summary of what Masterson terms the "borderline triad." In effect, the failure of the borderline individual to separate successfully leads to sadness and depression. In Masterson's frame, borderline behavior and cognitions become a defensive style masking the very real and profound pain of the underlying depression. Masterson also gives attention to the narcissistic and antisocial styles, pointing out that, like the borderline person, individuals exhibiting these styles also have developed their personality styles as a defense against underlying depression.

Atkinson and Goldberg (2003) have given extensive attention to issues of attachment and how this theory relates to psychopathology and specific treatment interventions. Their careful review of the literature and clear explanation of attachment theory provide a solid foundation for further study and applied practice. In addition, they are among the first to recognize the vital importance of attachment theory as a basis for treatment. This chapter is in full agreement with their concepts and you will find many treatment parallels between the DCT approach and their methods. Attachment theory provides a sturdy theoretical/practical base for counseling and psychotherapy.

Separation and attachment concepts, however, can be criticized from a culture-centered framework as the "center" or balance point is not defined. In the DCT frame, each family and culture is seen as having different ideas of the appropriate balance. The Native American tradition, for example, focuses on *interdependence* and *holism* as the focal point of relationships. LaFromboise (1996), Trimble and Fleming (1989), and McCormick (1997), as well as Garrett (1999) and Garrett and Myers (1996) have all addressed the holistic frame of reference while criticizing autonomy and independence as often inappropriate goals for counseling. Speaking from a Native American perspective, McGaa (1989, p. xv) states:

> Interdependence is at the center of all things. The separation between nature and us is a mirage. The perception of separation is the result of ignorance that stems from the arrogant belief that a human being is unlike animal beings and rock beings and plant beings.

From this orientation to life, it can be seen that locating issues *in the individual* is an example of cultural imperialism and colonialism (see, especially, Duran & Duran, 1995).

Flaherty (1989) studied 20 borderline inpatients and found that 19 of them had experienced sexual abuse or incest. This is a clear example in U.S. culture of how external experience relates to what happens in the person. While we give Masterson high compliments for his theoretical conceptions, we again raise the question: *Is the problem in the individual, or is it in the system?*

Medication tends not to be effective for the borderline client, but may be useful when underlying depression appears. Borderline clients find depression so painful that their constantly varying behaviors and emotions are preferred to mask the underlying sadness. When we view it from this framework, we realize that the borderline style is a logical result of environmental insult.

DCT expands the Masterson model. The several diagnostic categories of Axis II remind us that depression is an underlying component of all the severe personality "disorders" or styles (see *DSM-IV-TR*'s comments about associated features of each Axis II diagnosis in Table 9-3). The counseling task, of course, is to unravel the developmental history and logic underlying personal style and to help the client write a new, more positive narrative with accompanying behavioral change.

Table 9-3   Developmental Personality Styles Related to Axis I Diagnoses

Axis II Personality Style	Examples of Axis I Diagnoses Related to Failure of Defensive Structures
Paranoid	Schizophrenia, paranoid type, delusional disorder
Schizoid Schizotypal	Schizophrenia, catatonic, disorganized type, undifferentiated, schizoaffective disorder, delusional disorder, childhood disintegrative disorder, Asperger's disorder, *child attachment disorder*
Antisocial	Strong tendency for concurrent substance abuse, post-traumatic stress, depression, attention deficit disorder, oppositional defiant disorder, conduct disorder
Borderline	Mood disorders, *depression,* post-traumatic stress, substance abuse, *child attachment disorder*
Histrionic	*Depression,* anxiety disorders, separation anxiety disorders (child and adult), *child attachment disorder*
Narcissistic	*Depression,* anxiety disorders, panic disorder, manic, hypomanic episode, *child attachment disorder*
Avoidant	*Depression,* anxiety disorders, social phobia, panic disorder, *child attachment disorder*
Dependent	Social phobia, *depression,* anxiety disorders, panic disorder, agoraphobia, mood disorders, *child attachment disorder*
Obsessive-compulsive	Obsessive-compulsive disorder, *depression,* anxiety disorders, phobias, addictive disorders, *child attachment disorder,* stereotypic movement disorder
Passive-aggressive	Dysthmic disorder, *depression,* oppositional defiant disorder (children), *child attachment disorder*

The following developmental model, an expansion of Masterson's basic triad, has explanatory power both for understanding the client's past and present and for planning treatment options. Briefly summarized, the model is the paradigm presented earlier:

1. Environmental or biological insult (may lead to)
2. Stress and physical/emotional pain, which is a threat to attachment and safety (which, in turn, may lead to)
3. Sadness/depression (which may lead to)
4. Defense against the pain and, in severe cases, Axis II personality styles (which may lead to)
5. Axis I defensive structures

For example, the borderline style might evolve in the following fashion: (1) Biological vulnerability coupled with the environmental trauma of abuse and/or incest leads to (2) severe stress with impact on physiology and immune system functioning as well as deep emotional scars (see, for example, Sherbourne, Hays, & Wells, 1995). These, in turn, lead to (3) deep sadness and depression. (4) The depression itself is so painful that the personality style of the borderline person becomes a defense mechanism against the depression. (5) Finally, a borderline individual under severe stress may decompensate to severe clinical depression, mood disorders, and substance abuse.

In our developmental history, most of us suffer a variety of environmental insults challenging our balance of separation and attachment tasks. We generate behaviors, cognitions, and emotions to defend ourselves from these attacks. Traditional psychodynamic defense mechanisms (sublimation, identification, continuation, projection) are examples of *behavioral complexes* we have learned in our personal experience, our families, and our cultural surround. When these defensive structures become inadequate or rigid, we see the arrival of Axis II personality styles (see Ivey et al., 2002, for a more complete discussion of the relationship between defense mechanisms and Axis II).

We stress that there is a developmental logic to any client's thought, emotion, behavior, or meaning organization. We believe that knowing how to treat depression and sadness is a central dimension for all counselors and therapists (a later section explores the issue of treatment in more detail). There is a distinction between depression at stage 3 above and clinical depression. The first is a sadness specifically (and normally) related to environmental insult or trauma. Clinical depression exists in a set of diagnostic categories within Axis I.

Clinical depression manifests itself more fully and completely when stress and environmental conditions break down Axis II defensive personality postures. One important route toward remediation and prevention of the trauma's becoming fixated intrapsychically is early intervention in which the trauma is openly focused on and discussed as soon as possible (Foa, Rothbaum, Riggs, & Murdock , 1991; Foa, Hearst-Ikeda, & Perry, 1995).

Masterson points out that underlying the antisocial personality is a depression so painful that the individual may run from therapy rather than deal with this foundational pain and sadness. Most antisocial personality diagnoses reveal a history of abuse and neglect. But this, of course, does not deny biological issues. At the same time, however, we would point out that child-rearing procedures and life experiences affect the child biologically as well as psychologically. Are we dealing with "wiring" or environment or, more likely, some combination of the two?

In the DCT view, the several developmental personality styles of Axis II are seen as learned ways of defending oneself against depression and underlying pain, particularly when early intervention has been absent or has failed. Table 9-2 presents the DCT developmental conception of Axis II. Note that the DCT framework suggests that each personality style has a positive, survival function that we need to respect and honor. Client behavior in the session will manifest the characteristics listed in *DSM-IV-TR*. And from this behavior we can conceptualize and anticipate client personal and family developmental history. We can also predict what is going on in their lives here and now in terms of relationships and vocational success or failure.

Our view of Axis II was the result of working with a practicum student who was counseling a high school–age client; this client showed many signs of classical dependency. The student came to the practicum student counselor several times daily pleading for advice and assistance on multiple issues. At first the student counselor was flattered and gave extensive support and nurturance, even suggesting some decisions to the client. But this only resulted in more dependency and the client came to spend almost every possible minute with the counselor. Finally, the student counselor became frustrated and started rejecting the client, at which time the client became more insistent. Then the student counselor became guilty and started reassuring the client and meeting her dependency needs again. This continued in a cycle of support and rejection. Neither the client nor the student counselor was satisfied with the situation.

Vocationally, the dependent high school student had been fired from three out-of-school placements because of her inability to take responsibility and act on her own. She relied extensively on her mother and a few remaining friends for the decisions she did not make without the counselor. Discussion of the family history revealed a dominating father and a mother who modeled the dependent style herself. An extensive history of learned dependent behavior in the home emerged. It seemed that the client's mother behaved toward her daughter as the counselor did, with an alternating pattern of support and rejection.

The dependent client was repeating her family developmental history in the interview, with her friends, and in the work setting. This discovery was made when the case was reviewed on videotape and the practicum student realized that the client was repeating client family patterns in the interview. And the practicum student saw that she, herself, was in many ways repeating behavioral and emotional styles from the client's family of origin. The resolution and eventual improvement of the dependent client revolved around treating her differently from the way she had been treated in the past by members of her family (see a later portion of this chapter for elaboration of treatment issues). Supervision for the practicum student focused on helping her become aware of her own developmental history. We often find that so-called blocks in the counseling relationship are really blocks and impasses in the counselor or therapist.

The case example above is important for reminding us that personality issues exist not only in mental health centers but also in our schools. The overly dependent child or adolescent is often seen by counselors and teachers as a nuisance and they too often offer little in the way of understanding and treatment. And overly dependent young women are most vulnerable to narcissistic and antisocial males who have a strong possibility of abusing them on dates or treating them violently in longer-term relationships. Paniagua (1998) examines Axis II of *DSM-IV* for cultural awareness and comments that cultural observations are too broad to be clinically helpful. One example is the histrionic style—"Norms for personal appearance, emotional expressiveness, and interpersonal behavior vary widely across cultures. . . . It is important to determine whether these symptoms cause clinically significant impairment or distress to the individual in comparison to what is culturally expected" (American Psychiatric Association, 2000, p. 712).

But what of Axis I?

AXIS I AS THE FAILURE OF AXIS II DEFENSIVE STRUCTURES

The personality styles of Axis II have been presented as defensive structures created by the individual to protect her or him from underlying depression and sadness. We have suggested that the healthier individual maintains a balance, and that one sign of danger or imminent breakdown is extreme reliance on one personality style. In this section we suggest that Axis I disorders are the result of Axis II personality style failure in defending the person from underlying trauma and distress. Fortunately, we know how to treat Axis I problems far more effectively than the more deeply rooted Axis II conditions. There is a problem, however. *When we have success at the Axis I level, the client often returns to Axis II defensive structures where our treatment efforts are often less effective.* For example, it is common for a client with a borderline or narcissistic style to break down under stress into Axis I depression. We can treat the depression fairly effectively, but when the depression lifts, the client returns to the original problematic personality style. The underlying family history and attachment style remain. The route toward resolving Axis II issues usually requires longer-term therapy, but it also permits more developmentally oriented treatment procedures.

Many Axis I issues can be related to Axis II. Table 9-3 presents some key relationships composed from differential diagnostic issues in *DSM-IV-TR* and DCT theory. As you review Table 9-3, note that most personality styles have some obvious or underlying depression. And, equally important, we can predict which Axis I category is likely to occur if the Axis II personality style fails and decompensates. The paranoid, schizoid, and schizotypal personality styles are expected to be primarily related to schizophrenic features, the antisocial and borderline personalities to substance abuse and severe post-traumatic stress. The histrionic, narcissist, avoidant, and dependent styles are generally related to mood disorders and anxiety, the obsessive compulsive to OCD disorder, and the passive-aggressive to dysthmia and, in children, oppositional defiance.

Perfectionism or self-criticism is an important dimension of several Axis II issues (particularly the obsessive-compulsive style). It was noted as a predictor of unsuccessful treatment for depression by Blatt, Quinlan, Pilkonis, and Shea (1995). Our history of attachment to others relates to our feelings of relation to self and other people. These authors present data and review literature indicating that severe self-critical behavior can lead to suicide attempts, particularly as related to external standards. Particularly difficult to treat are depressed clients whose feelings of self-criticism are based on an external orientation to others. On the other hand, perfectionism based on feelings of low self-worth and low self-definition was more amenable to successful treatment. These data suggest that an examination of developmental history and the specific nature of depression and personality style can be useful in adjusting treatment plans.

As you read Table 9-3, note how often "attachment disorder" appears in the *DSM-IV-TR* diagnoses. (These words have been placed in italics so that the importance of attachment issues can be more fully appreciated.) This observation may be useful to you as it links Bowlby's attachment theory and the general area of social learning theory and/or object relations theory to *DSM-IV-TR*. This table illustrates how individual styles of relating are connected to issues of separation and attachment in the family of origin. The words *attachment disorder* appear frequently in *DSM-IV-TR* descriptions, but the diagnosis could be made more precise with clearer reference to work stemming from Bowlby's theoretical foundation.

Attachment theory has considerable explanatory power for helping clinicians understand and treat emotional distress. What we see in client behavior before us is the logical result of developmental history (biological "wiring" plus environmental experience). Bowlby's attachment theory is strongly supported by research by Ainsworth (1967, 1977, 1979, 1985) and others (cf. reviews by Ainsworth & Bowlby, 1991; Ivey et al., 2002). We have good evidence that solid early attachments lead to better mental health in later childhood. These data also show strong cross-cultural agreement. Moreover, the data increasingly indicate that these early positive or negative childhood attachments relate to later adult accomplishments or adult difficulties.

Shortly before John Bowlby's death, Allen Ivey had the good fortune to meet with him in London. In a few short, powerful statements, he summarized key points of his theoretical frame. "*Expect the client to treat you as he (or she) was treated*" was Bowlby's summary of how past attachment history affects the client. In the here and now behavior of the interview relationship, the client's past experience will be manifested. Recall the practicum student and the dependent student client who repeated her family relationship in the here and now of the interview. In effect, expect the abused borderline or antisocial client to abuse you as therapist in some way. Anticipate that the client brought up in a family or cultural environment that fostered paranoid behavior will be suspicious of you. From this, you can see that Axis II personality styles are defensive structures representing clients' past experience. The issue is made somewhat more complicated since personality styles can be viewed as complexes of traditional defense mechanisms of isolation, projection, sublimation, and so on (also see Ivey et al., 2002).

When he was queried about treatment implications of attachment theory, Bowlby's first response was equally to the point. Paraphrased, he said, "*Treatment involves treating the client differently from the way he (or she) has been treated in the past.*" *Relationship,* that critical counseling word, becomes even more central, but *precision relationships* are often required. It makes little sense to treat or relate to a dependent client the same way you would a borderline personality. While both may benefit from Rogerian core conditions of empathy and respect, the way we manifest these dimensions must be unique and appropriate to the client's developmental history.

Moreover, we also need to include more awareness of cultural variations that will affect the way we meet the core relationship conditions in the helping interview.

Space does not permit a full account of Bowlby's treatment concepts, but the essence could be summarized informally in the word *reparenting*. For example, the dependent client (overattached) needs acceptance and boundaries but will benefit from a consistent supportive relationship that later builds support for separation attempts. The more difficult borderline client also needs empathic acceptance and boundaries in the relationship, but for you to demonstrate acceptance may be more challenging with this client, and the establishment of boundaries may need to be even clearer. On this foundation, confronting borderline behavior becomes more feasible, and using the microskills of feedback and limited interpretation may be helpful.

The current trend in treating so-called pathological issues is differential treatment without any central conceptual framework. DCT's developmental frame takes the risk of suggesting that a more integrative developmental approach may be feasible. Attachment theory needs to take a central place in a developmentally sophisticated counseling and therapy.

POST-TRAUMATIC STRESS AS A CENTRAL ISSUE

The term *post-traumatic stress* (PTS) rather than *post-traumatic stress disorder* is used in this section. This decision reflects the belief that PTS is a logical internal response to an insane, illogical external situation. The position does not deny the importance of biology or internal cognitions. What is critical, however, is recognizing that PTS is not just internal "wiring." External stress changes internal biological functioning (see, for example, Carter, 2003) and, of course, the pressures of the external world often become internalized psychologically. In the DCT frame, PTS is not considered a "disorder." Rather it is a complex response, based on internal biology and personal psychological history, to external situations. To use the word *disorder* is to locate the problem in the person rather than to recognize that environmental concerns are a central part of the issue. "Atypical" human behavior is again a logical response to environmental contingencies.

Fullerton and Ursano (1997) present a comprehensive view of PTS. Acute stress in multiple forms (war, weather disasters, criminal assault/rape) often results in chronic diagnosable issues known as post-traumatic stress "disorder." Counselors working as volunteers after a disaster such as a plane crash or as crisis counselors with war survivors often demonstrate multiple signs of PTS. Fullerton and Ursano estimate that up to 7% of the U.S. population is exposed to trauma yearly while 1 person in 100 may be affected by PTS throughout her or his life. Post-traumatic stress may be even more common than suggested here. There is evidence that clients who present with depression, anxiety, and other severe problems often have underlying post-traumatic stress that remains undetected (Sheeran & Zimmerman, 2002).

At the same time, trauma experts note that trauma and loss can help some people move to health. The trauma can become a new center for a disorganized life—it can provide meaning and feelings of self-worth as one overcomes distress and/or helps others. Frankl's (1946/1959) *Man's Search for Meaning* immediately comes to mind as illustrative of how healthy and positive intrapersonal and interpersonal strengths can help us find personal power in even the most impossible of situations. Frankl wrote that book in two weeks shortly after his release from a German concentration camp. No doubt the writing was helpful for his own process of recovery, as journaling and bibliotherapy (see Chapter 12) have been shown to be positive supplements to treatment.

Let us return to the five-step model:

1. Environmental or biological insult (may lead to)
2. Stress and physical/emotional pain, which is a threat to attachment and safety (which, in turn, may lead to)
3. Sadness/depression (which may lead to)
4. Defense against the pain and, in severe cases, Axis II personality styles (which may lead to)
5. Axis I defensive structures

Trauma represents a major physiological and psychological insult. The extreme pain of the trauma, if not worked through in a timely fashion, results in depression and an array of severe Axis I and Axis II difficulties. The traumas we most often think of are living through extreme violence, such as the 9/11 attack on the World Trade Center or the war in Iraq, or experiencing rape, abuse, or incest. *DSM-IV-TR's* discussion of trauma wisely includes those who have suffered from social unrest and civil unrest. The abuse and neglect so often experienced by borderline or antisocial clients is another form of common and severe trauma, but this is not part of the formal trauma definition. Moreover, it is increasingly clear that survivors of severe accidents, cancer survivors, people with AIDS, and those who are suddenly disabled experience many of the symptoms of PTS (e.g., distressing recollections of the event, intrusive thoughts, flashbacks, physiological reactivity).

The DCT approach extends the definition of trauma to include repeated sexual or racial harassment, a physical beating as a result of homophobia, poverty, and repeated issues of discrimination for reasons of physical disability or challenge. Many children and adults who experience divorce or growing up in an alcoholic family also experience many of the signs of PTS. Some might respond by pointing out that *DSM-IV-TR's* acute stress disorder needs to be considered from this frame. However, *DSM-IV-TR* limits acute stress disorder to a period of two days to four weeks. The repetition traumas (racism, sexual, verbal harassment from family and/or peers) and their lifetime effects occur daily before and after treatment. At issue for the client is learning how to cope with trauma and realizing that the problem is not her or his issue; rather, it is an external oppressive issue.

Victor Frankl's approach to life in the death camp reminds us how positive meanings can be used to overlay negative experience. When confronted with sadism, hunger, and death, Frankl might notice a brilliant sunset, think of his beloved wife, or rethink how he would rewrite the book destroyed by the Germans when he arrived at Auschwitz. The DCT approach would suggest that Frankl's past attachment history and Jewish cultural strengths enabled him to cope with the stressors and pain of the concentration camp. We should also recall the word *spirit:* Frankl transcended himself and impossible daily conditions through a holistic connection with a something larger than himself.

The positive meaning-making approach of Frankl is very much in line with the positive developmental orientation of wellness and DCT. Our task is to help survivors of various types of trauma get in touch with their strengths as well as helping them work through the negative. What is it that leads a Viktor Frankl to new levels of strength? Why does one child succumb to the grinding humiliation of poverty while another child develops unique strengths to overcome impossible conditions? The five-stage model thus has important prevention implications. By working developmentally with individuals, families, and communities, we can help build a framework of attachment enabling individuals to live more effectively with the inevitable stressors and trauma of their lives.

The wellness approach of Chapter 2 should be considered a part of treatment for those who experience trauma. Their physical selves need to be nurtured (nutrition, sleep, exercise) as their body needs have often been severely disrupted. War veterans, in particular, speak of the noise and trauma of intense battle entering every single orifice until one's insides seem to explode. Gaining control of one's body is an important first step. Experiencing spirituality (see Chapter 13) and learning how to care for one's psychological needs will be basic for many. Wellness assessment (see Chapter 2 and Figure 2-1) can be an integral part of treatment.

If this expanded view of trauma is considered, then it follows that personality styles are often a defense against a history of trauma and a wide variety of Axis I issues may be better reconceptualized as a variant of PTS. Their "disorders" are really logical responses to painful situations and experiences. We as counselors need to recognize that each client's attachment history will deeply affect how trauma is conceptualized and lived in the physiology and psychology of each individual. And the wellness orientation can be a vital part of holistic treatment.

MULTICULTURAL ISSUES

What occurs in the external environment relates to what occurs inside the person and can be the major causative factor for trauma reactions. Evidence for this is provided by Savin-Williams (1994), who discusses how gay, lesbian, and bisexual youths experience repeated verbal and physical abuse. This constant harassment all too often becomes internalized, leading to depression and self-hatred. Running away from home, substance abuse, prostitution, and suicide are possible results of the constant daily press of environmental stressors. Carter (2003) has noted the same issues in regard to racial harassment.

Vietnam veterans made a breakthrough for the helping field when they met in groups discussing their reactions to the war. This sharing of stories led them to name the commonality of the problems. It was their war experiences that led to much of their distress, not an inherent fault in themselves. This realization rapidly led to a new "disorder" in the *DSM* series—post-traumatic stress disorder. This is an example of how consciousness liberation can be co-opted by the helping profession, for here we see how professionals have taken external problems and placed them in the client. It will be a challenge for the helping professions to recognize that a disorder may be in the context or environment and only showing its face in problems of the individual.

Bullying in schools is one example of external harassment that can lead to internalized oppression and severe emotional stress. In a sample of 760 12- to 17-year-olds, 6% of disabled children were bullied, 4% of African Americans, 3% of Whites, 3% of Asians, 2% of Latinas/Latinos, 11% of those who were overweight, and *25% of those who were gay or thought to be gay!* (Tomsho, 2003). Despite these statistics, conservative groups have fought anti-bullying laws and programs in the schools, claiming that these programs of teaching tolerance might promote a gay lifestyle.

Smart and Smart (1997) outline five useful and important changes found in *DSM-IV* and continued in *DSM-IV-TR.* There has been a gradual evolution toward awareness that culture interfaces with diagnostic issues. *DSM-IV-TR* now reminds us of specific cultural features related to various "disorders." It now contains a glossary of key syndromes related to culture, and cultural considerations are suggested for formulating diagnoses; Axis IV is now related to multicultural dimensions; and the "V" codes provide a useful new direction. *However, we note that cultural issues remain located primarily in Appendix 1 of DSM-IV-TR.*

Smart and Smart point out that 79 of 400 "disorders" now contain some cultural description, but nonetheless, most cultural descriptions are brief and incomplete. Particularly, the new discussion of depression has moved toward more cultural awareness. For example, *DSM-IV-TR* comments (p. 353):

> Culture can influence the experience and communication of symptoms of depression. . . . For example, in some cultures, depression may be experienced largely in somatic terms, rather than sadness or guilt. Complaints of "nerves" and headaches (in Latino and Mediterranean cultures), of weakness, tiredness, or imbalance (in Chinese and Asian cultures), of problems of the "heart" (in Middle Eastern countries), or of being "heartbroken" (among Hopi) may express the depressive experience.

Nonetheless, depression remains "located in the person" and we see little discussion of contextual issues and potential trauma. Certainly, no attention is given to culturally relevant treatment. For example, a Puerto Rican woman suffering from "nerves" or depression may be reacting to cultural pressures of being a woman in Latino society or to issues of poverty and past experiences of abuse as a child (Riviera, 1991). *DSM-IV-TR* talks about depression associated with the onset of menses but gives insufficient attention to how ongoing issues of gender discrimination may lead to depression. Paniagua (1998) comments clearly that professionals have considerable work ahead of us if we are to successfully encounter the complexity of culture and its ramifications in many settings.

Particularly useful for a developmental approach are the revisions in Axis IV—"Psychosocial and Environmental Problems." Axis IV, nonetheless, remains secondary and insufficiently addressed by practicing clinicians and insurance agencies. The culture-centered developmental approach would give Axis IV central attention while Axes I and II move to a secondary position. The new Axis IV outlines critical environmental problems such as housing, discrimination, migration, access to health care, and problems with the legal system. Smart and Smart state that addressing these dimensions will help us avoid "blaming the victim."

Finally, acculturation and religious/spiritual issues have been added to the "V-Codes." These contextual issues enrich, and eventually, we hope, will come to take a more central place in future revisions of *DSM-IV-TR*. Smart and Smart strongly endorse this last point and conclude by citing the American Psychiatric Association's comments on their own work: "It is hoped that these new features will increase sensitivity in how mental disorders may be expressed in different cultures and will reduce the possible effect of unintended bias stemming from the clinician's own cultural background" (American Psychiatric Association, 1994, p. xxv; 2000, p. xxxiv).

One important future direction will be to recognize that certain Axis II personality "disorders" are really developmental blocks and issues. Each cultural framework will have unique reasons for generating certain styles of being. The dependent style, for example, may be more functional in an interdependent culture but less so in an individualistic society. Depression and other Axis I issues need to be seen as possible responses to contextual issues instead of just as an internal problem. A developmental orientation seems highly appropriate to the challenges of redefining "disorder" and moving toward a positive orientation to human growth.

INSTITUTING DEVELOPMENTALLY APPROPRIATE TREATMENT PLANS

Whereas *DSM-IV-TR* leaves the client with only a diagnosis, the DCT paradigm encourages counselors and therapists to conceptualize the client's likely developmental history and current significant relationships, and to anticipate and understand behavior apparent in the here and now of the interview. Equally important is DCT's emphasis on generating treatment plans. The current direction in counseling and therapy is on diagnosis-specific treatment options. While we would agree that ultimately treatment must be tailored to the unique individual, we also believe that a generic framework for conceptualizing treatment planning will be useful. From this broad view, we can work with the individual client to co-generate diagnostic and treatment alternatives.

Let us begin with an expansion of Gordon Paul's (1967) classic statement, "What treatment, by whom, is most effective for this individual with that specific problem, and under which set of circumstances?" We suggest a rephrasing and expansion of Paul's framework:

> What set of treatments, by whom, is most effective for this individual or family, with what set of developmental issues or concerns, with what specific culturally and individually appropriate goal(s), and under which set of relationship conditions and treatment alternatives?
>
> Additionally, how can relapse of treatment be prevented, and how can we involve the client (or family) in treatment planning in a co-constructed egalitarian and culturally sensitive fashion?

We recognize that "single-shot" treatments (for example, medication, a specific cognitive-behavioral intervention) may indeed be useful and effective in promoting change. However, these by themselves are often insufficient to maintain change. Furthermore, clients are unique and may respond differently to the same treatment, no matter how efficient it is generally. The DCT frame suggests that we need to have multiple treatment interventions available. Instead of calling the client "resistant" to change, we need to work with the client to co-generate treatment alternatives that are personally meaningful and comprehensible to that client (see Table 9-4).

DCT theory and research reveal that four primary client information processing styles can be identified: sensorimotor, concrete, formal, and dialectic/systemic. The sensorimotor processing system focuses on here and now sensory "reality." What does the client see, hear, feel, smell, taste? Emphasis is on holistic immediate experience. The concrete-operational client tends to describe her or his world in linear specific fashion and tell concrete, descriptive stories. The formal-operational client is more reflective, epistemologically removed from the "here and now" to thinking about self and situation. The information processing orientation of the dialectic/systemic client tends to be multidimensional and multiperspective. This last dimension focuses on self-in-system and is particularly important in conceptualizing how internal and external events relate to so-called pathological conditions.

The construct validity of the concepts has been demonstrated in several research projects ranging from clinical measures of actual patient language with depressed clients (Rigazio-DiGilio & Ivey, 1990) and teenage substance abusers (Boyer, 1996) to a factor analytic study of over 1,600 college students (Heesacker, Prichard, Rigazio-DiGilio, & Ivey, 1995).

None of the four styles is considered superior. Rather, for full human functioning, development in all areas is to be desired. For our clients, the developmental is-

Table 9-4   Depression: Treatment Interventions Organized Around DCT's Information Processing Systems

DCT Information Processing System	Example Treatment Alternatives
Sensorimotor	Medication, meditation, bodywork (relaxation, nutrition, exercise, yoga), imagery, Gestalt, holistic work with traditional healers
Concrete	Skills training, drawing out client concrete narratives via listening skills, desensitization hierarchies and training, positive strengths and stories from the narrative and DCT perspectives, assertiveness training, completing an automatic thoughts inventory or REBT A-B-C-D-E-F analysis, thought stopping, ethnic/racial or feminist narratives
Formal	Reflection on any of the above sensorimotor or concrete methods. Person-centered theory, psychoanalytic/psychodynamic treatment, cognitive portion of CBT, logotherapy, psychoeducational workshops focusing on self-esteem
Dialectic/systemic	Reflection of how any of the above may have been developed in a family, cultural, or gender system, trauma work that focuses on how the external world relates to internal experience, feminist therapy, consciousness-raising groups, examination of countertransference and/or projective identification, psychotherapy as liberation, involvement of traditional healers in counseling process, social justice action

sues vary; a client's development may be incomplete or he or she may have encountered serious issues or trauma. For example, Beaver (1993) has reviewed the literature on incest survivors and has discovered that they generally have four types of memories and reflections on their trauma. Any one client may utilize one or more methods of processing his or her developmental history. At the sensorimotor level, these trauma survivors talk of body memories, random images, and verbalizations. Flashbacks, script memories, and specific stories of the incest represent the concrete survivor. At the formal level, more complete and reflective narratives appear, while at the dialectic/systemic orientation, a multiperspective and contextual discussion may be manifested.

In treating survivors of incest or other traumas, the DCT framework suggests the need to work through the issue at multiple levels. These clients need to recover their body memories, tell their stories concretely, reflect on them, and discover how they may be systemic in nature, thus enabling them and us to take multiple perspectives. Each client style requires a different theoretical/practical strategy that, in turn, must be applied to the specific needs of the client. For example, an incest survivor or Vietnam veteran may be embedded in sensorimotor and concrete experience. Using formal-operational treatment strategies with this person obviously will be ineffective. It is vital to meet the client where he or she is. Other trauma survivors, however, may be quite formal and reflective, thus avoiding a present-tense concrete experience.

We need to join the client where he or she is cognitively and emotionally, but we also need to encourage the client to explore the issues at other levels. Sensorimotor and concrete clients need to learn to reflect and think about themselves from other perspectives. Formal and dialectic/systemic clients may be using reflective thought to avoid experiencing and taking concrete action on their issues. The counselor or therapist needs to be ready to work with clients where they are *and* to help them explore the world from differing vantage points.

From a narrative perspective, our clients need to experience their stories from the sensorimotor perspective, tell us concrete narratives, reflect on these narratives via formal operations, and view their stories from multiple perspectives and a social historical context. This multiple storytelling leads to new and often contextual understanding of how the self exists in a social environment—the "self-in-relation" rather than the totally autonomous self.

Depression has been presented here as a central issue in *DSM-IV-TR* personality styles and as underlying many Axis I issues, including anxiety disorders (for example, Zlotnick, Warshaw, Shea, & Keller, 1997). And, of course, depression is a major issue in itself. Despite its prevalence, there is one positive dimension: We have considerable clinical and research evidence that many approaches to treating depression are available. And there seems to be increasing awareness that depression, like PTS, is related to external conditions. Rigazio-DiGilio and Ivey (1990) found that 17 of 20 inpatient depressed clients had severe histories of trauma. Moreover, they found that when clients were interviewed via the systematic DCT assessment plan, virtually all depressed inpatients were able to see their issues in social context rather than blaming themselves alone for their difficulties.

Table 9-4 presents the multiple treatments available for depression—and by extension to many, perhaps most, Axis I and II issues. The listed treatment alternatives are categorized in terms of their predominant DCT information processing style.

However, we should recall that any action within any part of the human system reverberates through the total system. For example, medication, clearly a sensorimotor intervention, affects cognitions and emotions throughout other information processing systems. One of these "ripple effects" throughout the intrapersonal system may be self-blaming for the "disorder" and a failure to deal with external contextual and developmental issues. Thus, a single intervention may be sufficient for truly significant client understanding and change. In addition, for maintenance of change and prevention of relapse, the DCT approach recommends multilevel treatments, particularly stressing the importance of helping the client become aware of how issues are developed in a systemic context.

The DCT framework encompasses the paradox of the "four-in-one." While the categories of DCT have held up well in empirical terms, we have discovered that each information processing system contains metaphoric aspects of all the other systems. Thus, in its more complex presentation, DCT has specific questions and assessment strategies to identify ways in which, for example, concrete information processing styles contain aspects of sensorimotor, formal, and dialectic/systemic styles. In that sense DCT is holistic and postmodern, recognizing that there is an infinite number of categories for considering human experience.

The DCT view implies both an alternative and a supplementary treatment. If underlying most so-called disorders is depression, then it is possible to generate a unifying treatment plan, suitable for conceptualizing treatment for many types of issues. In that sense, our approach to treatment is an extension of Beck's (1976) pioneering work with depression and mood disorders. Within the DCT framework, it remains important to select specific treatments to meet the client's information processing capability where the client is at the moment. At the same time, we need to explore alternative treatments from other dimensions that may help the client tell the story and find new solutions from new perspectives.

Many of our existing therapeutic and counseling interventions are multilevel in intent and practice and involve strategies from several information processing styles. An effective stress management program will typically use strategies from all orientations but likely will give less attention to dialectic/systemic issues. Specifically, meditation and relaxation training offer effective modes of sensorimotor treatment, and concrete skills training and linear analysis of thought patterns are also important. Stress management is also helpful in enabling the client to reflect on her or his life through cognitive/emotional self-management and personal reflection. DCT gives more consideration to how systemic issues such as intergenerational family patterns, the stress of racism and sexism, and other external issues relate to internal stress.

When Aaron Beck works with a patient with panic "disorder," we can anticipate that he will often (a) draw out the client's story, which may be presented primarily at any of the four information processing levels or at multiple levels; (b) ask the client for a sensorimotor image; (c) draw out the story of the image through concrete, linear narrative; (d) work with the client to reflect on the story and image through formal operations on thoughts, emotions, and behaviors; and (e) construct a treatment plan that will involve a variety of concrete (e.g., automatic thoughts chart), sensorimotor (e.g., relaxation techniques), and formal (e.g., reflecting on information gained through the chart and the interview) thought. In addition, we can anticipate that concrete strategies for homework and reflective thought after the session will be part of treatment. However, missing from Beck's cognitive orientation, and most treatment programs, is the dialectic/systemic orientation in which the client examines how her or his issues were generated in a family and social context.

The psychoeducational approach to treatment and prevention, while often beginning with a focus on concrete issues, soon opens clients to direct experiencing, reflective thought, and dialectic/systemic multiple perspectives. LaFromboise (1996) has developed a life-skills curriculum for suicide prevention among Native American youth. Adolescents are involved in a number of holistic experiential activities and are encouraged to share their concrete narratives of life experience. Later, they reflect individually and in groups and learn how oppressive systems can be met with personal and cultural pride. Ivey's (1973, 1991) work with long-term inpatients in a VA hospital began with concrete skills training in listening skills, followed by experiential activities to help patients get in touch with their bodies; this approach resulted in a quicker release from the hospital treatment program than had been recorded for other patients. Reflective and systemic thought, as in the LaFromboise example, was encouraged through group work and family interventions. Kerstein (2003) reports on a successful psychoeducational program to help families and friends of veterans cope with "mental illness." The program taught skills and methods to help both the family and the patient. Evidence is clear that such psychoeducational programs, usually oriented to wellness, make a significant difference in patients' gaining release from the hospital and in keeping them from returning.

From a cultural frame, there is need to consider the place of traditional healers in any treatment program. Achebe (1986) has outlined the relationship of traditional healing to Western systems (also see Ivey et al., 2002, pp. 348–350). Structurally, traditional healing has much in common with Western psychotherapy methods, particularly as we think about belief systems. Cognitive/emotional issues are deeply involved with a person's beliefs. Both traditional and Western healers rely on social influence dimensions; if the client believes that the counselor or healer is attractive, competent, and powerful, treatment is much more likely to be effective. Again, we see the importance of *relationship* in the interview. The methods of traditional and Western healers may be widely different, but in important ways they are more alike than we might ordinarily think. Ritual and storytelling, for example, are becoming more fully recognized in modern healing, but they have been used by traditional healers virtually since time began. Increasingly, today's counselors and therapists are working with, rather than against, traditional healers.

Psychotherapy as liberation, as presented in the chapter on multicultural issues, is an example of a multilevel treatment designed to center on systemic issues. The word *liberation* is used as the emphasis is on facilitating the discovery by clients of how their personal issues were generated in a sociocultural framework. Liberation occurs as the client learns a new balance of external and internal responsibility for problems and concerns. Whereas most theories and practices focus on individual resolution of issues and thus place the problem in the person, the liberation emphasis is on the client's transactions and relationships with the world. *But psychotherapy as liberation does not deny traditional methods.* As appropriate, medication, asssertiveness training, and cognitive formal reflection on the nature of the traditional "self" would be part of a broad-based treatment plan. What is different in this system is the importance of helping the client see self-in-context, self-in-relation. Specific questioning strategies are presented, enabling the expansion of client awareness, emotion, cognitions, and behaviors around the issues.

Psychotherapy as liberation does not deny other theories but welcomes them as appropriate to client needs and wishes. For example, medication, cognitive behavioral therapy, family strategies, and other approaches become an important part of a comprehensive network treatment plan.

The psychotherapy as liberation approach asks us to move to a culture-centered framework in which we balance our diagnostic formulations between the individual and the individual's context. Our next step may be to move toward consciousness-raising in ourselves and in our clients of how person and environment are related, much as Paulo Friere did (see Chapter 8). In this way, *DSM-IV-TR*'s Axes IV and V can take a more central place in our work and help us move toward new, more satisfactory formulations of issues faced by our clients. The multicultural competencies (Arredondo et al., 1996; Sue et al., 1982) become especially relevant as we move to this new culture-centered frame of reference.

SUMMARY

DCT's developmental view of DSM-IV-TR *may be useful in helping us take a more positive, proactive view as we work with so-called pathology.* We have suggested that considering individual biological, psychological, and social history in a developmental context can be a viable alternative to the pathological model. The DCT framework implies that much greater attention needs to be paid to environmental and contextual issues. A so-called disorder is a logical response to biological and developmental history.

DSM-IV-TR *Axis II personality "disorders" can be reconceptualized as developmental personality styles.* The logic of each style was presented in Table 9-2, which summarizes positive aspects of each style, behaviors and thoughts that you might find in the session, possible family history, the predicted nature of current relationships, and a possible treatment approach.

Axis I severe emotional distress categories (e.g., depression, schizophrenia, obsessive-compulsive) are presented as the breakdown of developmental defensive structures. The developmental frameworks of Masterson and Bowlby are presented as particularly helpful in the positive integration of ideas presented in *DSM-IV-TR*.

- Environmental or biological insult (may lead to)
- Stress and physical/emotional pain, which is a threat to attachment and safety (which, in turn, may lead to)
- Sadness/depression (which may lead to)
- Defense against the pain and, in severe cases, Axis II personality styles (which may lead to)
- Axis I defensive structures

Post-traumatic stress is presented as a central developmental issue in the breakdown of internal defensive structures supporting the person. The importance of finding positive meaning and encouraging client awareness of environmental context (dialectic/systemic thinking) can be important in helping clients work through serious stressors.

DSM-IV-TR has gradually reflected increased awareness and incorporation of multicultural issues. Nonetheless, further work is necessary for a broader inclusion of contextual issues.

With an understanding of developmental aspects of severe emotional distress, counselors can institute developmentally appropriate treatment plans. In this chapter, we gave special attention to the issue of depression, considering it an underlying issue in many other diagnostic dimensions of *DSM-IV-TR.* Specifics of DCT were presented as a way to integrate treatment planning using a broad array of theoretical methods and strategies (Table 9-4).

Philosophically, the chapter also draws from psychotherapy as liberation of consciousness, presented in detail in the multicultural chapter (Chapter 8). The liberation aspects of a developmental view of severe emotional distress are focused on liberating the client to see her or his problems ("disorder") in a new way. Through naming things more positively, counselors can develop a more optimistic developmental treatment plan in concert with the client.

Challenges: While the developmental approach makes sense and is an effective alternative and supplement to the traditional pathological view, it requires major reframing of your thinking and practice. What is presented here, of course, is at best a beginning, a start toward a new future. Furthermore, you will note that this approach also asks you to learn and eventually become expert in multiple theories and strategies. The most challenging dimension of the developmental approach is perhaps the hard work and continued study that it requires.

Research issues: Note that DCT is an integrative framework that utilizes past and present research, both medical and biological, in any treatment plan. DCT serves as an organizing tool for existing systems of therapy. As a new and often psychoeducational approach, the developmental system itself has not been fully tested or researched, although some efforts in this direction are cited and they certainly are promising. Countless issues of effectiveness need to be examined as well as how the developmental approach can supplement traditional systems.

THEORY INTO PRACTICE: DEVELOPING YOUR PORTFOLIO OF COMPETENCE

Self-Assessment Exercise

Exercise 1. Identifying your own developmental history

Most of us have favorite types of clients—those with whom we can most easily develop rapport and understanding and with whom the interview goes well. But we also have certain clients who are difficult for us. Think of specific clients you know whom you have had an easy relationship with. Then think about those who are more challenging and difficult. List below your difficult clients and those you look forward to meeting with. If you are not yet in counseling practice, think back on the types of people you get along well with and those who are more troublesome for you. These personal relationships may reappear in the helping interview.

Who are the clients or people you enjoy working with? What are their characteristics?

_____

_____

_____

Who are the clients or people you find more difficult? What are their characteristics?

_____

_____

_____

Review Table 9-2 on developmental personality styles. Do any of your clients fit these categories or at least show some elements of that type of behavior? Regardless, what types of personality styles do you find more difficult and challenging for you?

_____

_____

_____

As you think about your developmental history, what in your past relationships might be reflected in some of your answers above? How might you transcend your past experience and work more effectively with some of these more difficult clients? It would also be helpful to have a friend or colleague take you through the four-level DCT questioning sequence to discover what is going on in more challenging depth.

_____

_____

_____

_____

_____

_____

Identification and Classification Exercises

Exercise 2. Examining your developmental history in relationship to the dependent personality style

The client affects you the therapist as you affect the client. You have knowledge, skills, and experience that can be helpful to the client. You need to be aware of these strengths. At the same time, you must be aware of blind spots that can hurt the interviewing interaction. One way to get in touch with your own developmental history, past and present, is to go through key developmental sequences of awareness.

This exercise focuses on your identifying some of your own history and how it might relate to your clients. One common issue among clients is dependency. We suggest you work through the exercise using this one personality style; if you prefer, however, you may work with another.

Take a moment to think of a specific dependent person you have known (or other personality style if you prefer). Or perhaps think of a time when you felt dependent on others and needy. If you have a current client who represents the dependent style, you may want to focus on your feelings and thoughts about that client. Relax and concentrate on getting a clear visual image of *one* of these times. Or, you may get an image of a voice or a sound. Now, try to locate, in your body, the feelings you associate with dependency. Locating feelings in specific parts of the body is particularly helpful in generating deeper understandings of present and past developmental issues.

Can you locate a specific feeling in your body? Describe it here.

_____

_____

_____

_____

It is wise to repeat the above exercise from a positive standpoint. Did you have a positive experience of having someone dependent on you or of being dependent on someone? These positive frames are important in helping you avoid blind spots in the session.

Can you locate a specific feeling in your body?

_____

_____

_____

_____

Next, stay with one of the feelings and think back to a specific situation in your own life when you experienced that feeling. This can be a current or a past situation, perhaps in adolescence or childhood. Describe the situation in your own words. What were you thinking? What were you feeling? What happened before? What happened afterward?

_____

_____

_____

_____

Is that situation a recurring pattern in your life? Does it occur in other situations? Reflect on your own feelings about yourself and issues of dependency.

_____

_____

_____

_____

Where did your patterns of feelings about dependency come from? Particularly, where did they come from in your family history? What was your family attitude toward dependency? Where did your family learn that attitude and the behaviors that go with it? What are some of the strengths in your developmental history surrounding this issue? What are the weaknesses?

_____

_____

_____

_____

Now review the above exercise. Did you focus on a positive experience of dependency or on one that was less positive? Whatever the focus, think about your choice and its implications for your own work with dependent clients. Then repeat this exercise using the opposite experience. What did you learn?

_____

_____

_____

_____

Given the above information, what potential difficulties might you have with the dependent client? What strengths do you have to offer? Some people don't like dependent styles and, because of their developmental history, become impatient with such clients. Others, because of their own personal style, may take over for the dependent client and offer too much nurturance and support. In either case, it is possible to repeat with the client the client's past developmental history. You as counselor can end up acting like a parent, sibling, or other important figure from the client's past history. Another term for this is *countertransference*; you as helper repeat your own developmental history with the client and fail to recognize the client as a unique individual.

Exercise 3. Generating a long-term treatment plan for the dependent client

Develop a comprehensive treatment plan for a dependent client (or your own selection of personality style), using what you know about the dependent developmental personality style in combination with your own counseling and therapy knowledge and other resources available in your work setting or community. The exercise asks you for two different treatment plans. The first assumes a client who is willing to spend a year or possibly more in the process. Here you can employ all the knowledge, experience, and referral sources available to you. In addition, think about how the client presents. Is he or she primarily sensorimotor, concrete, formal, or dialectic? Use the strategies presented in Chapter 5 to help develop a treatment plan appropriate to your client's primary cognitive style.

However, few clients have the luxury of unlimited time and resources. Thus, the second part of the exercise asks you to assume that you have only 10 sessions to work with the client. Your mode of treatment should be designed to accommodate this limitation.

Read and work through this exercise using as your "client" either a case you are aware of or an individual or friend who has aspects of the dependent style.

1. *Positive assets and wellness strengths.* How will you develop a positive base for treatment both in each interview and over the longer period? What does this client bring as internal and external assets and strengths? How do these assets present in terms of the client's cognitive style?

_____

_____

_____

2. *Key relationship issues.* What is your personal history and attitude toward dependency? What type of relationship with the client will you strive for? How will you change that relationship as the client develops? What balance of attachment and separation behaviors does this individual need? How can you promote this balance using your knowledge of the client's cognitive/emotional styles?

_____

_____

_____

_____

_____

_____

_____

3. *Treatment possibilities with each developmental style.* These treatment options must be based on your own personal competence. You may want to refer to the list of suggested treatment alternatives at each developmental level presented in Table 9-4. On the following, list only those treatments that make sense to you for this particular client. Also, recall that taking the dependent client through the DCT systematic questioning sequence is a viable treatment alternative.

Plan for sensorimotor treatment. What techniques and theories will you use?

_____

_____

_____

_____

Plan for concrete-operational treatment. Which techniques and theories will you use?

_____

_____

_____

_____

Plan for formal-operational treatment. Which techniques and theories will you use?

_____

_____

_____

_____

Plan for dialectic/systemic treatment. Which techniques and theories will you use? Will you include some family interventions?

_____

_____

_____

_____

_____

4. *Client/counselor contract for the treatment plan.* Should a treatment plan be shared with the client? Traditionally, professionals have kept their ideas about treatment from the client on the theory that they may be more effective if the client is not told about them. However, the DCT approach suggests that you consider sharing your treatment plan with the client and jointly develop a plan oriented toward mutual responsibility and accountability. By sharing information, you may discover that what the client needs or wants is a good program of jogging, relaxation training, and nutrition. Assertiveness training is often considered a treatment of choice for the dependent personality style. Those clients desiring long-term therapy might want to pursue psychoanalytic work. Family systems therapy in conjunction with the individual treatment plan may be critical.

How much would you involve your clients in decisions about the nature and length of counseling and therapy?

_____

_____

_____

_____

5. *The 10-session treatment.* Completing all of the above treatments might take a year or more. In some case, many years of treatment are warranted. More often, your agency, health insurance company, or client constraints indicate brief therapy and counseling. In the helping field, the trend is increasingly toward treatment programs that aim to achieve specific goals in a certain length of time.

Given 10 interviews, what would be your treatment plan? How would you present the plan to the client? How much will the client participate in decisions about that treatment plan?

_____

_____

_____

_____

_____

_____

_____

Toward Multicultural Competence

Exercise 4. Multicultural harassment

It is clear that racial, gender, sexual orientation, physical ability, or other minority harassment can lead to constant instances of bullying, whether one is a child or an adult. Many of those who are harassed blame themselves for their problem rather than environmental stressors and they may even try to be invisible.

Revisit the RESPECTFUL multicultural cube in Chapter 8. What has been your personal experience with harassment? Where have you been oppressed and where have you perhaps engaged in harassment?

_____

_____

_____

_____

_____

What actions are you going to take when you observe the results of harassment and bullying in your own practice?

_____

_____

_____

_____

Interviewing Practice Exercise

Exercise 5. Practice with DCT in a role-played interview

The following exercise has been especially helpful in making clear and concrete the concepts of DCT for Axis II developmental personality styles and more severe Axis I problems. In this exercise, the client adopts one of the personality styles (dependent, narcissistic, and so on) or a more severe disturbance (conduct disorder, depression, agoraphobia). Follow your usual ethical guidelines.

Most of us have had certain incidents or periods in our lives when we have been especially dependent or mistrustful (paranoid), have acted out (antisocial or conduct disorder), or have been overly self-focused (narcissistic). Most of us also have experienced at least mild depression, slight phobias, and some part of the total confusion of schizophrenics.

Role-play a client and identify the part of yourself that represents a particular developmental personality style. Enlarge on that part of yourself and allow it to take over the role-play. This exercise will give you an opportunity to learn about the personality style.

Discussing your own issues can be a powerful experience. It is particularly important that you work with a group you trust and that a qualified supervisor be immediately available. During the sensorimotor questioning sequence, this exercise can become highly emotional. You may prefer to role-play a client you have had. If so, be sure to inform your interviewer that you are role-playing a client.

When you provide immediate feedback (Step 6 in this exercise), the focus is on the counselor and his or her feelings and thoughts during the role-played interview.

Step 1: Divide Into Practice Groups

Step 2: Select a Group Leader

Step 3: Assign Roles for the Practice Session

- *Role-played client.* The role-played client will present an Axis II developmental personality style or an Axis I personality problem as discussed above.
- *Interviewer.* The interviewer will ask the DCT four-level questions. Alternatively, you could use the introspective developmental counseling framework of Tamase and conduct a review of this part of the client's life. Remember to use listening skills frequently and help the client organize information through reflection of feeling and summarization.
- *Observers 1 and 2.* The observers will provide specific feedback on the relationship between the client and counselor at each part of the interview.

Step 4: Plan the Session
The interviewer and client first need to agree on the topic to be reviewed. This is an informal miniversion of the DCT counselor/client contract. The two observers can examine the feedback form.

Step 5: Conduct a 30-Minute Interviewing Session
Again, it is helpful to videotape and/or audiotape practice sessions.

Step 6: Provide Immediate Feedback and Complete Notes (5 to 20 Minutes)
Allow the client and interviewer time to provide immediate personal reactions to the practice session. After this has been done, the observers and the role-played client can focus on the thoughts and feelings of the counselor. Ask the counselor to generate a specific visual image of the interview and then go through the specific four-level questioning strategies with the counselor. It is important during this process to ask the counselor for his or her bodily feeling when the image of the client was called to mind. This part of the exercise is particularly helpful to the counselor's understanding of how personal issues may affect the counseling process.

Step 7: Review Practice Session and Provide Feedback (15 to 30 Minutes)
The interviewer should be the one who asks for feedback rather than receiving it without having asked. The observers can share their observations from the feedback form and from their observations as the session progressed. Avoid judgmental feedback.

Generalization: Taking Chapter Exercises Back Home

Exercise 6. Generate a treatment plan for one of your own clients

If you are not working with a client currently, select one of the Axis II or Axis I categories discussed in this chapter and work through the specific steps of a DCT treatment plan, paying special attention to how your own developmental history relates to that particular client in the interview. As you begin (perhaps even now), focus on one visual image of your client, locate a feeling in your body, and see where that leads you.

If you are working with clients, select one client with whom you are currently working and generate a treatment plan using the concepts of this chapter.

Portfolio Reflections

Exercise 7. Your reflections on a developmental approach to DSM-IV-TR

What stood out for you from this chapter? What sense do you make of what you have read and experienced? What are your key points from this chapter? Write your thoughts here and add them to your Portfolio Folder in your computer.

_____

_____

_____

_____

_____

REFERENCES

Achebe, C. (1986). *The world of the Ogbanje.* Enugu, Nigeria: Fourth Dimension.

Ainsworth, M. (1967). *Infancy in Uganda: Infant care and the growth of love.* Baltimore: Johns Hopkins University Press.

Ainsworth, M. (1977). Social development in the first year of life. In J. Tanner (Ed.), *Developments in psychiatric research.* London: Hodder & Stoughton.

Ainsworth, M. (1979). Attachment theory and its utility in cross-cultural research. In P. Leiderman, S. Tulkin, & A. Rosenfeld (Eds.), *Culture and infancy: Variations in the human experience* (pp. 47–67). San Diego: Academic Press.

Ainsworth, M. (1985). Patterns of infant-mother attachment: II. Attachments across the life-span. *Bulletin of the New York Academy of Medicine, 61,* 771–812.

Ainsworth, M., & Bowlby, J. (1991). An ethological approach to personality development. *American Psychologist, 46,* 333–341.

American Psychiatric Association. (1994). *Diagnostic and statistical manual of mental disorders.* Washington, DC: Author.

American Psychiatric Association. (2000). *Diagnostic and statistical manual of mental disorders: Text revision.* Washington, DC: Author.

Arredondo, P., Toporek, R., Brown, S., Jones, J., Locke, D., Sanchez, J., & Stadler, H. (1996). *Operalization of the multicultural counseling competencies.* Washington, DC: Association for Multicultural Counseling and Development.

Atkinson, L., & Goldberg, S. (2003). Attachment issues in psychopathology and intervention. Mahwah, NJ: Erlbaum.

Baker Miller, J. (1976). *Toward a new psychology of women.* Boston: Beacon.

Beaver, A. (1993). *Delayed memory of childhood trauma: Models of memory and therapeutic practice.* Unpublished comprehensive examination, University of Massachusetts, Amherst.

Beck, A. (1976). *Cognitive therapy and the emotional disorders.* New York: International Universities Press.

Beck, A., Freeman, A., & Associates. (1990). *Cognitive therapy of the personality disorders.* New York: Guilford Press.

Blatt, S., Quinlan, D., Pilkonis, P., & Shea, M. (1995). Impact of perfectionism and need for approval on the brief treatment of depression: The National Institute of Mental Health Treatment of Depression Collaborative Research Program revisited. *Journal of Consulting and Clinical Psychology, 63,* 125–132.

Bowlby, J. (1969). *Attachment.* New York: Basic Books.

Bowlby, J. (1973). *Separation.* New York: Basic Books.

Bowlby, J. (1988). *A secure base.* New York: Basic Books.

Boyer, D. (1996). *DCT and adolescent drug abuse.* Unpublished doctoral dissertation, University of Massachusetts, Amherst.

Carter, R. (2003). *Racism: The unidentified trauma.* Presentation to the 20th Annual Teachers College Winter Roundtable on Cultural Psychology and Education. New York: Columbia University.

Davis, L. (1997, February). *Diagnostic and Statistical Manual of Mental Disorders* (4th ed.). (Book Review). *Harper's Magazine,* pp. 61–64.

de Shazer, S. (1982). *Patterns of brief therapy.* New York: Guilford Press.

Duran, E., & Duran, B. (1995). *Native American postcolonial psychology.* Albany: State University of New York Press.

Flaherty, M. (1989). *Perceived differences in early family relationship and parent/child relations between adults diagnosed as borderline personality or bipolar disorder.* Unpublished doctoral dissertation, University of Massachusetts, Amherst.

Foa, E., Hearst-Ikeda, D., & Perry, K. (1995). Evaluation of a brief cognitive-behavioral program for prevention of chronic PTSD in recent assault victims. *Journal of Consulting and Clinical Psychology, 63,* 948–955.

Foa, E., Rothbaum, B., Riggs, D., & Murdock, T. (1991). Treatment of posttraumatic stress disorder in rape victims: A comparison between cognitive-behavior procedures and counseling. *Journal of Consulting and Clinical Psychology, 99,* 715–723.

Frankl, V. (1959). *Man's search for meaning.* New York: Pocket Books. (Original work published 1946)

Fullerton, C., & Ursano, R. (1997). *Posttraumatic stress disorder.* Washington, DC: American Psychiatric Association Press.

Garrett, M. T. (1999). Understanding the "medicine" of Native American traditional values: An integrative review. *Counseling and Values, 43,* 84–98.

Garrett, M. T., & Myers, J. E. (1996). The rule of opposites: A paradigm for counseling Native Americans. *Journal of Multicultural Counseling and Development, 24,* 89–104.

Heesacker, M., Prichard, S., Rigazio-DiGilio, S., & Ivey, A. (1995). *Development of a paper and pencil measure on cognitive-developmental orientations.* Unpublished report, Department of Psychology, University of Florida, Gainesville.

Ivey, A. (1973). Media therapy: Educational change planning for psychiatric patients. *Journal of Counseling Psychology, 20,* 338–343.

Ivey, A. (1991, October). *Media therapy reconsidered: Developmental counseling and therapy as a comprehensive model for treating severely distressed clients.* Paper presented at the Veterans Administration Conference, Orlando, Florida.

Ivey, A. (2000). *Developmental therapy: Theory into practice.* San Francisco: Jossey-Bass. (Original work published 1986)

Ivey, A., D'Andrea, M., Ivey, M., & Simek-Morgan, L. (2002). *Counseling and psychotherapy: A multicultural perspective.* Boston: Allyn & Bacon.

Ivey, A., & Gluckstern, N. (1974). *Basic attending skills.* North Amherst, MA: Microtraining.

Ivey, A., & Ivey, M. (2003). *Intentional interviewing and counseling: Faciliating client development in a multicultural society.* Pacific Grove, CA: Brooks/Cole.

Ivey, M., & Ivey, A. (1993). Network interventions and DCT. In A. Ivey (Ed.), *Developmental strategies for helpers: Individual, family and network interventions.* North Amherst, MA: Microtraining.

Jongsma, A., Jr., Peterson, M., & McInnis, W. (1996). *The child and adolescent psychotherapy treatment planner.* New York: Wiley.

Kerstein, K. (2003, April). Psychoeducational programs help families cope with mental illness. *Monitor on Psychology, 16.*

Kjos, D. (1995). Linking career counseling to personality disorders. *Journal of Counseling and Development, 73,* 592–596.

Koerner, K., Kohlenberg, R., & Parker, C. (1996). Diagnosis of personality disorder: A radical behavioral alternative. *Journal of Consulting and Clinical Psychology, 64,* 1169–1176.

LaFromboise, T. (1996). *American Indian life skills curriculum.* Madison: University of Wisconsin Press.

Larson, D. D. (1999). The conceptualization of health. *Medical Care Research and Review, 56,* 123–136.

Levers, L., & Maki, D. (1994). *An ethnographic analysis of traditional healing and rehabilitation services in southern Africa: Cross-cultural implications.* Durham: University of New Hampshire, World Rehabilitation Fund.

Littrell, J. (1998). *Brief counseling in action.* New York: Norton.

Mahler, M. (1975). *The psychological birth of the human infant.* New York: Basic Books.

Masterson, J. (1981). *The narcissistic and borderline disorders.* New York: Brunner/Mazel.

McCormick, R. (1997). Healing through interdependence: The role of connecting First Nations in healing practices. *Canadian Journal of Counselling, 31,* 172–184.

McGaa, E. (1989). *Mother earth spirituality: Native American paths to healing ourselves and our world.* San Francisco: Harper & Row.

Muñoz, R. (2001). On the road to a world without depression. *Journal of Primary Prevention, 21,* 325–338.

O'Hanlon, W., & Weiner-Davis, M. (1989). *In search of solutions.* New York: Norton.

Paniagua, F. (1998). *Assessing and treating culturally diverse clients: A practical guide* (2nd ed.). Newbury Park, CA: Sage.

Paul, G. (1967). Strategy of outcome research in psychotherapy. *Journal of Consulting Psychology, 31,* 109–118.

Rigazio-DiGilio, S., & Ivey, A. (1990). Developmental therapy and depressive disorders: Measuring cognitive levels through patient natural language. *Professional Psychology: Research and Practice. 21,* 470–475.

Riviera, M. (1991). *Attaques de nervios.* Unpublished comprehensive paper, University of Massachusetts, Amherst.

Rush, A. (1995). *Strategies and tactics in the treatment of mood disorders.* (Video). Washington, DC: American Psychiatric Association.

Savin-Williams, R. (1994). Verbal and physical abuse as stressors in the lives of lesbian, gay male, and bisexual youths: Associations with school problems, running away, substance abuse, prostitution, and suicide. *Journal of Consulting and Clinical Psychology, 62,* 262–269.

Seem, S., & Hernandez, T. (1997, September). *Teaching the DSM-IV-TR system: Feminist and cross cultural perspectives.* Presentation at the Conference of the North Atlantic Regional Association of Counselor Educators and Supervisors, Plattsburgh, New York.

Sheeran, T., & Zimmerman, M. (2002). Screening for posttraumatic stress disorder in a general psychiatric outpatient setting. *Journal of Consulting and Clinical Psychology, 70,* 961–966.

Sherbourne, C., Hays, R., & Wells, K. (1995). Personal and psychosocial risk factors for physical and mental health outcomes and course of depression among depressed patients. *Journal of Consulting and Clinical Psychology 63,* 345–355.

Smart, D., & Smart, J. (1997). *DSM-IV-TR* and culturally sensitive diagnosis: Some observations for counselors. *Journal of Counseling and Development, 75,* 392–398.

Stiver, I. (1991). The meaning of "dependency" in female-male relationships. In J. Jordan, A. Kaplan, J. Baker Miller, I. Stiver, & J. Surry (Eds.), *Women's growth in connection* (pp. 143–161). New York: Guilford Press.

Sue, D., Bernier, J., Durran, M., Feinberg, L., Pedersen, P., Smith, E., & Vasquez, E. (1982). Position paper: Cross-cultural counseling competencies. *The Counseling Psychologist, 10,* 45–52.

Tomsho, R. (2003, February 20). Schools' efforts to protect gays face opposition. *Wall Street Journal,* p. B1.

Trimble, J., & Fleming, C. (1989). Providing counseling services for Native American Indians: Client, counselor, and community characteristics. In P. Pedersen, J. Draguns, P. Lonner, & J. Trimble (Eds.), *Counseling across cultures* (3rd ed.). Honolulu: University of Hawaii Press.

Twinge, J. (2000). The age of anxiety? Birth cohort change in anxiety and neuroticism, 1952–1993. *Journal of Personality and Social Psychology, 79,* 1007–1021.

White, M., & Epston, D. (1990). *Narrative means to therapeutic ends.* New York: Norton.

Zlotnick, C., Warshaw, M., Shea, M., & Keller, M. (1997). Trauma and chronic depression among patients with anxiety disorders. *Journal of Consulting and Clinical Psychology, 65,* 333–336.

CHAPTER 10
Early Recollections

Using DCT With Early Memories to Facilitate Second-Order Change

CENTRAL PRACTICE OBJECTIVE	Mastery and practice of concepts in this chapter will enable you to use the theoretical/practical Adlerian approach to early recollections as (a) a positive support base for your clients and (b) a way to help clients understand how their past relates to the present and how it can help them build toward the future.

U sing Adlerian theory (Adler, 1927/1954) and DCT (Ivey, 1986/2000; Ivey & Ivey, 2003) as the theoretical bases of understanding and intervening, early recollections help disclose the rules about life that guide one's actions, emotions, and thought processes. Further, methods for bringing about change desired by the client flow out of these approaches and empower clients to make new choices and experience more positive emotions. This chapter provides an introduction to these concepts and methods using early recollections as a gateway.

Knowledge of and skill in the concepts of this chapter can enable you to:

1. Explore Adlerian concepts of development and functioning, with special attention to the importance of early recollections in establishing metaphors for coping with life tasks and challenges.
2. Apply the concepts of this chapter in real life through reflection and practice exercises and develop a portfolio of competence. Special attention will be paid to Adlerian early recollections through integration of developmental counseling and therapy strategies.
3. Conceptualize human development and wellness holistically, thus avoiding reductionistic strategies common in the physical and medical sciences influencing contemporary theory.

INTRODUCTION: THE MEANING OF EARLY MEMORIES

Before you begin, you may want to return to Chapter 2 and review the major principles of Adlerian theory. In particular, an understanding of the *socio-teleo-analytic* concepts that underlie discovering one's *private logic* will help provide a context for applying these methods in a more positive, wellness orientation to helping (see Chapter 2; Sweeney, 1998; Mosak & Dreikurs, 1973). Early memories may contain emotions, behaviors, and/or themes that thwart positive self-assessment and coping with life's tasks. No responsible practitioner would deliberately uncover such discouragement without a plan for helping a client overcome the consequences of these experiences. The combination of Adlerian and DCT approaches helps ensure that the skilled practitioner has the means to provide effective counseling.

Early memories are a rich source of insights related to current and future responses to life's requirements and opportunities (Clark, 2002; Sweeney, 1998). Contrary to what one might expect, however, the *past* is not the determinant of future behavior. Rather it is a person's *expectations* for the future that shape her or his responses to life's daily activities. The *anticipation of what will happen* influences the choices each of us makes in both large and small decisions related to work, friendships, love relationships, self, and spiritual matters (Dreikurs, 1967, 1971).

Behavior that was appropriate for a young person in a dysfunctional situation can be maladaptive in later life. Both Adlerian and DCT methods provide the means to help clients loosen the bonds of faulty reasoning and emotion learned in earlier times. More important, they help clients learn new ways of responding that can be liberating.

EARLY RECOLLECTIONS

Early recollections are metaphors to which each of us assigns meaning (Clark, 2002; Sweeney, 1998; Ansbacher, 1969; Ansbacher & Ansbacher, 1956). The meanings are our unique "biased apperceptions" about self, life, and others. They are a source of themes that guide us in our daily activities and emotions. Integrating early recollections with DCT offers another alternative for helping individuals in their search for a more satisfying life.

Developmentally, human beings are among the most dependent of all creatures at birth. They must be cared for if they are to survive. As a consequence, knowing about their early interactions with others can be a major source of understanding their expectations and present behavior. Through early impressions as children, we develop rules about life that we use to understand and manage unique perceptions of ourselves and the world (Sweeney, 1995, 1998). Out of these early experiences, we develop a private logic that becomes a part of our unconscious guiding principles for daily living.

Adler believed that individuals behave "*as if*" circumstances were absolutely true—for example, life is threatening, I am inadequate, or others are more able than I. Some ideas people have are clear to them and held as firm beliefs; other ideas are more subtle but still powerful in their influence on the person's behavior. Adler (1927/1954) referred to all such beliefs as *fictive notions*. Within DCT, many of these are examined as "rules" adopted from life's experiences. Themes related to these fictive notions can often be discovered through a lifestyle assessment that includes exploration of early recollections—specific events the client remembers as happening before he or she was 6 to 8 years old, including sensorimotor, concrete, cognitive, and emotional content. This process of self-discovery allows clients to explore their private logic and motivations in ways that generally go unexamined. The combination of early recollections and DCT assessment can be very effective in practice.

EARLY RECOLLECTIONS: INTEGRATING ADLERIAN INDIVIDUAL PSYCHOLOGY WITH DCT

Adlerian theory is particularly helpful as it shows how our functioning now relates to our total developmental history. We build our future on our past life and our many connections with others—socio, teleo, and analytic. Whereas Freud gave prime attention to negative issues and pathology, Adler emphasized how we can utilize our past strengths in the present. Many would argue that he was the first to emphasize positive psychology. In fact, some Adlerians extended Adler's concepts to incorporate wellness beginning in the1980s and they continue with that work in the present (Myers & Sweeney, in press; Myers, Sweeney, & Witmer, 2000; Sweeney & Witmer, 1991; Witmer & Sweeney, 1992). Likewise, DCT seeks to facilitate wellness over the lifespan from a developmental perspective and provides both a theoretical framework and a structured methodology for assessment and intervention.

A basic Individual Psychology (IP) exercise centers the client on early life recollections that can help you assess and understand the client more fully. In the following exercise, you will examine *early recollections (ERs)*. Work through this exercise using your own experience. A detailed exercise for using early recollections with volunteer or real clients appears in the interviewing practice exercise at the conclusion of this chapter.

As a beginning, let us start with you. What are your earliest recollections? You might well wonder how these are affecting your thoughts, feelings, and behavior today. Some people have difficulty connecting with their early life experiences. In most cases, it is simply a matter of reconnecting by successive approximations in which we help individuals start with a broad area and then focus on details and specific events. Metaphorically, clients save memories much like subjects in file drawers in a cabinet. As they think back to their childhood home, neighborhood (some people prefer the outdoors!), siblings, games, pets, favorite stuffed animals, and similar trigger associations, one memory seems to lead to another. For example, right now select one of those topics as an entry "file drawer" and notice what comes to mind. A chain of memories and associations usually follows.

What occurred for you in this brief introduction? What are *your* earliest personal recollections? Write these as if telling a story to someone else including all the details of who was there, what you were doing, in what location, with sounds, sights, colors, and feelings as they unfold much as in a film or video.

_____

_____

_____

_____

_____

The difference between a significant early recollection and a report is important. Many people recall family routines or general descriptions of early experiences. For example, one individual reported that every summer her family made ice cream as a pastime. Another remembered a constant pattern of family arguments around alcohol. Others have talked of early experiences with oppression such as racism, sexism, or heterosexism. DCT would call these types of recollections examples of formal operations as they represent a pattern rather than a single concrete and specific event. Even with more detail, this formal/pattern type of memory is not to be confused with a recollection unless a specific episode is reported.

A useful recollection brings attention to a particular *concrete* incident. For example, at one ice cream–making session, the client may recall in great detail what a grandparent did that was particularly important to her or him at that time. Another client might talk about what occurred during one particularly traumatic evening with a drunken father. A client who experienced an early oppressive incident will describe it concretely. Often the early recollection will be so vivid that it easily takes on a "here and now" sensorimotor quality with a strong affective reaction. This immediate expression of the "here and now" abreaction to the experience can be both powerful and revealing.

Although negative early recollections are, of course, vital for understanding clients and working through both daily problems and severe distress, we strongly suggest that you encourage clients to start with positive and comfortable recollections. On this positive or strength base, they can later deal more effectively with difficult memories and related issues that they bring up. With a wellness approach to the client who recalls a severe evening with the drunken father, our task is to search out strengths and resources that enabled the client to survive. These might include active emotional distancing, going out with friends, or even balancing the negative experience with some good qualities of the parents themselves. Those who experience oppression also have positive early recollections that can facilitate their dealing with these challenges. In each case, concrete and sensorimotor recollections of the positive experiences are most likely to be helpful. Frankl (1946/1959) has noted that mere survival and continuing on is an important strength.

As a next step, relax in a comfortable, quiet place and image your early childhood. Call up a positive early recollection. Many people can remember an "earliest" recollection in early childhood. Others may start with the teen years, then move back to elementary school, and finally to preschool years. The earlier the recollection, the more foundational it is to the present. If you happen to start with a negative recollection, notice it briefly and realize that you can come back to this later. Move on to a positive recollection. You may find it helpful to think and record how old you were when this recollection occurred as well as specific events such as sibling births, deaths, and other events that may later prove to be connected in some manner (some individuals remember their crib experiences!).

Summarize your recollection here:

_____

_____

_____

_____

_____

Sensorimotor/concrete recollections tend to be the most powerful whereas abstract/formal remembrances are often used by clients to distance themselves from their experiences. What DCT cognitive/emotional styles do your recollections represent? Supply specific evidence to back up your impressions.

Sensorimotor here and now evidence (look for bringing the past into the present, often along with bodily feelings):

_____

_____

Concrete evidence (look for the aspects of your early recollection that focus on specifics of what happened; it is important that you describe it in detail and sequentially to discover meaning—e.g., consequences of specific behaviors):

_____

_____

Abstract formal or dialectic/systemic evidence (look for patterns and reflections on the experience; if you find yourself doing this, seek to return to a here and now recollection of the early *immediate experience*):

_____

_____

All recollections have the potential for being understood in relation to present behaviors and feelings. You are also likely to discover socio (the way you connect with others), teleo (your present goals), and analytic (discovery of new unconscious reasons that you behave as you do) explanations through this exercise.

After you have experienced your early recollection as deeply and fully as possible, move to abstract reflection on what you experienced and record here some of your major discoveries. (See p. 42 for a review of socio, teleo, and analytic.)

Socio: _____

_____

_____

_____

Teleo: _____

_____

_____

_____

Analytic: _____

_____

_____

_____

As you examine early recollections, themes and patterns become important as metaphors for helping understand behavior. These themes become apparent as we examine three types of self-statements: *I am . . .* , *Others are . . .* , and *Life is . . .* The first set of statements incorporates both our actual self-concept and our ideal self-concept. For example, our self-statements based on our ERs might include "I am gentle in nature," "I am short," or "I am honest." While these may or may not be objectively true (i.e., a very short person may not feel short while a tall person may feel short), it is the subjective evaluation that is most important and must be understood. It is important to look for missing and implied unspoken modifiers in the recollections, such as I am *only* a woman, I *must* be honest, or I am *very* short.

When looking for statements that reflect the ideal self, look for declarative statements about what one *should* or *must* be or do—for example, I *should* work hard, I *must* work hard, I *should* be strong *because* I am a man/woman. Family and cultural values and home atmosphere can be seen to have an influence on the self-ideal—for example, you must get a good education to get ahead, always work to win, love cures all, men are more important than women, Black is beautiful.

As you look at statements concerning perceptions of other people, both general and specific statements may be apparent. For example, ERs may clearly imply that "others are generally kind and trustworthy" or "others are not predictable and can be dangerous." Specific statements might include "Women are good servants," "Men are strong," or "Children should be seen but not heard."

Convictions about life also will be both general and specific. For example, general statements might include "Life is full of dangers," "Life is a great big circus," or "Life is a challenge to be met." Specific statements would be like these: "Things are exactly as they seem." "Nature is very unforgiving of a weak person like me." "Each day is a new opportunity for me."

By observing combinations of *I am, others are,* and *life is,* you can make inferences about how an individual meets the basic life tasks as defined by Adler. Study the following example to learn more about understanding and interpreting early recollections.

EXAMPLE OF EARLY RECOLLECTION AND INTERPRETATION

Early Recollection. I remember one Sunday afternoon it was very hot outside and the older kids and adults were all busy doing something even though the sodas were supposed to be put on ice. I decided that I would cool the sodas and began putting the cans into the ice chest. No one particularly noticed that I had seen the job to the end. When they enjoyed the cold sodas later so did I. I really felt pleased with myself and have enjoyed a cold soda on a hot day ever since (laugh).

Interpretation. We might hypothesize from this recollection the individual's belief that "when others shirk their responsibility, I can be depended upon to see that the job gets done. Among life's greatest satisfactions is seeing a job to the end, even when others may not know about it. I can and do enjoy contributing to others' pleasure."

Possible life rules (Adlerian "fictive notions") or self-statements that may be discovered through further examination and discussion of this recollection include the following:

Other people can't be counted on when a job needs to be done; I need to do it myself.
For me, the joy is in the doing (activity).
Doing for others is a source of pleasure for me.
I need to be responsible and help others in order to feel good.

While all of these rules may be seen as appropriate to the individual (as well as others), the *degree* to which they are believed may be a problem at times, such as I will be happy *only* when I serve, am responsible, and so on. Each of us can do a "good thing" too much or otherwise expect too much from ourselves and others. As we have noted over the years and in keeping with Adler and Dreikurs's theory, individuals revert to their earliest interpretations about life, themselves, and others whenever they perceive themselves in a new and potentially unpredictable situation (stressful). Our need to understand and manage change seems to call on prior experience as a source for coping with new situations.

True mastery of the early recollections strategy will not occur until you have experienced it fully yourself. Then, through the practice exercises at the end of this chapter, you can gradually learn to master and utilize this important strategy. Once you have experience with the model from a positive frame of reference, you may then consider using the strategy to explore negative early recollections. However, when working with stressful early recollections, we strongly recommend that you proceed cautiously and seek supervision when this is indicated (Clark, 2002). Even then, we urge that you frequently refer to positive strengths from early recollections as it is the strengths that will help the client deal with difficult challenges. Think in terms of positive psychology and wellness rather than a problem-focused psychology and illness.

USING ERs WITH DCT: A WELLNESS CASE ILLUSTRATION

The client, Rashida, is a 38-year-old African American female. She is the oldest of six children, raised in a predominantly Black neighborhood in a large metropolitan area in the South. She was reared by her mother and grandmother, both of whom held fundamentalist religious beliefs. Spirituality is a very significant part of her life. She is a single mother of three children—an oldest daughter, 19 years old; a son, 17 years old; and a daughter, 15 years old. She has worked all her adult life. Her husband died in a car accident shortly after the third child was born so she has been the sole support for her family. She attended a community college in order to keep her present office job but has not completed a degree.

She sought help through her employee assistance program at work because of stress. Her presenting problems were related to work, her children, and her mother. Her work is increasingly dependent on computer knowledge and skills that she does not possess. Family responsibilities make it difficult for her to seek further education although her employer would pay for her credits and books. She has been coming to work tired and increasingly error prone.

She reports that her son is a constant worry because he has lied to her about his activities, friends, and progress in school. While she thinks his friends are fairly nice, she worries about their occasional sneaky night antics. She is concerned that they may get mixed up with some of the rough boys in the community who like to start fights and carry weapons. She has begun staying up late or waking up during the night to be sure her son has not climbed out the window to meet his friends.

Her girls are doing fine; the oldest is in junior college with financial aid and the youngest is doing well in school, although she worries about her being sexually active and not protecting herself. With all of this happening, the client's mother is talking about moving in with her to help out, and she is trying to view this as positive and helpful. Nothing could be further from the truth; her mother's meddling and criticizing will just make matters worse. In addition, there would be an expectation that she would cover her mother's living and health expenses, and Rashida's budget is hardly adequate for her current obligations. Rashida, however, finds standing up to her mother difficult. In fact, she rarely speaks up to anyone when she disagrees with that person's opinions or behaviors. Her son seems to understand this about her and takes advantage of her unwillingness to engage in confrontations.

Early Recollection and DCT Assessment

As an Adlerian counselor, the author uses specific earliest recollections to help clients discover how their earliest developmental attitudes, beliefs, and expectations shape their behavior and emotions as adults. In this case, Rashida disclosed one of her earliest memories. She recalled that when she was 6 years old her mother came home from the hospital with her brother. She and her younger sister were standing near the front door as their new baby brother was carried into the house by her father. She was so excited that she jumped up and down and began asking to hold him but both mother and father scolded her saying that she might scare the baby. She felt very hurt and never asked to hold him again. She was emotionally moved when recounting this memory, as though it had happened only yesterday.

Using the DCT process of having the client recount the event in the here and now, Rashida closed her eyes and relived the scene again. She was asked what she heard: the car door closing, her parents coming up the steps. What she was seeing: father holding a bundle cradled in his arms, mother holding his arm as they climb the steps. Rashida swings the door open and begins jumping up and down, clapping her hands and asking to see and hold the baby. Father briskly pulls away from her scowling; at the same time, mother slaps her arm and pushes her back. At this point, Rashida is physically pulling back in her chair and sitting upright, almost stiff. When asked how she is feeling, she replies, shocked, hurt, disappointed, and unprepared for the rebuke that she received. She just wants to celebrate her new brother's coming home, but no one cares or seems to trust her to be careful. No one cares how she feels. That's where her recollection ended.

When asked where these feelings are located in her body, she replies in her hands and her heart. Her hands are tightly held together and she moves them to her chest where she says her heart, too, feels tight. The full scenario is summarized and reflected in the same tone, words, tense, and order to Rashida with a view to reflecting what she has just shared. Rashida is fully attentive and apparently comfortable with the accuracy of the reflections.

DCT Assessment With a Current Scenario

Following the guided imagery that evokes a sensorimotor experience, Rashida is asked, have you ever felt this way before? Oh, yes, she said. One such incident happened when visiting with her mother recently. Rashida expressed concern about her son's behavior and her mother attacked her as being too lax in parenting her children. She was asked to describe the scene in a concrete, linear, detailed manner.

A *concrete* description of what is happening resulted in the following description: Her mother got up and turned toward the sink without comment. At first her mother said nothing so Rashida became more expressive about her concerns when suddenly her mother turned, put her hand on Rashida's arm, gave her a slight but firm shove, and with a stern face said that she always knew Rashida was not a firm enough parent and now she would have to see the fruits of her lax guidance for her children. Again Rashida was sitting upright in the chair, hands clasped firmly, with tears coming to her eyes. When asked what followed, Rashida said only that she left as soon as possible and that she felt crushed by what her mother had said to her.

At this point, we again summarize verbatim each scene from both sensorimotor and concrete perspectives, and then Rashida is asked, using the *formal-operational* style, whether she could see any similarities in these two scenes. After a pause, she said that she realized her mother's rebukes were harsh and in each case they hurt her so deeply that she found it hard to speak. In each case, her competence to act responsibly was challenged. Her expression of enthusiasm or any emotion was quickly squelched. She felt totally bound by the experiences, physically and emotionally.

When asked what rules guided her in these instances, she responded: rule number one, don't share your excitement, and rule number two, be responsible but don't expect support. Rashida then said that it wasn't just her mother who made her feel this way. She feels "bound up" at work although no one there is as harsh to her as her mother is. It is that she anticipates a rebuke or challenge to her competence. This brought forth the questions (*dialectic*), *so where did these rules come from? Are these rules good rules for today? Are they good rules in most life situations?*

Rashida expressed surprise at how the connection between these seemingly unrelated events with her parents, her mother in particular, have affected her attitude and behavior at work and likely elsewhere. Having said this, she could see how such "rules" are not valid in other situations. The next question addressed the consequences of using such rules in all situations: Rashida, *at what price to your physical and emotional health do you hold these rules?* She concluded "at a considerable price," especially now as she finds dealing with her son and mother more challenging.

Based on the interview as well as both DCT and Adlerian theory constructs presented earlier, we note that Rashida grew up believing that she was to make her place in her family and community by being responsible, compliant, and uncomplaining. When everyone else was happy, she thought that she was doing her part. However, not everyone can be made happy, and worse, when they are not happy, she felt she was responsible for that, too. Her rules about life, her private logic for making her place, had been unexamined and basically unchallenged. She was ready for change.

Co-constructed intervention: At this point Rashida was asked, do you want to change how you feel and behave? She immediately said "yes." Naturally, with such deeply held experiences and expectations, change will require new thoughts and experiences to reinforce them. To help in this process, Rashida was introduced to the concept of wellness using Figure 2-2 and the descriptors of the components. She was invited to complete a self-assessment of the components and note those on which she scored highest and lowest.

Wellness assessment: During her intake process, Rashida completed a wellness inventory (the Five Factor Wellness Inventory; Myers & Sweeney, 1998) based on the 5 factors and 17 components of wellness described in Chapter 2. Her highest scores were in the Essential Self (spirituality, self-worth, cultural identity, self-care). Her lowest scores were in the Coping Self (realistic beliefs, stress management) and Creative Self (emotions, positive humor).

Not surprisingly, she was fairly accurate with the exception of her realistic beliefs and positive humor. She thought of herself as "realistic"! These items relate to the desire to please others, to be perfectly competent, and to be generally self-effacing to maintain an agreeable demeanor. Once she understood the content of the realistic beliefs items in the assessment, she smiled agreement. Likewise, she thinks of herself as having a "good" sense of humor although she doesn't make jokes or see much humor in her life. In short, she enjoys a "good" laugh but doesn't laugh often and makes no effort to find humor in situations around her, not even by reading the comics in the daily newspaper.

At this point, Rashida was asked what she would like to focus on first. She chose "stress management." Note that no matter what component is chosen, it can be the "correct" one with which to begin. Self-efficacy is developed in increments and when the client chooses the activities and extent of her involvement, success is more readily assured. Small steps can lead to large gains. From a holistic perspective, success in one area will have benefits in others. This can be seen in Rashida's case. As a beginning, she was invited to practice the "push button" technique for relaxation: She was asked to relax and imagine herself in control, safe, and at peace in whatever environment she chose. With some clients—predominantly concrete ones—we can practice initially with a toy "cricket clicker" for them to use as a button to press when they want to change visual images and emotional states. Rashida was invited to experience the change of pushing the button metaphorically and seeing, for example, her son "talking back" to her (or another image if we had determined that such an image was too emotionally stressful). The objective was to have her practice taking charge of her own images and, consequently, her emotions. A practice audiotape was made and she continued using it until she was able to experience a relaxation response with her own signals.

She also was asked if she could make time to walk for a half hour or more every other day to establish an exercise routine as a part of her stress management practices. A suggestion that made this more effective was inviting a friend and on occasion one of her children to join her during these walks. Surprising to her, even her son agreed to join her when he understood it was to help her improve her health. Clearly, the time they spent together had a positive impact on her relationship with him and opened new avenues for effective and meaningful conversation for both Rashida and her son.

Subsequent individual and family counseling helped her achieve greater communication, respect, and cooperation with the children. As Rashida experienced a greater sense of control over her thoughts and feelings, her mirth response improved as well. Her son agreed to help restore his mother's confidence in him so that she could rest at night and could go back to school to complete a degree program that would enhance her position at work.

Rashida's relationship with her mother continued to be contentious at times. Rashida, however, decided not to let her mother move in and, equally important, not "to let her push my buttons!" Rashida also decided to change the church that she attended. She found a need for a different grounding for her spiritual beliefs from the orthodoxy that she grew up with as a child. Her desire for a closer relationship with a loving Creator was a prime motivation. In short, Rashida began taking charge of what she thought, how she felt, and how she would be behave, and not everyone was going to agree with her in all matters—and that was going to be okay!

SUMMARY

Early recollections and DCT assessment and intervention are complementary theories with specific implications for practice. Adlerian use of early recollections involves an understanding of both the philosophical foundations and psychology of Alfred Adler (Adler, 1927/1954; Dreikurs, 1967; Sweeney, 1998). Because both DCT and Adlerian psychology have, as their basis for intervention, respect for the individual as well as the cultural context in which the individual exists including the family, they complement one another's theory, methods, and practices. The case of Rashida is illustrative of the several ways that DCT, Adlerian, and wellness approaches can be blended in practice.

Early memories disclose expectations for the future that shape one's responses to daily life tasks. The anticipation of what will happen when influences the choices each of us makes in both large and small decisions related to work, friendships, love relationships, self, and spiritual matters. Helping clients uncover the meaning and purpose associated with these early recollections empowers them to make new choices, exercise new behaviors, and discover new emotions associated with familiar life experiences and relationships.

Contrary to what might be expected, early recollections can and do change to fit one's expectations. Adlerians distinguish between first-order and second-order change through the use of early recollections. What is commonly referred to as counseling addresses first-order change—for example, helping clients modify behaviors in order to meet their life tasks related to work, friendship, love, self, and spirit (Sweeney, 1998). Psychotherapy, however, results in second-order change that can be validated by noted changes in the content, affect, and themes of early recollections. Adlerians thus distinguish motivation modification (purposiveness of behavior) from behavior modification to distinguish psychotherapy outcomes from counseling outcomes: It is the life goals one seeks that are modified in psychotherapy, thus resulting in changes in the recollections that fortify them in shaping future responses to action.

By using DCT assessment and intervention strategies with early recollections, clients can be helped to more quickly uncover mistaken expectations that they hold for self, others, and life in general. Unrealistic expectations found in early recollections such as "If it is to be, it is *always* up to me!" or "Whatever I do must be done the very best it can be done!" are types of rules that become guiding notions toward life easily associated with stress, emotional turmoil, and physical consequences. Through DCT, we deconstruct such rules in order to help clients delete or change completely expectations that do not serve them or others well. New or modified rules offer more flexibility and less stress.

Wellness as a deliberate guiding orientation to life empowers clients to create new interpretations of what they need and want—for example, from relationships, work, and themselves as participants in their own life story. From both an Adlerian and a DCT perspective, clients are involved in a creative process of becoming throughout their lives. Through purposeful planning and deliberate action, they can learn to modify behaviors and even reorient their most fundamental life goals in positive, life-enhancing ways.

Challenges: Early recollections in the abstract can be no more than interesting stories or seemingly unimportant moments in another's life. The challenge is to help connect the *meaning and purpose* behind the recollection to understand how it is helpful to a client in coping with present and anticipated tasks in that individual's life. If, for example, you can relate the meaning within one of your early recollections to how you cope in present-day circumstances, you will be better able to see how early recollections have relevance for others as well. By participating in a DCT assessment using one or more of your own recollections, you will be able to discover the relatively simple but important connection between early memories and present behavior and the anticipated future.

Research issues: The research on early recollections is substantial (Clark, 2002). The usefulness of such recollections in counseling and therapy remains subject to criticism, however, because so much depends on the experience, orientation, and skill of the practitioner. We believe that much of this criticism can be ameliorated by using the combination of the Adlerian and DCT approaches as illustrated in this chapter and Chapter 2. Nevertheless, there is much room for validation of this position by further research.

Future research to assess the value of these approaches and their methods would do well to incorporate a qualitative analysis of a client's early recollection context and themes before, during, and after intervention. Successful counseling should show early recollection changes also in a wellness direction. Clients will remember different events and/or remember the same events with different content and emotion after successful intervention—for example, someone else is present and helps them when previously they reported being alone and feeling lonely. Psychotherapy, however, should result in clearly distinguishable early recollections from those noted prior to intervention. In fact, some clients may be unwilling to believe they reported earlier recollections unless they hear audiotapes of their own voices that can assure them these were indeed their own self-reports.

THEORY INTO PRACTICE: DEVELOPING YOUR PORTFOLIO OF COMPETENCE

Self-Assessment Exercise

Exercise 1. Examining your early recollections from the DCT perspective

Using the following format, examine your earliest recollections through the DCT questioning process. What rules or expectations seem to be underlying these specific experiences? Look for corroboration of these rules in recent life experiences. (Note: These rules are most easily found in events that were especially pleasurable or stressful because desires and expectations for life were being met or challenged.)

a. Early recollection—specific, verbatim detail (before the age of 8):

_____

_____

_____

_____

Feelings associated with this early recollection:

_____

_____

Specific location and types of feelings in your body:

_____

_____

_____

b. Describe in detail another event with a similar experience of bodily feeling:

_____

_____

_____

_____

_____

c. What do these two events have in common, that is, how are they similar?

_____

_____

_____

_____

What rules seem to be guiding your thoughts, feelings, and behavior?

_____

_____

_____

Are there times and circumstances when these rules do not serve you well? In what ways?

_____

_____

_____

_____

What are the origins of these rules (e.g., parents, teachers, friends)? Are they good rules in all or most circumstances (e.g., how do they help or hinder you in achieving educational or career goals, sustained relationships, or personal positive health)? Do they help you get along better with other people (e.g., understand others' thoughts and feelings, negotiate better relationship agreements)? Do they help you solve problems more effectively? Do they help you to feel better about yourself, others, and life more often than not? Do they help you have more positive feelings (e.g., happiness, joy, satisfaction, contentment) than others (e.g., anger, guilt, disappointment, hurt)? Answering these questions and pondering their significance for how you cope with and transcend life challenges in work, friendship, love/family, self, and spiritual development can lead to new insights, positive feelings, and alternative behaviors.

As long as individuals function fairly well in their daily lives, their fictive notions remain unexamined. When their notions are challenged or proved ineffective at maintaining feelings of security, an emotional crisis develops (Sweeney, 1998). At these times, clients are most open to seeking counseling or psychotherapy. At such times of readiness for change, the issue of "where we are going" becomes essential to the focus and outcomes sought in counseling.

Toward Multicultural Competence

Exercise 2. Understanding life experiences of persons from other cultures and backgrounds

Interview one or two individuals from different gender, ethnic, religious, or sexual orientations. Ask them to identify specific early memories associated with their gender, ethnicity, religion, or sexual orientation. Using the format provided above, examine these early memories from Adlerian and DCT perspectives. What can you identify as the major life themes and rules relative to these multicultural issues? How do they affect the person's current behavior?

_____

_____

_____

_____

_____

Interview Practice Exercises

Exercise 3. Interpreting early recollections

Interview a partner or an actual client. Ask the person to spend a few moments reflecting on her or his earliest memories, being sure to think about those that happened before the age of 8. Write down two or three of these memories below (or more using an additional sheet of paper). Be sure to note (1) the age at which the memory occurred, (2) what happened as if it were happening now, and (3) how the person felt.

You may find it helpful to audiotape what the person sees, hears, and feels. Try to get the client to be as specific and detailed as possible. Ask questions such as these: Who else (if anyone) is with you in the early recollection? Who is doing what (if anything)? What are your surroundings? Report the events in the here and now as if they are occurring at this very moment.

If the person is writing or typing the recollection, ask him or her to record the story in the same order, detail, and use of terms as if he or she were speaking. Ask where in the body these feelings are specifically located.

_____

_____

_____

_____

_____

_____

_____

_____

_____

_____

After recording one or more early recollections, you may study them by asking your client some additional questions. In these recollections,

Are you active or passive?
Are you an observer or participant?
Are you giving or taking (sharing, caring, other)?
Are you alone or with others?
Are you concerned with people, things, or ideas?
What emotional and physical position are you in with others?
    Inferior (below)? Superior (above)?
What feeling tone is attached to the event or outcome?
What emotions do you use to feel comfort in relation to others (if any)?
What details, smells, sounds, and colors are present (if any)?
Do stereotypes of authorities, subordinates, men, women, old, and young reveal themselves?

Next, look for themes and an overall pattern if more than one ER is used. Try to complete the following sentences:

I am _____

Others are _____

Life is _____

Exercise 4. Group practice with early recollections

Step 1: Divide into practice groups.

Step 2: Select a group leader.

Step 3: Ask each member of the group to recall a specific early recollection related to her or his gender, ethnicity, or religious/spiritual background.

Step 4: Discuss how these recollections help us develop unique perceptions of the world around us.

At this point be sure that all individuals have time to present their reflections and obtain feedback from others in the group. Feedback should be strength-based and positive.

Generalization: Taking Adlerian and Wellness Concepts Home

Exercise 5. Practice and observation with individuals in daily life

During the next week, observe individuals as they talk about themselves and their experiences. Listen for statements that describe key life themes about self, others, and life. Try to imagine what kinds of early life memories led to their current beliefs about themselves, life, and others.

Portfolio Reflections

Exercise 6. Reflections on your early memories and wellness

What stood out for you from this chapter? What sense do you make of the exercises on your early memories? What are the key points you want to remember from this chapter? Record your thoughts below and in your Portfolio Folder.

_____

_____

_____

_____

_____

_____

_____

_____

REFERENCES

Adler, A. (1954). *Understanding human nature* (W. B. Wolf, Trans.). New York: Fawcett. (Original work published 1927)

Ansbacher, H. L. (Ed.). (1969). *The science of living: Alfred Adler*. Garden City, NY: Doubleday.

Ansbacher, H. L., & Ansbacher, R. R. (Eds.). (1956). *The individual psychology of Alfred Adler*. New York: Harper & Row.

Clark, A. J. (2002). *Early recollections*. New York: Brunner-Routledge.

Dreikurs, R. (1967). *Psychodynamics, psychotherapy, and counseling*. Chicago: Alfred Adler Institute.

Dreikurs, R. (1971). *Social equality: The challenge of today*. Chicago: Regnery.

Frankl, V. (1959) *Man's search for meaning*. New York: Pocket Books. (Original work published 1946)

Ivey, A. (2000). *Developmental therapy: Theory into practice*. North Amherst, MA: Microtraining. (Original work published 1986)

Ivey, A., & Ivey, M. (2003). *Intentional interviewing and counseling: Facilitating client development in a multicultural society*. Pacific Grove, CA: Brooks/Cole.

Mosak, H. H., & Dreikurs, R. (1967). The life task III, the fifth life task. *Individual Psychologist, 5*(1), 16, 22.

Mosak, H. H., & Dreikurs, R. (1973). Adlerian psychotherapy. In R. Corsini (Ed.), *Current psychotherapies*. Itasca, IL: Peacock.

Myers, J. E., & Sweeney, T. J. (1998). *Five factor wellness inventory*. Greensboro, NC: Authors.

Myers, J. E., & Sweeney, T. J. (in press). The indivisible self: An evidence-based model of wellness. *Journal of Individual Psychology*.

Myers, J. E., Sweeney, T. J., & Witmer, J. M. (2000). The Wheel of Wellness counseling for wellness: A holistic model for treatment planning. *Journal of Counseling and Development, 78*(3), 251–266.

Sweeney, T. J. (1995). Adlerian theory. In D. Cappuzi & D. Gross (Eds.), *Counseling and psychotherapy* (pp. 171–206). Columbus, OH: Merrill.

Sweeney, T. J. (1998). *Adlerian counseling: A practitioners approach*. Philadelphia: Accelerated Development.

Sweeney, T. J., & Witmer, J. M. (1991). Beyond social interest: Striving toward optimum health and wellness. *Individual Psychology, 47*(4), 527–540.

Witmer, J. M., & Sweeney, T. J. (1992). A holistic model for wellness and prevention over the lifespan. *Journal of Counseling and Development, 71*, 140–148.

CHAPTER 11
Using Developmental Counseling and Therapy With Families

Jane Myers, Sandra Rigazio-DiGilio, and Allen Ivey

CENTRAL PRACTICE OBJECTIVE | Mastery and practice of concepts in this chapter will enable you to understand and work with families at various stages of the life cycle and to apply DCT questioning strategies to facilitate family development.

Lifespan developmental tasks are more complicated when family and systemic issues are considered. Coordinating multiple developmental tasks and needs of family members in an intact, nuclear family is in itself quite complicated. Other factors, such as differing cultural and family types and the continuing impact of our complex, postindustrial society, add further complications and challenges. Developmental counseling and therapy provides a useful way to map the family life cycle and is an important therapeutic tool for working effectively with family systems.

Family work by its very nature is dialectic/systemic. We are always working on issues of relationships and systems. However, once we enter family counseling work, we still can rely on DCT's sensorimotor, concrete, and formal strategies. Thus, as you read this chapter, keep in mind that ideas of dialectic/systemic thinking are behind all that is presented here.

Sandra Rigazio-DiGilio has adapted DCT for family work. Entitled systemic cognitive developmental therapy (SCDT), this system is an integrative metatheory of family helping and family process. See Rigazio-DiGilio (2002) for a summary of this work and Rigazio-DiGilio, Ivey, Kunkler, and O'Grady (2004), who expand these ideas in their presentation of the community genogram. For additional reading to supplement the information in this chapter, the following may be useful: Carlson and Kejos (2002), Gladding (2002), Carter and McGoldrick (1999), and Nichols and Schwartz (2001a, 2001b).

Knowledge of and skill in the concepts of this chapter can enable you to:

1. Understand the family life cycle and how to integrate lifespan and family life-cycle theory in your practice.
2. Use DCT to facilitate family development and wellness.
3. Apply DCT in simulated and real family counseling situations.

INTRODUCTION: THE FAMILY LIFE CYCLE, A DELICATE BALANCE

Just as individuals move through the life cycle, so does the family unit. A teenager seeking a sense of identity may have a 35-year-old mother starting work for the first time and a 43-year-old father going through a mid-life crisis. The father faces a life issue of maintaining generativity in the face of declining physical ability. The mother, for the first time in her life, may be just beginning to gain a sense of her identity and competence in the work world. The teenager's stress in developing an identity may be intensified by the stress in the family, as each family member attempts to resolve possibly conflicting developmental needs.

Developing an individual identity is highly related to the developmental stage and needs of each family member and the family as a whole. Each person in the family has personal developmental tasks, which may not always be in accord with those of other family members. In addition, the parents may not have worked through their own developmental tasks adequately and thus may never have established their own identity or sense of trust. All these factors deeply influence the developmental path of the child and adolescent. The first life-cycle theory for the family was developed by Haley (1987, 1991, 1996). This theory pointed out that many family problems occur during transitions in the life cycle; for example, when a couple marries (or lives together), major adjustments in life style have to be made. Transitions continue through retirement and old age.

The DCT approach to the family life cycle presented in Figure 11-1 is based on Haley's original work but portrays additional complexities and interactions. The outer circle represents the family's life stages ranging from the parents' young adulthood through marriage to retirement. The inner circle represents one child's life stages within that family. The birth of the child, of course, is a major developmental transition for the couple. As the young adult separates and leaves home for a job or college, the developmental task of the parents is to adapt to the change or loss. When the child marries, the parents take on new challenges, just as their child does, but each is facing a very different stage in the life cycle. The separation and attachment tasks and needs of parents and married children are very different.

Each of these family life stages brings with it special problems relating to often difficult transitions. Be prepared to search for developmental family issues in all your clients. The family issues may not be central to their reasons for contacting you, but often family life-cycle issues will exacerbate the individual's difficulties—or transitions in the family life cycle may be the most important underlying issue.

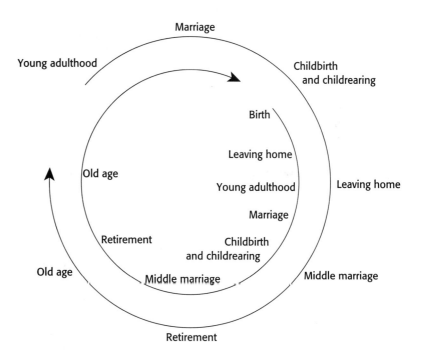

Figure 11-1 The Family Life Cycle
The outer circle represents the parents, the inner circle the child. Note that separation and attachment needs will vary markedly for each. Divorce, death, single parenting, cultural differences, and major events in society will change the nature of the family life cycle.

Each stage of family life has key separation and attachment tasks (see Table 11-1). For example, when children leave home, the couple faces this separation from their children as well as their own need to reattach to each other in a new way. Sometimes families become too enmeshed and the result is a lack of boundary definition. In such cases, when children leave home, the event can be traumatic enough to trigger a severe family crisis. If the family was too separate and detached, with rigid boundaries, the parents may have problems during this time reattaching to each other. Also, the couple may need to support aging parents, who are becoming increasingly dependent. A delicate balance is required of individuals and families as they negotiate their way through the life cycle. Not only do these issues affect families; you will also encounter many in individual counseling who face these issues.

Table 11-1   The Family Life Cycle and Issues of Separation and Attachment

The model below clearly does not represent the vast array of family types, but in each stage we illustrate common issues that may cause the nature of separation and attachment issues to vary.

Developmental Stage	Developmental Tasks and Issues of Separation and Attachment
Young adulthood	Increasing attachment to peers; separation from parents; courtship and selection of mate; choice of career and job initiated. *Example life-stage variation:* Early pregnancy may bring the mother back to the home and a new form of attachment.
Marriage	Attachment to mate and new friends; further separation from parents as a "child" and reattachment to parents as an adult; need to attach to in-laws; establishing a home and career fully initiated. *Example life-stage variations:* Couple may live together and not marry or be a married gay or lesbian pair.
Childbirth and childrearing	Separation from a couple relationship built up over several years and attachment to the infant. Establishment of new relationship with parents, in-laws, peers; as child starts school, the first of many separations occurs between parents and child; balancing of work and home responsibilities. Possible job crises. *Example life-stage variations:* The child comes before marriage, difficulty in becoming pregnant, adoption, or no child at all.
Leaving home	Separation of child from parents as he or she leaves for school or job; reattachment of marital dyad; establishment of new relationships with friends. *Example life-stage variation:* Divorce is common at this stage and may result in a whole new set of attachments and separations.
Middle marriage	A period of time for the couple to firmly establish themselves as a couple or as separate individuals; financial resources often at a high; mid-50s crisis as they realize that major goals are not to be achieved; reattachment to one's own aging parents; attachment to grandchildren. *Example life-stage variations:* One's own parents and/or one's children return home.
Retirement	Separation from careers, more attachment as a dyad; reattachment of adult children as friends. *Example life-stage variations:* Difficulties in using leisure time, concerns about health, finances, and worry about children and grandchildren.
Old age	Separation from friends and/or life partner through death; increasing concerns over illness; dependency and attachment to children; spiritual attachments become more important; financial and health difficulties may be central. *Example life-stage variations:* Healthy lifestyle through early 90s, serious illness such as blindness, deafness, and inability to walk, abandoned by disinterested children.

Retirement and old age are separated in the DCT approach to the family cycle, as the developmental tasks between the two are very different—for example, the transition from work to leisure as contrasted with the transition to old age and being cared for by others, usually family members. In early retirement, some couples may find themselves helping older children and/or caring for grandchildren. In late retirement and old age, the couple often encounters ill health and the loss of one spouse, and they may find they need care from their families.

The meaning and content of the life cycle vary with culture and family type. Table 11-1 shows the many possibilities for differing experiences in the family life cycle. Also, there are fewer intact nuclear families than there were 20 years ago. Figure 11-1 thus should be modified to fit each culture and family type; for instance, the separation and attachment patterns of fundamentalist Christian, Jewish Orthodox, and conservative Muslim families will obviously differ considerably. Americans of Irish, Chinese, Puerto Rican, and Mexican backgrounds will also differ in the patterns, particularly depending on their degree of acculturation. Regardless of such differences, all families must in some way work through the developmental tasks associated with the family life cycle, although the tasks may be sequenced differently with varying degrees of importance, according to the culture.

Of course, the increasing complexity of family structures, including blended families, extended blended families (see Myers & Schwiebert, 1999), stepparent families, multigeneration families, gay and lesbian families, grandparent-headed families, and grandparents raising grandchildren, results in considerable diversity in family development beyond the life-cycle paradigm. Creativity and dialectic perspectives are required to help families cope with these changing structures, particularly as demands of these structures will be different depending on the developmental stage of the individual members of the family system.

INTEGRATING LIFESPAN AND FAMILY LIFE-CYCLE THEORY

All members of the family have their own lifespan issues—and, of course, they are different for men and women. Men and women often see the meaning of marriage differently—especially if one member of the couple is older than the other. A 34-year-old woman who marries a man 16 years her senior (who already has children) may want to become pregnant and raise a family whereas the husband resists. Then, when the child has left home, the husband may be nearing retirement age whereas she may be reaching the height of her career. Differences in ages, lifestyles, and cultural backgrounds can create immense challenges and needs for counseling and therapy. Lifespan theory and past patterns of attachment and separation deeply affect the family life cycle.

Families are also affected by lifespans beyond their own. You may wish to develop a family chart, genogram, or family tree to map the extended family. Here you may find intergenerational issues that have been passed down over time. The basic source for developing a family genogram is McGoldrick, Gerson, and Shellenberger (1999).

As this point, a useful exercise is to identify one lifespan developmental stage that was or is of particular interest to you—for example, adolescent identity development. As you developed your own personal identity, other family members were struggling with their life issues. What happened to your parents inevitably affected your sense of self and ability to be both connected with others and autonomous. At this critical stage of development, divorce or the absence or death of one parent can be especially difficult. At times, your need to establish a separate identity may have clashed with needs of other family members grappling with their life issues. As you were working through your issue of identity, what Eriksonian developmental tasks were your family members facing? Did your parents achieve a sense of intimacy or of generativity? You may find it useful to review the theories presented in Chapter 3 as you think about your own development.

_____

_____

_____

_____

Outline your own personal struggle with the issue of identity. How might the individual developmental needs of each family member have conflicted with your gaining a sense of identity and affected you as the person you now are?

_____

_____

_____

_____

_____

Consider those early events that affected your later life patterns of thinking, feeling, and behaving. What patterns in your present life have continued from these events?

_____

_____

_____

_____

_____

As discussed earlier, cultural and sexual differences affect how you develop a sense of trust, autonomy, industry, and identity. How did your gender and cultural differences affect your development of these qualities?

_____

_____

_____

_____

DCT AND FAMILY PERSPECTIVES: A CASE STUDY

In the family life cycle, family difficulties are considered within a developmental framework. Family and individual symptoms are seen as indicators of uncompleted life stages and difficult transitions rather than as signals of pathology. Similar to DCT, Haley's (1987, 1996) view is that dysfunctional behavior and cognitions result from unfinished developmental tasks and are not just caused by interpersonal conflict or environmental stressors.

From the DCT perspective, the counseling and therapy process is similar to family development. The therapeutic process reflects the family life cycle. Working therapeutically with a family, for example, may be compared to a marriage in that trust is essential and a contract is important. For a short time, the therapist functions almost as a family member. The process of understanding the presenting problem follows, and a new way of seeing and working with the problem evolves. As the family develops and grows, the therapist separates from the family. The therapeutic cycle has many parallels to the family life cycle, as is shown in the following list (adapted from DeFranck-Lynch, 1986, p. 56):

The Life Cycle of Family Therapy

1. Joining, engagement, attachment, and assessment	The therapist becomes a metaphorical family member, but one with clinical distance and defined boundaries.
2. Cognitive and behavioral interventions	The therapist participates in family life, affecting and being affected by the family.
3. Integrating, consolidating change, separation, and termination	The therapist and family separate, taking with them new views of the developmental process.

Stage 1: Joining

The counselor or therapist must accommodate to the family in the joining process. All family members need to feel that they are accepted as valuable contributors to the process. By asking open-ended questions of each individual and the family as a whole, the therapist can help each person feel comfortable and participatory. In addition, the responses to these questions enable the counselor to assess cognitive/emotional styles of the individual and of the family as a unit.

The following example (altered to disguise identifying data) shows how to assess developmental styles in a short period of time. In response to therapist inquiries, the Cachet family members introduced themselves as follows:

Ray: As you can probably tell by the accent, I'm French-Canadian. My parents came here from Montreal. I work as a cabinetmaker for a living and took over my dad's business because I was the oldest son. I make a good living. It's harder now that I'm sick, but the doctors say I will recover OK. (Predominantly concrete)

Stephanie: I'm French-Canadian, too. I have the same accent, only a little less. Let's see . . . well, I'm a mother. Lisa is my only child. I have lived in Carthage almost all my life. My sister lives around the corner from me. (Predominantly concrete)

Lisa: (Withdraws and whimpers. Mother spoke for her, but the child was asked again and the mother's help was blocked.) I don't want to be here. It's scary. Why did we have to come? I know I'm bad. I'll be good (cries again). (Predominantly sensorimotor)

The goal in this first stage of family intervention is for the helper to attach to, or join with, the family to establish a working therapeutic system. It is important to help the family arrive at a consensual view of the problem. This can be done by asking the whole family "What do you want changed?" and then working out an answer with which all can agree. Again, the process of defining the problem gives the counselor an opportunity to observe how the family operates and what its rules, perspectives, and organizational arrangements are.

Although family members will vary in cognitive/emotional style as they describe the problem, the family as a whole will usually define it in a single cognitive/emotional style. Some families present the issue in a confused, illogical, sensorimotor fashion, a mode often characteristic of those in chaos and trauma. A formal family will usually define the issue abstractly ("We need to learn how to solve problems and talk about things more openly" or "We always seem to be avoiding the issue"). A family who uses a concrete style will usually describe a specific event or problem needing solution ("Susie needs to start eating properly" or "John is depressed and can't work"). As discussed in earlier chapters, the predominantly formal style family needs to work more at a concrete style, and the more concretely oriented family needs to examine larger patterns (but only after concrete issues are dealt with, resolved, and understood). It may not be necessary to take a family through the full cognitive/emotional sequence.

The Cachet family described their problem to the therapist as follows:

Stephanie: I just want my daughter to behave—to stop acting or being sick, to go back to school every day and get good grades.

Ray: That's right. I can't be bothered with these disruptions. I have to get well so I can get back to work. You have to buck up and fly right, Lisa. That's why we are here.

Stephanie: That's right, Lisa. Tell the therapist what's wrong. We keep getting letters from school.

Lisa: I don't know. I don't understand. I try to be good. I just keep getting sick. I don't know why. I don't want to be sick anymore. (Whimpers and withdraws)

One can assess here that the Cachet parental authority is predominantly concrete while the daughter is using a sensorimotor style. The general cognitive/emotional style of the family as a whole appears to be concrete.

Many families will hold one individual, the "identified patient" (IP), responsible for the problem. In such cases, the family frames the problem in a linear, causal way: "If only so and so would change, then everything would be fine." A key objective of family therapy is to help the family move to a dialectic/systemic frame of reference—that is, to help family members expand their view of the problem so they can see more options for change. If, with guidance and support of the therapist, the family can learn to look at itself as a system, family members will begin to understand how their interactions affect one another and how these interactions can exacerbate or alleviate the problems.

Box 11-1   DCT Questioning Strategies for Families

Sensorimotor	■ At this moment, what are the two of you feeling in your body?
	■ What are you feeling as you see Samantha cry?
	■ Tell Deryl how what he just said produced changes in your body.
	■ You say "fear of harm" . . . could you go further with that?
	■ Both of you, please sit in silence—note what occurs for each of you in reaction to what just happened.
	■ Did you see Chloe's body jump when you said that?
	■ What, specifically, did you hear your parents say, Chloe?
	■ What does eating at the dinner table feel like to each of you?
Concrete	■ Could you give me a specific example of how (the presenting problem—bulimia, acting out, fighting) occurs?
	■ Would the two parents discuss what happens just before Chloe vomits? What happens afterward?
	■ Deryl and Samantha, what did the two of you say to each other about the incident.
	■ How did the whole family feel after the last vomiting incident?
Formal	■ Is this style of interaction a repeating pattern for you?
	■ How often does it happen? What are the variations?
	■ Does the pattern bring the two of you and the family closer together or more apart?
	■ Stop for a moment and reflect on what's happened here and now in this session. What has stood out for you?
Dialectic/Systemic	■ Looking at all this, how would you describe this family?
	■ Could you talk about the family from another perspective or point of view?
	■ What type of rule is this family operating under?
	■ What are the flaws in that rule?
	■ What would you as a family like to do with that rule?
	■ What role does religion/ethnicity play in the ways your family interacts?
	■ How are you similar to or different from your families of origin?

Using the DCT questions from Box 11-1, the counselor can help the family view the problem from different perspectives. The family's responses allow the therapist to identify the family's ability to function within each cognitive/emotional style. Is the family overwhelmed by emotions? Does it see events as isolated or as connected by patterns? The questions are posed to dyads and triads within the family. The therapist's responsibility is to ensure that these dyads and triads discuss and answer the questions without assistance from other family members.

By such questionings, the therapist gains an idea of the family's sense of reality at different cognitive styles and helps to foster interactions among family members.

The Cachet family then went through the Standard Cognitive/Emotional Developmental Interview (see Appendix 3). This process took about an hour. Some example responses from each of the developmental styles, in abbreviated form, are shown on the following pages:

Sensorimotor exploration, brief example:

Therapist: As the two of you (parents) see your (daughter) being so confused, how are you feeling right now?

Stephanie: I just think my daughter is out of control, and it makes me feel depressed. I'm at my wit's end. I just don't know what to do. My husband . . . (emotional tone is sad and confused)

Ray: I can't stand my wife being so sad. It bothers me to see her so upset. (Emotionally flat)

Therapist: Talk to each other about how you are feeling right now.

Stephanie: You know it makes me sad and it makes me angry. (Anger shows in vocal tone and flashing eyes)

Ray: I just wish you could snap out of it and take control of the situation. (Angry)

Concrete exploration, brief example:

Therapist: Can you give me an example of how this sickness of Lisa's and refusal to go to school occurs?

Stephanie: Well, what happens is that Lisa starts feeling sick at night and has difficulty sleeping. I try to comfort her and calm her down, but it doesn't work. In the morning she usually feels just the same. I try to get her to go to school, but many times it won't work. I talk to her . . .

   I plead with her to go . . . if I take the time and trouble to force her to go, the nurse calls me and says I have to come and take her home because she's feeling ill.

Ray: I just watch it all happen. She should be more firm and take control. Pleading doesn't work. They have to straighten out their relationship. They used to be so close; I never had to worry about either of them. Things were more relaxed then.

Stephanie: I do what you suggest, but it doesn't work. She is so obstinate lately. (Angry)

Ray: You really need to enforce the rules, like you used to. (Angry)

Lisa: I feel sick in the morning. I just want to stay home. It starts at night. I get headaches and my tummy hurts. But I don't say nothing until morning. I don't even eat breakfast. It's hard to go to school.

   The therapist moves to late concrete questions to obtain the sequence of Lisa's behavior. Stephanie describes a scene at home where Ray is working hard even though recovering from a heart attack. She tries to get Lisa to school, but Lisa stays home in bed. The sequence ends with another angry exchange.

Formal exploration, brief example:

Therapist: Has anything like this ever happened before?

Stephanie: When I was a girl, I never acted this way. I listened to my mother and I stayed out of my father's way.

Ray: I took care of myself, too. I left high school to work with my father. That's the only time I saw him, in fact. He was always working, working. We never had this problem.

Therapist: And what's going on between the two of you now?

Ray: Well, ever since my attack, I've been home more and I see what the two of them are doing. Stephanie says that Lisa used to do what she said, but I surely don't see it.

Stephanie: Well, Ray, you have trouble resting and you need a lot of rest. When Lisa and I argue he has difficulty resting.

Ray: That's right. And you seem to get depressed when you can't keep things under control. It's like when Lisa's bad you seem to get depressed. I guess there's too much happening in the family right now. We need to get on track.

Stephanie: Yes, this can't go on (pause) . . . Ray sick, me depressed, and Lisa not going to school.

Ray's new presence at home appeared at the same time as Lisa's symptoms and Stephanie's depression. The family begins to understand the issue as a repeating pattern of interaction. The therapist notes that Ray is continuing his father's pattern of constant work.

Dialectic/systemic, brief example:

The therapist summarizes the family pattern and she asks for the family rule. Again, all the exchanges in this transcript are greatly abbreviated.

Therapist: Well, given all this, what do you imagine the rule to be that you are operating under?

Ray: Well, practically speaking, a smooth running show is what we need. Everyone on track and getting their job done.

Stephanie: That's the way it is supposed to be, but Lisa is not fitting in and I'm angry at her. Ray shouldn't have to hear all this turmoil.

Therapist: So the rule seems to be that a smooth running "on-track" show with all the family members doing their job is best.

Ray: Yes.

Therapist: Can you give me some idea about where you learned this rule about everyone doing his own job and keeping on track?

Ray: Well, we both come from French-Canadian families. Work was the way we survived. It was hard making it in Carthage in those days. Everyone had to sacrifice. Everyone always pulled their load, but we are at wit's end with Lisa.

Therapist: So dads worked, and moms always took care of the home, and the children were always good. Sounds perfect. But nothing is ever really perfect. What were some things that you may have missed working under those rules?

Stephanie: Well, I guess my mom was kind of sheltered. I guess I am, too. I mean, my husband's illness has really thrown me for a loop. I wish I could help more.

Ray: She was asking if we missed out on things as kids. I guess I missed out on being a kid. When I watch Lisa have fun I feel it in my heart. She's so pretty when she's happy. My dad worked hard and after he died, I missed out on having fun with him.

Stephanie: Me too, me too. I never got to know my dad.

Lisa: (sniffles) I don't like to see Daddy sick.

The DCT questioning sequence started with an emotional base at the sensorimotor style followed by concrete description of the interaction around the child. At the formal orientation, the family is beginning to see its repeating patterns; and at the dialectic/systemic style, they are beginning to see how they have recreated old intergenerational family patterns, some of which they regret.

Stage 2: Cognitive and Behavioral Intervention

The first stage of family therapy may involve from one to three interviews. The key developmental intervention in stage 2 is to help the family state the consensual family problem from a new frame of reference. This reframing (or reframe) synthesizes family data and the therapist's clinical framework into a new gestalt.

In order for the reframe to be effective, it must be accepted by all members of the family, show no judgment or blame, incorporate the developmental context of the family, and be understandable at the cognitive/emotional style of each member. Particularly important, the reframe must expand possibilities and provide opportunity for new solutions, thus engendering hope and focusing on concrete goals. An abstract dialectic/systemic reframe may be theoretically elegant but will be of little use if it is "over the family's head."

The reframe often comes near the end of the joining process and may be as simple a statement as "This is not a problem of your daughter Jane; rather, it is an issue of family interaction that all of us can work on. Jane is not the problem." Another approach is the positive reframe: "Jane's behavior seems to bring the family back together. Until she had her problem, you were all going separate ways. But now you are working together again." Providing a variety of perspective changes is often useful: "Another way to look at the problem is that Jane protects the family from arguments. Every time her behavior draws attention to herself, the family must put all other issues on hold."

The purpose of reframes is to help the family look at itself as a system. The system can be examined concretely or abstractly. Interventions at this stage are most effective if matched to the cognitive/emotional style of the family. Most reframes involve formal dimensions and thus may require both interpretation and concrete behavioral enactments, or role-plays, and homework so that families oriented to concreteness can understand and work through the new concepts.

DCT helps the therapist design interventions at appropriate cognitive/emotional styles to facilitate vertical or horizontal movement in the development of the family. A behavioral approach or Haley's (1987, 1996) problem-solving family theory method may be especially effective when a therapist is beginning to work with a family with a concrete style. Chaotic families may approach a sensorimotor style of functioning, in which case the therapist may need to take a stronger role in interventions.

Formally oriented DCT questioning techniques and psychoeducational methods can help families become aware of repeating patterns. The communications approach to families (e.g., Satir, 1967; Satir, Dengo, & Peck, 2001) seeks to help families reflect on their interactions while simultaneously supporting concrete skills of accurate communication. The best known dialectic/systemic family style is Bowen's (1985/1990) intergenerational approach, which helps individuals and families understand how present behavior is derived from past rules. The classic book *Ethnicity and Family Therapy* (McGoldrick, Giordano, & Pearce, 1996) provides the therapist with a wealth of detail about issues of culture and family development and remains a standard of the field.

More difficult to classify in terms of DCT are Minuchin's (1998) structural approach and therapies of the Milan group (see Minuchin & Fishman, 1981; Carlson & Kejos, 2002), which can be described as multistyle interventions—a combination of specific concrete interventions with elements of formal pattern recognition.

The systematic questioning strategies of DCT can themselves be used as a treatment intervention. The structured interview of Appendix 3 can be used effectively with families, although the sequence of questions must be modified to accommodate the multiple styles of development within the family. DCT encourages us as helping professionals to accept the various cognitive/emotional styles in the family and view these differences as resources rather than as sources of tension. Retrospective family analysis of both concrete events and patterns could involve Tamase's introspective developmental counseling methods of Chapter 3 and Appendix 1 although, again, with modification for multiple developmental styles. Specific questions could be derived from Haley's life-cycle approach to enable families to examine themselves and their development.

With the Cachet family, the therapist focused on the family construct of doing things well, with the following major reframe. (Note that she starts with a highly positive reframe of the family's difficult situation.)

Therapist: I commend both of you for keeping the family rule of doing things well, even in the difficult time of Ray's illness. I commend your strength and loyalty to each other. I commend Ray for continuing to try even though he feels so tired much of the time. I commend Stephanie for trying not to interfere and doing her best. I also commend Lisa for knowing just how to be sure that her mother's sadness and worry over Ray could be helped. Your behavior, Lisa, keeps you and your mom fighting. And until you, Stephanie, believe it is okay to discuss your sadness with your husband, your daughter will help you stay disappointed in her.

The difficult part is that the rules about keeping on track and not showing that you are scared or angry are not working for you right now. Changing the rule to go with your present situation may be difficult. Stephanie, you say you are depressed. Ray, you say you cannot rest. Lisa, you say you are sick and unhappy. This is proof that the rules aren't working.

You both said you missed your own fathers while you were growing up and that your mothers missed much of the world. Perhaps we can look at this crisis as an opportunity rather than a burden. You may be able to use this time to rethink how you share responsibility for Lisa so that you don't have the regrets you had about your own parents, and the three of you might be able to have a little more fun.

I could help you in the next few months to try some new ways that will help your daughter know what's expected of her and allow her to feel less anxious about her mom and happier having a little time with her dad, which she's never had.

Stephanie and Ray, I'm going to ask you to try some things you've never tried before. I'm sure if you try these things, Lisa will know what she's supposed to do.

The data for this reframe obviously came from the DCT questioning sequence, and the therapist used issues of emotional importance in the past and present to motivate the family toward change. With the help of the therapist, Ray was able to recognize his withdrawal from the family in work, and Stephanie was able to find a part-time job in the community to help with the financial burden. With less attention from her mother and more from her father, Lisa's difficulties with attending school ceased. Most of the therapist's interventions were paced at the concrete style so that the Cachet family had new alternatives for action. However, emotional thoughts about their own family history helped Ray and Stephanie change some very old patterns in their relationship. As the family interaction improved so did Ray's health, and thus the therapist was able to withdraw after 10 sessions spread over four months.

Effective family developmental intervention can take many forms, but the main goal is to reframe the problem from a new perspective and help the family look at issues from a systemic context. In an individualistic society, thinking of oneself or one's family as a system is often difficult. However, the systematic approach of DCT is logical and appealing and offers much for family and individual counseling. Applying a systems approach such as DCT represents a major theoretical shift in the helping field.

Stage 3: Separation and Support for Change

As the family takes more responsibility for achieving the goals of therapy and for confronting the consequences of change, the therapist can begin the process of separation. The counselor does this by firmly reiterating the reframe, accepting and encouraging the family's new way of acting, and reinforcing the family's developmental growth patterns.

In two to five sessions, the therapist can help the family review the therapy process and their expanded behavioral and cognitive repertoire. During this time, the family becomes more secure about their newly acquired problem-solving skills. The temptation for the formal-operational therapist may be to analyze and review, but concrete action and discussion are very important. Homework and behavioral enactment procedures help reinforce concrete achievements.

The final objective at this stage is to assist the family and its members reorient to life without therapy. Sessions become less frequent, and the therapist may adopt a role that is more a listener and consultant. Respect for the various cognitive-developmental styles of family members is stressed, and this helps the family learn to accept their own and others' styles of cognitive development. This acceptance and understanding of our need for support in working through life-cycle tasks is the most positive and helpful reorientation toward life problems that the family can acquire through DCT.

SUMMARY

Expect both individual and family clients to present many issues in counseling and therapy that are based on life-cycle changes and transitions. The family life cycle provides a framework for the many developmental transitions couples face throughout their lives. In addition, the birth of a child starting her or his own life's journey brings a new person with unique developmental transitions to the couple. The intersection of one or more children with the family life cycle complicates the many transitional issues faced by all.

Alternative family organizational types and multicultural issues need to be central considerations as we review the family life cycle. Single-parent families, divorce, gay/lesbian couples with and without children, and many other types of families exist. Each of these requires sensitivity to its uniqueness.

Lifespan theory intersects with family life-cycle theory in important ways. While it is clear that the family life cycle and its transitions bring about many issues, the intersection of individual lifespans greatly complicates the issue. It is important that you be able to take a multiperspective view of any individual or family that comes before you.

DCT questioning procedures and strategies are equally effective in family counseling and family therapy. Example questions and interventions were presented along with a case study illustrating the process.

A three-stage model of family intervention was presented—joining; cognitive-behavioral intervention; integrating change, separation, and termination. In a sense, your task in joining the family is an attachment issue, followed by virtual membership in the family, and completed through successful separation and termination.

Challenges: Your first sessions with a couple or family are likely to be sufficient challenge in themselves, as another level of alertness and expertise will be required of you beyond that needed to work with individuals. Further challenges include the complexity of the family life cycle and individual differences as they occur throughout the lifespan.

Research issues: Assessment of family members' presenting issues is an essential first step in family counseling. In this chapter, the importance of assessing the differing cognitive styles of family members was also stressed. Design and implement a research project to help counselors identify cognitive styles in family sessions and evaluate the differential impact of working with families with and without the DCT assessment. How are family interventions made easier when the cognitive/emotional styles of individual family members are known as well as the general cognitive/emotional styles of the entire family?

THEORY INTO PRACTICE: DEVELOPING YOUR PORTFOLIO OF COMPETENCE

Self-Assessment Exercises

Exercise 1. Identifying cognitive/emotional styles in your family of origin

Family members present themselves at varying cognitive-developmental styles. Think about your own family of origin. Examine family interactions to see the interplay of these concepts with individuals. For each family member, recall positive interactions and memories. What cognitive styles were evident for you and for the other family members during those interactions? What does this tell you about your own style of comfort in relating to family members?

_____

_____

_____

_____

_____

Exercise 2. Identifying your family interaction patterns based on cognitive/emotional styles

Perhaps you are a predominantly formal-operational individual and you may have had conflicts with a family member who uses a concrete style. For each family member, try to recall a time when you felt you were not communicating well and one or both of you were frustrated or angry. What cognitive/emotional styles were evident for you and for the other family members during those interactions? What does this tell you about your patterns of relating to other family members?

_____

_____

_____

_____

Toward Multicultural Competence

Exercise 3. Examining cultural differences in family communication

Take a few moments to think about and write down your thoughts about possible cultural differences in family communication. Interview members of ethnic minority groups about communication patterns in their families of origin. Are there differences you can detect relative to culture? What are those differences? You may find it useful to review the multicultural issues discussed in Chapter 8 as you complete this exercise.

Interviewing Practice Exercises

Exercise 4. Interviewing others to determine family cognitive styles and communication patterns

Interview a peer about their patterns of family communications. Ask for specific examples of communication with each member of the family. Try to identify the cognitive/emotional style for each family member in the specific interactions. Are there identifiable patterns of relating to specific family members (it is fairly typical for patterns to exist within dyads in a family system)? In addition, you will find that some families operate predominantly at one style, despite individual differences in cognitive/emotional style.

Exercise 5. Client and counselor developmental style in a role-played family counseling practice session

An extension of the preceding exercise can be done in a role-played family counseling session. Experience reveals that groups of six work best in this situation. Given the complexity of the many personalities, using video- or audiotape is very helpful. As always, follow usual ethical guidelines, established in your class or workshop.

As a first step in family practice, it is useful to do a family demonstration while the rest of the class or workshop watches the session. Approximately one hour will be required for development and debriefing of the family session. Before beginning, make a copy of the form in Box 11-2. During the session, make notes that will help you complete this form once the session has ended.

Step 1: Select Six Willing Participants
Two of these will be co-therapists and the other four will be the family. The remainder of the members of the class or workshop will observe the entire process and later serve as process consultants who reflect on the session.

Box 11-2   Feedback Sheet for Family Development

After you have completed summarizing the individual cognitive/emotional styles, review the session and place here the predominant overall family styles with comments on special issues (for example, the family may be mainly formal, but one member is very concrete and out of synchrony with others).

_____

Place the name and then the main words of each family member's comments below and classify each comment.

1. Main words of member's comment _____
   Classification: SM C F D/S
2. Main words of member's comment _____
   Classification: SM C F D/S
3. Main words of member's comment _____
   Classification: SM C F D/S
4. Main words of member's comment _____
   Classification: SM C F D/S
5. Main words of member's comment _____
   Classification: SM C F D/S
6. Main words of member's comment _____
   Classification: SM C F D/S
7. Main words of member's comment _____
   Classification: SM C F D/S
8. Main words of member's comment _____
   Classification: SM C F D/S
10. Main words of member's comment _____
    Classification: SM C F D/S
11. Main words of member's comment _____
    Classification: SM C F D/S
12. Main words of member's comment _____
    Classification: SM C F D/S
13. Main words of member's comment _____
    Classification: SM C F D/S
14. Main words of member's comment _____
    Classification: SM C F D/S
15. Main words of member's comment _____
    Classification: SM C F D/S
16. Main words of member's comment _____
    Classification: SM C F D/S

Step 2: Have the Workshop Leader Assume the Leadership Role

Due to the complexity of the process, the workshop leader or teacher should assume the leader role and ensure that the group follows the specific steps of the practice session.

Step 3: Assign Roles for the Practice Session

Role-played family: For this first session, a "typical" family should probably be used (that is, a couple having an intact first marriage and family consisting of father, mother, daughter, and son). Later, other common family patterns—such as blended, single-parent, and gay/lesbian—can be used.

Interviewer: The family will be cooperative, talk freely about the topic, and not give the interviewer a difficult time. In later practice sessions, however, it is critical that difficult problems and families be selected. A useful first topic is family fighting or a teenager who is acting out.

Therapists: Two therapists/counselors can work together in this session.

Workshop/class observers: All remaining individuals in the session will sit in a circle around the family.

Step 4: Plan the Session

The family members can leave the room and define their roles and the problem they wish to present. The nature of the problem will be a surprise to the therapists. The family needs to define a problem or reason for coming to the family session.

The two therapists may wish to think through their relationship briefly. One way to start the session is by an informal "joining" with the family through conversation. Other therapists prefer to start immediately. A useful way to start the process is to employ a form of circular questioning in which the therapists ask the family members if someone can answer the question "Why are you here?" This same question is then asked of each family member. Elicit each family member's perception of the problem. In this way, family therapists learn about different perspectives on the same problem. Follow cultural norms by asking who is in charge and having that person speak first.

After each member of the family has spoken, one or both of the therapists may wish to summarize the family as a whole. Many families will hold one member responsible for the problem. In many family therapy sessions, the therapist at this point often will reframe/reinterpret the individual problem as an issue of family interaction: "What is going on with Jane/John is not an individual problem but a family issue we are going to examine."

Again, the task of the two therapists is simply to draw out four different (or similar) interpretations of the problem. Using questioning, listening, and summarization skills is helpful. Avoid giving advice and making interpretations; try to see the family as it sees itself.

The family observers have several roles: (1) They all can be participants or observers; the therapists should feel free to stop the interview in mid-session and ask the observers for help and suggestions. (2) Four observers should be assigned to various members of the family. Their task is to identify the cognitive/emotional style of one family member. Two observers may watch the therapists and assess the style of their questions. The rest of the group should note the cognitive/emotional style of the family as a whole. Use the same feedback forms for the individual practice session as in the preceding exercise.

You will find, for example, that some families present at the concrete style and others at the formal style. In addition, different members within the family may be talking about the problem from different styles.

Step 5: Conduct a 5- to 10-Minute Interviewing Session

The therapists and family will discuss the varying perceptions of the problem for 5 minutes while the observers keep track of their progress and classify the statements of each. Again, you will find it helpful to videotape and/or audiotape practice sessions.

However, family dynamics often confuse even the most effective therapists. Thus the therapists should feel free to stop for a moment in the middle of the session and ask the external observers for their reactions and suggestions. Family therapy specialists may note the similarity of this training procedure to the "reflecting team" concept in which experts view a family session through a one-way mirror and contact the therapists by telephone with specific suggestions for action.

Step 6: Provide Immediate Feedback and Complete Notes (5 Minutes)

This is a highly structured session, and there is often immediate need to personally "process" and discuss the session. In particular, it is helpful for the therapists to ask the family "What stands out for you from this practice session?" Allow some time to provide true personal reactions to the practice.

At this point, the observers should sit back and let the participants take control. Use this time to complete your classification and notes.

Step 7: Review the Practice Session and Provide Feedback (15 Minutes)

When giving feedback, allow the therapists and the family receiving the feedback to be in charge. At this point, the observers can share their observations. Again, feedback should be specific, concrete, and nonjudgmental and attention should be given to strengths of the interview.

Generalization: Taking Concepts of Family Development Home

Exercise 6. Examining family cognitive/emotional styles in your daily life

During the next week, pay close attention to interactions with your biological family or family of choice. What cognitive/emotional styles are evident during times of effective and ineffective communication among dyads in the family? How might communication be enhanced through matching or mismatching of cognitive/emotional styles?

Portfolio Reflections

Exercise 7. Reflections

What stood out for you from this chapter? What sense do you make of the exercises on family issues? What are the key points you want to remember from this chapter? Record your thoughts below and in your Portfolio Folder.

REFERENCES

Bowen, M. (1990). *Family therapy in clinical practice.* New York: Jason Aronson. (Original work published 1985)

Carlson, J., & Kejos, D. (2002). *Theories and methods of family therapy.* Boston: Allyn & Bacon.

Carter, B., & McGoldrick, M. (1999). *The expanded family life cycle: Individual, family, and social perspectives* (3rd ed.). Boston: Allyn & Bacon.

Combrinck-Graham, L. (1985). A developmental model for family systems. *Family Process, 24,* 139–150.

DeFranck-Lynch. (1986). *Therapie familiale structurale.* Paris: Les Editions ESF.

Gladding, S. (2002). *Family therapy: History, theory, and practice* (3rd ed.). Upper Saddle River, NJ: Merrill-Prentice Hall.

Haley, J. (1987). *Problem solving therapy* (2nd ed.). San Francisco: Jossey-Bass.

Haley, J. (1991). *Problem-solving therapy.* San Francisco: Jossey-Bass.

Haley, J. (1996). *Learning and teaching therapy.* New York: Guilford.

McGoldrick, M., Gerson, R., & Shellenberger, S. (1999). *Genograms: Assessment and intervention.* New York: Norton.

McGoldrick, M., Giordano, J., & Pearce, J. (1996). *Ethnicity and family therapy.* New York: Guilford.

Minuchin, S. (1998). *Family healing.* New York: Free Press.

Minuchin, S., & Fishman, H. (1981). *Family therapy techniques.* Cambridge, MA: Harvard University Press.

Myers, J. E., & Schwiebert, V. (1999). Grandparents and stepgrandparents: Challenges in counseling the extended blended family. *Journal of Adult Development and Aging, 1*(1), 50–60.

Nichols, M. P., & Schwartz, R. C. (2001a). *The essentials of family therapy.* Boston: Allyn & Bacon.

Nichols, M. P., & Schwartz, R. C. (2001b). *Family therapy: Concepts and methods* (5th ed.). Boston: Allyn & Bacon.

Rigazio-DiGilio, S. 2002. Family counseling and therapy: Theoretical foundations and issues of practice. In A. Ivey, M. D'Andrea, M. Ivey, & L. Simek-Morgan (Eds.), *Counseling and psychotherapy: A multicultural perspective.* Boston: Allyn & Bacon.

Rigazio-DiGilio, S., Ivey, A., Kunkler, K., & O'Grady, L. (2004). *The community genogram.* New York: Teachers College Press.

Satir, V. (1967). *Conjoint family therapy.* Palo Alto, CA: Science and Behavior Books.

Satir, V., Dengo, M., & Peck, J. (2001). *Self-esteem.* Berkeley, CA: Celestial Arts.

CHAPTER 12
Bibliotherapy, Metaphors, and Narratives

CENTRAL PRACTICE OBJECTIVE
Mastery and practice of concepts in this chapter will enable you to bring more creative and artistic processes into the stories surrounding the counseling and psychotherapy process, including the use of media and journaling.

This chapter provides both theoretical and practical perspectives to help you utilize bibliotherapy in your own work. Bibliotherapy, combined with DCT, provides a means of understanding client narratives, or the manner in which we
construct meaning through telling stories and listening to the stories of others
(DeRiveria & Sarbin, 1998; Myers, 1998; Sarbin, 1986). Bibliotherapy, in its many
forms (e.g., books, art, media, journaling, the Internet), brings uniqueness and the
creative process to counseling and therapy theory and methods. Bibliotherapy is particularly strong in its use of metaphor and images, thus helping clients generalize
important ideas and experiences to their own lives. In this chapter we focus on several strategies that can enrich a developmental approach to bibliotherapy and increase its use as an important tool in the mental health field.

Knowledge of and skill in the concepts of this chapter can enable you to:

1. Develop an understanding of metaphor, narrative therapy, and bibliotherapy
   as therapeutic processes.
2. Understand how these processes reflect powerful images that help clients
   make choices toward illness or greater wellness.
3. Integrate DCT with narrative approaches to promote and create therapeutic
   change.

INTRODUCTION: THE CREATIVE PROCESSES OF BIBLIOTHERAPY, METAPHORS, AND NARRATIVES

Images have been discussed throughout this book as central to the processes of
DCT. Creation of an image is an essential first step in developmental assessment,
followed by exploration of the image using each of the four DCT cognitive styles.
Often we are asked what to do if a client is unable to generate an image. At other
times we are asked to help clients generate therapeutic images as resources for
change. Bibliotherapy is a creative process through which we can help clients both
create and become aware of their images. These images often serve as metaphors (or
life scripts, as discussed in the chapters on Adlerian lifestyle and early recollections)
that guide our thinking and behavior. Using DCT helps make these metaphors conscious and available tools for intentional development and growth.

Images (visual, auditory, kinesthetic, taste, odors), in a sense, are or can be
metaphors that help to define our experiences. They serve this function by bringing
together in one place a holistic summary of experience. Further, we can use bibliotherapy to create new metaphors to promote change. DCT offers a structured means
of combining these two powerful approaches for working with a variety of clients.
When addressing issues of multiculturalism, in particular, narrative strategies such as
bibliotherapy are an important means for helping us enter the world of our clients
and achieve an in-depth understanding of their unique experiences and meaning-
making processes (Zuniga, 1992).

Bibliotherapy uses a focus on media, external stimuli, to evoke images in a manner similar to other projective techniques. The media are essentially neutral until the
client projects his or her internal experience onto them to explain what they mean.

Thus, bibliotherapy provides a structure for helping clients explain what happens for them, inside, when they focus on something external, such as a particular story. Because the media are external, the image or narrative that is created is "safe"—the client need not own the creation early in the process. Later, when the client is helped to own the co-constructed narrative, the process of connection promotes insight and often second-order change.

To a great extent, concepts such as metaphor, narrative, and bibliotherapy share common meanings. In counseling literature, these concepts are often used interchangeably, yet volumes have been written on each approach. Seminal writings for further study include Gordon's (1978) *Therapeutic Metaphor*, Hynes and Hynes-Berry's (1986) *Bibliotherapy: The Interactive Process*, Sarbin's (1986) *Narrative Psychology: The Storied Nature of Human Conduct*, and Gladding's (1992) *Counseling as an Art: The Creative Arts in Counseling*. Brief descriptions of metaphor and narrative are provided here, followed by a more extensive review of the key tenets of bibliotherapy. Strategies for integrating bibliotherapy with DCT are presented. These strategies can increase the power of narrative interventions. A case example demonstrating the use of DCT with bibliotherapy will be presented.

METAPHOR

Webster defined metaphor as "a figure of speech in which a word or phrase literally denoting one kind of object or idea is used in place of another to suggest a likeness or analogy between them" (http://www.m-w.com/cgi-bin/dictionary). Haley (1986) defined metaphors in counseling as communications that have more than one meaning. Further, they reflect our private logic as well as fictive notions (described in Chapter 2) that define how we make meaning in relation to ourselves, life, and other people (Sweeney, 1998).

Metaphors are useful in helping clients see similarities or patterns across events that are temporally separated but share certain common yet perhaps not well understood features. They can help very concretely oriented clients connect seemingly inexplicable events in their lives (Hendrix, 1992). Metaphors provide a powerful means of helping clients overcome strong defenses that prevent them from dealing effectively with problem situations. Finally, the use of metaphors may stimulate new learning and promote development by helping clients achieve new constructions of reality.

For example, one of our clients said that Mary Poppins was her childhood heroine. Mary Poppins was a character in a movie who had magical powers that allowed her to do such things as clean rooms by a swirl of her hand, create beautiful wardrobes instantaneously with a similar motion, take people on trips to fantasy realms, and heal physical and relationship hurts through song and caring smiles. As an adult the client was constantly finding herself in situations where she did not perform up to her own expectations and could not "fix things" and "make things right" for other people, especially her husband and children. After we discussed her feelings about Mary Poppins, we were able to use this metaphor to help her understand her own desire to *be* a Mary Poppins—clearly an impossibility for a mere mortal. When she presented yet another story of how powerless she was in a certain situation, a statement such as "Oh, there you are, trying to be Mary Poppins again" would bring perspective and allow her to both see her pattern and choose to try to change it.

Sensorimotor images of what we see, hear, feel, taste, and smell can be viewed as a type of metaphor. Images represent still frames of life experience that often distill many memories, thoughts, and feelings in one location. With your help, clients can then "unpack" the multiple meanings of the image and you as therapist will learn to understand the client's experiential world more fully.

Metaphors and their companion, similes, can also be used in briefer form to help clients describe what is occurring for them. For example, a client may be struggling to describe her feelings about a relationship. Rather than sad, mad, glad, or frightened, the client may say, I'm feeling "tight as a drum," "free as a bird," or "a lion caged." Each of these phrases serves as a metaphor for how clients are making meaning of their experiences. You as a therapist can provide metaphors that may help your clients sort out their lives. But this must be done with care as the client, not the therapist, is the person who must make sense of her or his world. When possible, take time to help define and then work with the client's metaphors.

Other examples might include the client who sees life as climbing a mountain or searching the sea for real meaning. Personal examples might be "eating like a bird," "proud as a peacock," "crashed like my computer," or "limp as a dishrag." Asking a client what animal he or she feels a close resemblance to can facilitate development of metaphors.

NARRATIVE

Narrative therapy is a phenomenological approach through which clients are encouraged to explore their subjective experience in social context. As described by White and Epston (1990), narrative therapy is based on the assumption that we experience problems when the stories of our lives, our narratives, do not sufficiently represent our lived experience. Importantly, these narratives may be created by ourselves or by others. In either case, they exert a powerful influence on our development and wellness.

The stories of our lives guide how we feel, think, and behave, and how we make sense of new experiences and challenges. Our stories are organizing forces that provide logic and meaning to our lived experience. Narrative therapy, then, is a process through which we story our lives, and, in a positive developmental manner, a process through which we re-story our lives to construct new meanings as a way of resolving sometimes painful issues. The essence of narrative therapy can be captured in the phrase or slogan "The person is never the problem; the problem is the problem." When we rewrite our stories, we change the nature of our problems. Through a second-order change process, we change our life script, lifestyle, or private logic (see Sweeney, 1998, and Chapter 2), our metaphors, and the powerful images through which we create meaning in our lives.

Concrete storytelling, of course, is the basis of much narrative work. Drawing out client stories is basic to most interviews. We can then turn to reflecting on the stories via formal-operational strategies. These reflections can lead to the writing of new stories about one's life. Dialectic/systemic strategies can further the process as we help clients take a multiperspective view of their issues.

For example, an African American male client explained how angry he became as an adolescent when he experienced discrimination from his peers or teachers. His feelings were intense; however, due to admonitions from his family to hide these feelings and ignore the discriminatory actions, he would smile and pretend not to notice the demeaning actions and comments of others. As an adult, he was finding it increasingly difficult to ignore even minor comments that could in any way be construed as having negative intent toward himself or his actions. In fact, he began to look for, and thus find, negativity in others in a variety of relationships. In effect, he began projecting hostile intent on people who likely meant him no harm. As he told the story of his life and experiences, he was encouraged to develop new stories and construct new endings to the many hurtful scenarios he had experienced. His new narratives increasingly placed him in the center of relationships as a potent force for positive change, through gentle yet persuasive comments to others that helped them confront and change their prejudicial attitudes. Through re-storying, he came to see himself as a change agent rather than a victim of circumstances.

BIBLIOTHERAPY

Norcross (2003) reports that 82% of psychologists refer clients to some sort of self-help book. He reviewed meta-analytic research in which bibliotherapy was compared to control groups and those receiving therapy. Marrs (1995) found that bibliotherapy was effective, with an effect size of .56 following treatment. This was only slightly less than for therapy itself. Norcross also noted that 93% of questionnaire respondents found that reading a self-help book was useful for them and 68% of those seeing a movie stated that it had moved them in a positive direction. Interestingly, 80% of Internet users are reported to have used the Internet searching for health information, and mental health issues figure prominently in that amount.

The above data provide a background suggesting that bibliotherapy is a potentially powerful form of therapy in itself. And, when conducted as an adjunct to traditional counseling, bibliotherapy can be an important strategy. We can help clients generate and change images as well as validate, change, and create metaphors through bibliotherapy. The roots of the word *bibliotherapy* lie in *biblio,* or books, and *therapeia,* or therapy. Bibliotherapy was first used in medical settings when staff observed that certain literature supported the healing process. In counseling, bibliotherapy is used to promote positive mental health and wellness. It is a therapeutic process that evokes and examines metaphors for life experiences as a means of helping clients verbalize their thoughts and feelings and learn new ways to cope with problems.

In practice, bibliotherapy has evolved to incorporate the use of virtually any medium (e.g., print, video) or creative process (e.g., writing, painting, movement) through which people tell their stories. Thus clients may be asked to consume media of various types (e.g., reading, viewing, observing) as well as to create literature or other products (e.g., writing/journaling, dancing). Emotional reactions evoked through the process of experiencing the various media are then explored. Through subsequent processing, conscious recognition of clients' ways of knowing and experiencing occurs. Both emotional and cognitive understanding of problems is enhanced.

Pardeck (1995) listed six major goals of bibliotherapy: (1) to provide information, (2) insight, and (3) solutions, (4) to stimulate discussion of problems, (5) to communicate new values and attitudes, and (6) to help clients understand that others have dealt with similar problems. He also cautioned that it is best used in conjunction with other counseling approaches, and that well-articulated treatment goals are essential when bibliotherapy is used. Books, especially, should be selected based on the reading ability of the client, and the theme, format, and believability of characters relative to the specific needs of the client. It is essential that the counselor be familiar with any resource or book used, having read it before providing the assignment to the client.

It is also important to consider the cultural issues and metaphors presented in the assignment. Books or media with multiple levels of meaning and multiple themes are most effective with a variety of clients. Children's books often have themes relevant to persons of all ages (Gladding, 1992) and have the additional advantages of being short and easy to read. The presentation of children's books, however, should always be made carefully and with consideration for possibly offending the adult client who may perceive these to be too simplistic. Accurate assessment of client needs is essential in selecting any intervention, including bibliotherapy.

In the follow-up to a homework assignment in which the client was asked to read a book, two guidelines may be helpful. First, always start the next session by asking the client if he or she read the book; next, ask for reflections on the book without requesting specific information or focus. This procedure allows the book to be used as a projective intervention, so the client *projects* his or her own meaning in the discussion. Second, be careful to allow the client to express his or her reactions and emotions. This is an important time for the client to determine and explain relevant themes, characters, and reactions. In constructing meaning, the client can express any metaphors stimulated by the reading that may be relevant. On occasion, clients may elaborate on themes counselors did not anticipate or intend. Or clients may "miss" themes the counselor had intended in assigning the reading. The counselor's task is to help clients process *their* reactions in an intentional manner. One way to do so that is particularly powerful is through the use of DCT.

USING DCT WITH BIBLIOTHERAPY

We have seen that images are central in DCT. The image created in the DCT process could be a metaphor generated by either the counselor or the client. Bibliotherapy provides an effective basis for presenting metaphors.

The DCT questioning sequence begins with the exploration of an image. When using bibliotherapy, the counselor's first question is also intended to generate an image. Begin by asking, "What happened for you when you (read the book/painted the picture/created your poem, etc.)?" Asking a variety of open-ended questions may be helpful with clients who need more guidance in exploring their reactions. Questions such as the following can help clients uncover personal meaning in what they have read. At the same time, responses to these questions provide an assessment for the counselor of the client's constructions of reality and ways of knowing:

Who were the main characters?
Who did you identify with most?
What about (the character) did you like most?
What happened in the story to (the character)?
Where did this happen?
When or how did it happen?

Following a summary of the client's responses, movement into sensorimotor experiencing may be fostered by asking a question such as "As you think about (this character), can you get an image of one particular part that stood out for you?" or "What image comes to mind as you think about (this character)?" As the client begins to explore the image, asking questions to facilitate sensorimotor experiencing (i.e., seeing, hearing, feeling) will be helpful (see Chapter 4).

Once the client has identified a physically embedded feeling (e.g., "I feel my arms tighten and my fists clench"), movement to concrete may be facilitated by reflecting feelings, then asking for a second example of a time when the client has felt the same way. Follow-up with open-ended questions helps the client explain what happened during that time. Questions concerning when the experience occurred, who was involved, and exactly what happened in a linear sequence of events are important to help uncover the client's understanding of the parallels between his or her life and the circumstances in the book.

Movement into formal-operational thinking is assisted by questions such as "What are the similarities between these two examples, the one from the book and your own?" "Is this a pattern for you?" Themes from the book often help clients identify patterns of which they were previously unaware. Talking about the book can help the client overcome defenses, since it is easier to identify and discuss metaphors in relation to external characters than one's own similar behaviors, at least initially. The behaviors of characters provide a "safe" focus for clients to examine patterns in a nonthreatening manner, because the pattern as first discussed really belongs to someone or something else.

Movement to the dialectic level occurs when clients are encouraged to view the situation and their own pattern from multiple perspectives. Co-constructing clients' rules and the origin of the rules helps lead clients to new ways of making meaning relative to the problem. By this point in the interview, the client has "owned" the problem and pattern, and further discussion of the book is usually unnecessary. However, in subsequent discussions and sessions, metaphors generated from reading the book can be used to remind the client of the links between the media used and her or his presenting concerns.

INTEGRATING BIBLIOTHERAPY AND DCT: A CASE EXAMPLE

A case example may help to clarify how bibliotherapy and DCT can be used in concert to help clients explore new ways of making sense of their lives. Shel Silverstein's (1986) book *The Giving Tree* was chosen as it is brief, has multiple themes and meanings, and is readily available. In fact, it is the best-selling book ever published by Harper and Row, and has been translated into more than two dozen different languages. The book tells the story of a tree that has a loving and intimate relationship with a boy. Over the course of his lifespan, the boy plays with the tree; brings his first love to the tree; uses the fruit, branches, and trunk of the tree to meet his tangible life needs; and finally returns when he is old to sit with the tree.

The client, Madeleine, was a 76-year-old widowed Jewish female with five adult children. Her relationships with most of the children were conflicted, as she clearly saw herself as the matriarch of the family and expected to make decisions and have them followed by others. The oldest daughter and two grandchildren lived with Madeleine. Another sibling was responsible for the referral for counseling, based on stories of overt conflict, bordering on physical abuse, between Mom and her oldest child. The cycle seemed to be one in which the daughter asked for help, or money, Mom gave the help, then Mom felt unappreciated and became angry. A fight ensued with each incident, and feelings were escalating over time for both Mom and her daughter. The daughter felt there was nothing she could ever do to make her mother happy, so she had quit trying long ago.

Madeleine was well-educated, with a master's degree in education and a commitment to lifelong learning through workshops, seminars, and classes at the community college. Other than her daughters and one brother who lived at a distance, she had little social support and was relatively isolated from contact with others. Her primary social activities included card playing with her daughter(s) and watching television.

After the first counseling session, an assessment of Madeleine's presenting issues clearly established her concerns relative to family conflicts, combined with a belief that she, like her own mother, should be the head of the family whose decisions would be unchallenged and willingly accepted. Madeleine was given a copy of *The Giving Tree* and asked to read it prior to the next session. At the start of the session, she was asked if she had read the book, and her response was affirmative; then she was asked, "What stood out for you when you read the book?" She was helped in processing her reactions by use of the DCT interview questions presented in Chapter 4. Key interactions during the session were as follows:

Co: What stood out for you when you read the book?

Cl: That's just the way life is.

Co: Can you tell me more about that?

Cl: You do everything for your kids; then they just use you.

Co: Can you tell me how this relates to the characters in the book?

Cl: Yes. The tree was like a mother. She gave everything to the boy. He was selfish and all he did was take from her.

Co: Did you identify with either of the two characters.

Cl: Oh yes! I am just like the tree. That's just the way my life is. I've given my kids everything and they just take, take, *take!* (said with great feeling and an angry glint in her eyes)

Co: (summarizing) So, you identified with the tree. Can you stop for a moment, close your eyes, and imagine you are the tree? What are you seeing? Hearing? Feeling?

Cl: I see the boy coming when he wants something. Then he is gone. I hear him always asking for what *he* wants. It's always what *he* wants. He never thinks about how *I* feel.

Co: As you see him coming to you when he wants something, and you hear him asking for what he wants, how are you feeling?

Cl: I feel used. I am angry. (Client looks away, and moves her hand to her chest.)

Co: (mirroring client's body movement) You feel used, and angry. Can you locate that feeling in your body?

Cl: Yes; it hurts in my chest, and my throat is tight.

Co: (moving from sensorimotor to concrete experiencing) As you see him coming to you, and hear him asking for what he wants, and you feel the hurt in your chest and the tightness in your throat . . . can you think of another time in your life when you felt this way?

Cl: Yes, lots of times.

Co: Can you pick just one, and tell me about that time?

At this point the client provided an example of a recent time when her oldest daughter asked to borrow money. She gave the money, knowing from experience that it would not be repaid even though the daughter promised, and knowing that she needed the money herself also. She again felt a pain in her chest, and tightness in her throat.

Processing at the formal-operational level led the client to understand that her pattern, when her children asked for help, was to give the help, but to do so grudgingly. Although an argument always ensued, she never discussed the reasons for her feelings and no doubt her children were confused about her anger.

Co: Is that a pattern for you?

Cl: Yes. I always give them what they want. And I always feel bad about it. I feel hurt because they don't think about what I want and need. Then I get mad because I have done it again. I'm just like that darn tree—I give and give and give, and now there isn't much left. They sure aren't trying to help *me!*

Further movement into dialectic processing led to the following interactions:

Co: What are you saying to yourself when this happens?

Cl: I'm saying, "I did it again. I did it again. I hate this. I'm *so* mad!"

Co: So, *if* you give your daughters money every time they ask for it, and you need the money yourself, *then* you get mad at yourself. Also, it really hurts that they think only about themselves and not about your needs.

Cl: That's right.

Co: Can we say this is a rule, something you say to yourself when asked for help?

Cl: Hmmm. I guess you could say that when my kids need help, I have to be there for them.

Co: So, your rule is "When my kids need help, I have to give them what they want."

Cl: That sounds right.

Co: As you think about your life and your family, where did that rule come from? Did anyone else in your family (growing up) have that rule?

Cl: Well, my mother was just the same way. She always said that mothers are supposed to help their kids when the kids need help. But she had lots of money, and I don't!

Co: So, could it be that the rule was good for your mother, but not for you?

From this point, the deconstruction of the client's rule led to a discussion about the need to take care of herself and to be sure she had enough money to cover her own needs for housing, food, and medical care now and in the future. Family counseling sessions were indicated, and bibliotherapy was again used with the family (the two daughters who attended read *The Giving Tree*). Processing of the book led to a frank discussion in which the expectations of the daughters for their mother's behavior and her expectations for them were processed openly. Eventually a compromise was reached relative to plans for sharing resources. No doubt the requests of her daughters and her response to them would continue in some familiar ways, but after the counseling sessions the client was much more willing to say "no" and able to do so without feeling an undue sense of guilt. She attributed this change to the new rule co-constructed in counseling, that parents do not always have to give their children what they ask for—at least once the kids are grown up.

As shown here, metaphors and narratives can be powerful sources of images that help us make meaning in life. Bibliotherapy was presented as an intervention to help clients tell their stories. This approach provides a nonthreatening way to help clients examine and own their metaphors and better understand the meanings underlying their thoughts, feelings, and behaviors. When used in concert with DCT, bibliotherapy can be a potent intervention to create second-order change.

SUMMARY

The creative process underlies much of counseling and therapy and we can use metaphors, narratives, and bibliotherapy to help clients find new ways of thinking, feeling, and behaving. DCT offers specific questioning strategies that may make the use of these methods even more useful and powerful.

Metaphors are imaginative comparisons between seemingly dissimilar things. The use of metaphors will often help clients link ideas that heretofore have been separate.

Narratives are stories that we tell about our life experiences. Using DCT strategies, we can draw out concrete stories, help clients reflect on the stories, and—using dialectic/systemic strategies—help them see the stories from multiple perspectives and perhaps even rewrite the stories in a new and more positive fashion.

Bibliotherapy uses media (books, television), journaling, movement, the Internet, and other activities to help clients in new and creative ways. You will find that children respond well to this approach, especially if you select media of special relevance to them. Bibliotherapy is quite often neglected in work with adults, but it can be especially beneficial to their personal growth.

The questioning strategies of developmental counseling and therapy can enrich the use of metaphors, narratives, and bibliotherapy. The systematic questioning procedures can help you and clients reach a great depth of understanding, thus leading to new and more creative results.

Challenges: The areas discussed in this chapter are very effective in practice and in engaging children, adolescents, adults, couples, and families in new and creative ways. However, their utility is often forgotten in a sometimes too linear and "practical" practice of counseling and therapy. As with all strategies that evoke sensorimotor responses, care must be used to help the client work through the emotions that are experienced.

Research issues: Are different kinds of media more or less useful with different clients? Review literature on cohort differences in lifespan development, and use this information to examine the potential usefulness of various media in counseling. For example, today's cohort of old-old persons (over age 85) likely learned poetry in their early school years as a way of practicing memorization as well as skills in interpreting poetry and prose. It is likely that teenagers and young adults today did not spend as much time learning poetry but may have spent many hours watching movies. What kinds of media would be most useful to you if you were a client?

THEORY INTO PRACTICE: DEVELOPING YOUR PORTFOLIO OF COMPETENCE

Self-Assessment Exercises

Exercise 1. Identifying resources for bibliotherapy

Review the research suggestion above. Within the media category or categories you mentioned, what are some specific resources that would be helpful if you were a client? What about these resources is most meaningful to you?

_____

_____

_____

_____

Exercise 2. Identifying your favorite childhood books

When you were a teenager or young adult, what were your favorite books? Who were the characters? Which characters did you identify with and why?

_____

_____

_____

_____

Exercise 3. Expanding your bibliotherapy resource list

Develop a list of favorite books and movies (preferably, brief movie segments) that can be used for bibliotherapy. Interview counselors who use bibliotherapy to find out what resources they use and add those to your list. Be sure to read/review each resource in detail before you use it with a client.

Interviewing Practice Exercises

Exercise 4. Individual bibliotherapy practice exercise

Choose a partner and interview the person about her or his favorite book or movie growing up. Ask the partner to explain the book or movie, describe the characters, then explain which characters he or she identified with most, and why.

Next, ask your partner to develop an image of a particular scene in the book or movie, and explain that scene. Proceed to process the image using the four sections of the developmental assessment interview. When you have finished, process with your client what this experience was like for her or him. What was it like for you?

Exercise 5. Group practice

For homework, assign each member of your group a particular book to read or movie to watch, or have someone read the book out loud to the group or watch the movie together. Assign one group member as the facilitator.

Process the group using the recommended steps above, exploring responses according to each of the four cognitive developmental styles for each group member.

Toward Multicultural Competence

Exercise 6. Multicultural interviewing practice

Interview people of different cultural backgrounds and ages. Ask them to identify the books and movies that affected them most during their development as young people. Explore, using specific DCT questions, the meaning of the books and movies. Add the media they talk about to your bibliotherapy resources list for use with future clients.

Exercise 7. Exploring media from a multicultural perspective

Choose a selection to read from a book or poem written by a popular minority author (e.g., Langston Hughes, Tony Morrison, Maya Angelou). Have each member of your group read the selection. Process your reactions in the group, noting your experiencing of the media through each of the four DCT cognitive styles. How does this help further your understanding of the stories of those who differ from you in terms of culture and life experience?

Generalization: Taking Concepts of Metaphor, Narrative, and Bibliotherapy Home

Exercise 8. Practicing bibliotherapy at home

During the next week, pay close attention to your responses to books, movies, and other media. How does your personal interpretation of the media contribute to your own sense of meaning? Your wellness? Your development? How do your responses differ from those of others? What does this mean to you?

Portfolio Reflections

Exercise 9. Reflections

What stood out for you from this chapter? What sense do you make of the exercises on your wellness? What are the key points you want to remember from this chapter?

Record your thoughts below and in your Portfolio Folder.

_____

_____

_____

_____

_____

REFERENCES

DeRiveria, J., & Sarbin, T. (1998). *Believe in imaginings: The narrative construction of reality.* Washington, DC: American Psychological Association.

Gladding, S. (1992). *Counseling as an art: The creative arts in counseling.* Alexandria, VA: American Counseling Association.

Gordon, D. (1978). *Therapeutic metaphor.* Capitola, CA: Meta Publications.

Haley, J. (1986). *Uncommon therapy: The psychiatric techniques of Milton H. Erickson, MD.* New York: Norton.

Hendrix, D. H. (1992). Metaphors as nudges toward understanding in mental health counseling. *Journal of Mental Health Counseling, 14,* 234–242.

Hynes, A. M., & Hynes-Berry, M. (1986). *Bibliotherapy: The interactive process.* Boulder, CO: Westview Press.

Marrs, R. (1995). A meta-analysis of bibliotherapy studies. *American Journal of Community Psychology, 29,* 834–870.

Myers, J. E. (1998). Bibliotherapy and DCT: Co-constructing the therapeutic metaphor. *Journal of Counseling and Development, 76*(3), 243–250.

Norcross, J. (2003, August). *Integrating self-help into psychotherapy: A revolution in mental health practice.* Presentation to the American Psychological Association Convention, Toronto.

Pardeck, J. T. (1995). Bibliotherapy: An innovative approach for helping children. *Early Childhood Development and Care, 110,* 83–88.

Sarbin, T. R. (Ed.). (1986). *Narrative psychology: The storied nature of human conduct.* New York: Praeger.

Silverstein, S. (1986). *The giving tree.* New York: Harper & Row.

Sweeney, T. J. (1998). *Adlerian counseling: A practitioner's approach* (4th ed.). Philadelphia: Accelerated Development.

White, M., & Epston, D. (1990). *Narrative means to therapeutic ends.* New York: Norton.

Zuniga, M. E. (1992). Using metaphors in therapy: Dichos and Latino clients. *Social Work, 37*(1), 55–60.

CHAPTER 13
Spirituality, Wellness, and Development
Applying DCT to Core Values in Clients' Lives

CENTRAL PRACTICE OBJECTIVE

Mastery and practice of concepts in this chapter will enable you to conceptualize and work comfortably with spiritual, religious, and meaning issues in the interview. You will be able to use DCT discernment processes to help clients find direction and make meaning in their lives.

Spirituality was presented as a central dimension of wellness for many people in Chapter 2. The literature on spirituality and its relation to counseling and psychotherapy has greatly increased in the last few years (e.g., Kelly, 1995; Miller & Thoresen, 2003; Myers & Williard, 2003; Nielsen, Johnson, & Ellis, 2001; Richards & Bergin, 1997; Shafranske, 1996). With the exception of William James, Alfred Adler, Carl Jung, and proponents of the transpersonal psychology movement, spiritual and religious issues have historically played little part in counseling and therapy theory. Even today, only minimal attention is given to this important area of life in counselor and therapist training programs.

The purpose of this chapter is to show how religion, spirituality, and meaning can be applied in the counseling and clinical session. As you read these pages, review key research, and engage in practice therapeutic strategies, our hope is that you will have a useful base for including these central life issues in your own interviewing practice.

Knowledge of and skill in the concepts of this chapter can enable you to:

1. Compare formal definitions of religion, spirituality, and meaning with your own perspectives.
2. Examine the process of discernment as a vital way to help clients find meaning and mission in their lives.
3. Explore stages of faith development and their relationship to DCT theory and practice.
4. Determine the place of religious, spiritual, and related issues in your counseling and psychotherapy practice.
5. Utilize special spiritually oriented strategies in the here and now of the therapeutic session.

INTRODUCTION: RESEARCH FINDINGS ON SPIRITUALITY

Religion and spiritual orientation form an important aspect of multicultural understanding and diversity (Ivey, D'Andrea, Ivey, & Simek-Morgan, 2002; Richards & Bergin, 1997). Clearly, multiplicity is as prominent in spiritual considerations as in race/ethnicity or socioeconomic areas. Moreover, helping fields have given insufficient attention to this core part of life. And even for those who find the words *religion* and *spirituality* uncomfortable, issues of meaning remain. For some of your clients, you may find that you can work with many of the concepts discussed in this chapter by substituting the words *meaning, purpose,* or *vision.*

Why are we seeing increased attention to spirituality and religious issues at this point in counseling and psychotherapy? Perhaps most convincing is the information found in polls taken of the U.S. populations over the past 10 years. Gallup (1996) found the following in the U.S. populace:

- 84% believe that God is involved in their lives
- 41% believe that they have personally experienced the miraculous
- 33% have had a profound mystical experience that has changed their lives
- 11% have seen a spiritual figure
- 90% of those who quit drinking say that they have had a spiritual experience

Miller and Thoresen (2003) report on more recent Gallup polls in which 95% state a belief in God or a higher power while 9 out of 10 pray. Sixty percent report that religion is important in their lives, a 7% increase in the last 10 years.

Research on spirituality has been increasing and a careful review by Powell, Shahabi, and Thoresen (2003) notes that religious participation clearly relates to physical health and even mortality. However, they comment that the relationship is made more complex, as those who have a spiritual orientation also have a healthier lifestyle and better social support systems, possibly due to the impact of church attendance and the social networking that results from participation in organized religious practices with others (e.g., the congregation's response to major physical illness). Religious participation and high academic performance were found to be correlated among 212 African American and European American students (Walker & Dixon, 2002). The African American students also showed a correlation between spiritual beliefs and academic success.

The body responds to religious and spiritual practices, according to a review by Seeman, Dubin, and Seeman (2003). While warning against overgeneralization and stating clearly the need for more research, they conclude that

> the evidence reported to date is generally consistent with the hypothesis that aspects of religiosity/spirituality may indeed be linked to physiological responses—including cardiovascular, neuroendocrine, and immune functioning. (p. 61)

Often-cited research has found therapeutic value in religious imagery and interventions within a cognitive behavioral therapy (CBT) framework (Probst, 1980; Probst Ostrom, Watkins, Dean, & Mashburn, 1992). Religiously oriented therapy with depressed clients proved more effective than traditional CBT approaches and the results were maintained over a two-year follow-up. Note that these clients already had a religious orientation. Virtually no research has examined the complex meaning of the words *religion* and *spirituality* and understanding how clients interpret these words. Yet, it is clear to many clinicians that this distinction is important.

With the prominence that spirituality and religion seem to have in the broad population, exploration of these issues will certainly be important and valuable to many of your clients. The purpose of this chapter is to direct you to specific avenues through which you can professionally and ethically bring this area to the counseling and psychotherapy session. Special attention is also given to the closely related areas of meaning and values (Bergin & Garfield, 1994).

DEFINITIONS AND PROMISE OF SPIRITUALITY IN COUNSELING AND PSYCHOTHERAPY

What does the word *religion* mean to you? Before going further, please spend a moment defining the term in your own words.

_____

_____

_____

_____

A common definition of religion is "an organized group, usually with a formal and commonly held story and beliefs and often with specific demands for membership." A revealed narrative from God (e.g., Bible, Qur'an, Torah) often forms the foundation for the beliefs.

Now, please define the word *spirituality* in your own language.

_____

_____

_____

A formal definition of spirituality tends to focus on an *interest* in spiritual and religious issues. This interest may be organized and become very similar to religion or it may be relatively unorganized and specific to a single person.

Now, our experience with clients and with groups is that the formal definition for religion provided above is satisfactory for most people. *But,* the formal definition of spirituality is a definite "no go" for many. We have found very few people who will allow someone else to define spirituality for them. We now believe that spirituality and spiritual beliefs are very close to the core of a person's meaning system. No longer do we attempt to define what spirituality means to any client. Rather it is our privilege to learn from and with them what spirituality means to them. We can then build on the unique strengths of each person and use spiritual dimensions as building blocks toward wellness.

Not all your clients will be comfortable with the words *spirituality* and *religion.* They may prefer *meaning* and *values*, words that may be more in keeping with traditional approaches to counseling and therapy. Shafranske (1996) has commented:

> In essence, we are calling for and envision a [counseling and therapy] curriculum that addresses the underlying value commitments that establish the canon of science and influence its application within clinical practice. Such an investigation will include a philosophic inquiry into the nature of facts, scientific practices, models of validation and falsification, and the assumptions on which clinical theories and treatments are based. . . . [It] would also include an investigation of the role of personal values of the clinician as they are expressed in clinical thinking and practice. (pp. 577–578)

Even if a client has no interest in spiritual issues, everyone is concerned with values and what has personal and central meaning. With changes in wording and helping style, all issues in this chapter can be viewed within the language system of values, meaning, and life purpose.

Viktor Frankl's logotherapy focuses on meaning. His most influential book, *Man's Search for Meaning* (1946/1959), was written in two weeks shortly after his liberation from the German concentration camp, Auschwitz. From Frankl's writing, we learn that having a firm sense of meaning and values was often central in survival through the most difficult times. Like spirituality, meaning focuses on belief systems and basic values. Thoughts, feelings, and behaviors are, of course, central to the helping process, but Ivey and Ivey (2003) argue that core values of meaning and

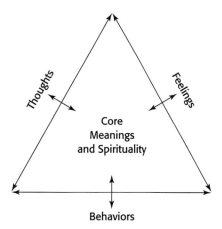

Figure 13-1   Meaning and Spirituality: Thoughts, Feelings, and Behaviors
Core meanings are often derived from cultural understandings with a
spiritual/religious base.

spirituality may be even more central. See Figure 13-1 for a diagram illustrating the
relationship of meaning and spirituality to thoughts, feelings, and behaviors.

As you review this chapter and think about the place of religion, spirituality, and
meaning in your approach to counseling and psychotherapy, it is important that you

■   Encounter the power of spirituality in counseling and psychotherapy for many
of your clients and be aware of your own search for meaning.

■   Discover yourself as a spiritual and meaning-making being so that you do not
mix your own thoughts and beliefs with those of the client. Be careful of
boundary issues.

■   Learn about and become sensitive to a multiplicity of meaning and value systems as well as religious and spiritual beliefs different from your own.

■   Be careful that you do not impose your spiritual, religious, or value preferences
on the client. Often as part of intake procedures, you can assess the importance
of these matters to clients, thus enabling you to build on their interests and belief systems. When you search out social support systems, it is wise to inquire
about clients' spiritual and religious interests. At any time, you can readily bring
up meaning and value issues that may allow some clients to talk about spirituality as well.

■   Never make an assumption about or stereotype an individual based solely on
spiritual or religious understandings. Always treat each person as an individual
as you seek to understand and empathize with his or her meaning making in
this central area of life.

CULTURE AND SPIRITUALITY

Spirituality and religious beliefs underlie core cultural values, and much of secular
life is deeply influenced by these traditions. The meaning of life and the personal
values a client holds can often be traced to spiritual roots, even if that client denies

the importance of religion. As an example of the power of religious values to affect personal meanings, let us compare two stories of creation. The first narrative represents the familiar Judeo-Christian heritage (and perhaps Islam as well); the second is drawn from traditional Australian Aboriginal culture (and this story has parallels in many indigenous traditions).

Aboriginal creation stories vary in details, but the example presented here is characteristic (Mountford, 1976, pp. 5–7).

> All was darkness. The earth was flat and featureless. . . . Suddenly, an old, blind woman, Kala, clasping three young children [at] her breast, rose miraculously out of the ground. . . . As she did so, a sea of water bubbled (in her steps creating the features of the land). . . . She decreed that the island of the Tiwi should be clothed with trees and inhabited with creatures and tiny spirit children, so that her own family, whom she was leaving behind, would have both sufficient food to keep alive and children to populate the land.

As the Aboriginal population grows, inevitable conflict occurs. After one of Kala's children dies, the people gather for the elaborate burial (still performed today by the Tiwi people). All descendants of Kala then transform themselves into one or another of the creatures, plants, or the heavenly bodies. The people are forever afterward guided toward *harmony* day and night by Tukimbin, the sun woman, and Japara, the moon man.

Many characteristics of both traditional and modern Aboriginal Australian culture may be found in this story. It is noteworthy that a woman formed the land by springing from the earth. Particularly important is the idea of harmony and consensus and living in synchrony with the land. Dirt (the earth) is not "dirty"; it is the very essence of life. Many Aboriginal people still visit the grove of trees, mountain, hillside, or valley feature where their people sprang from the earth. Aboriginal communities work on consensus decision making in a style somewhat similar to the Quaker meeting—not making a decision until full agreement is reached by the total community. The highest goal of a traditional Aboriginal person is to live in full harmony and accord with others—the self-in-relation, the person-in-community.

The first book of Moses, commonly called *Genesis,* presents a different creation story, with both interesting parallels to and important differences from the Australian Aboriginal story.

> In the beginning God created the heavens and the earth. The earth was without form and void, and darkness was on the face of the deep; and the Spirit of God was moving over the surface of the waters. And God said, "let there be light." . . . God created man in his own image. . . . "Be fruitful and multiply, and fill the earth and subdue it; and have dominion over every living thing that moves upon the earth."

Then follows the story of the Garden of Eden and the fall of Adam and Eve, as the pair are expelled to face the world.

In the Judeo-Christian tradition, a male God makes the world and gives dominion and ownership to man. The earth and its creatures are to be subdued. The resolution of the conflict is expulsion and individuals are to face the world and their relationship with the Creator. Words such as *self-actualization, autonomy,* and *self-realization* are logical outcomes of this creation legend. Much of modern psychology theory follows dimensions already outlined in this creation story.

Why might these two examples be relevant to you as a counselor or therapist? First, spiritual and religious issues are basic to multicultural understanding. Clients' definitions of effective resolution of problems can vary with their spiritual and cultural backgrounds. It is important is to realize that bedrock foundational meaning issues in life can be related to spiritual beliefs and understandings. African American and Native American Indian cultures, in particular, stress connectedness and community as contrasted with individualism.

The Native American and Japanese Shinto traditions give primacy to harmony with the land, much like the Aboriginal patterns presented here. A "good" and a spiritual client may have very different beliefs about what is right and correct, depending on their religious and cultural roots. A Muslim client, focusing on Allah's will, may conceive of personal responsibility in a very different fashion from a Southern Baptist client. A Hindu client, believing in reincarnation, views the purpose of life differently from a Buddhist, a Jewish client, or a member of the Church of Latter Day Saints.

The purpose of this brief section is not to promote any specific orientation to spirituality or religion but to stress its very deep importance to the vast majority of your clients. Given the vitality and centrality of spiritual issues to so many people, it seems indeed strange that only recently has the counseling field started to address spirituality and religion in any significant way. Spirituality and religion are either directly or indirectly involved in the way most people make meaning and sense of their lives.

We are aware that these brief comments have perhaps stirred up some thoughts and emotions in you, the reader. Please take a moment—breathe deeply and note your present emotions and feelings. What do you notice in your body (sensorimotor) as you think about what you've read here and the meaning of spirituality and religion to you? What concrete stories and narratives have you heard that stand out for you as you think about spirituality and religion? What are your formal reflections about these ideas? And in the dialectic/systemic integrative sense, what are your preliminary thoughts about the place of these important topics in your own counseling and therapy practice?

_____

_____

_____

_____

_____

_____

_____

DISCERNMENT: DISCOVERING OUR DEEPEST MEANINGS

He who has a why *to live can bear with almost any* how.

—Nietzsche

Discernment is about finding one's purpose and mission in life—*why* are you living and what difference do you want to make in the world? When a person has a sense of mission, a vision for the future, problem solving and action often can more easily follow. Perhaps the key questions in discernment are "What do you really want to give to the world?" and "How best can I spend my limited time on earth?" But answering these very open questions can be extremely difficult, particularly in an individualistic or "I-centered" culture. Discernment can focus on self or self-in-relation. The Native American tradition speaks of the "vision quest" in which an individual goes out in the wilderness alone to seek a higher purpose—and that purpose most often focuses on how to serve others and the broader community.

We live in a confusing and challenging world in which things are not always as they seem to be. Life throws us many things we do not expect and mere problem solving may not be enough. When clients are faced with a serious illness, a death, or other major life issue, usually effective helping strategies such as those used in cognitive behavioral therapy and other theories may not be sufficient. Counseling offers many helpful routes toward problem solving and goal setting, but we may need something more as we set about determining our life's purpose and how we want to live in the world.

Speaking more formally about discernment, Farnham, Gill, McLean, and Ward (1991) comment:

> *Discernment* comes from the Latin word *discernere,* which means "to separate," "to determine," "to sort out." In classical spirituality, discernment means identifying when the spirit is at work in a situation: the Spirit of God or some other spirit. Discernment is "sifting through" our interior and exterior experiences to determine their origin. (p. 23)

Victor Frankl (1978) speaks to these issues in *The Unheard Cry for Meaning.* He reports that 85% of suicide attempters speak of their lives as meaningless. Camus (1955, p. 3) stated, "There is but one truly serious problem, and that is . . . judging whether or not life is or is not worth living." Frankl attacks excessive focus on self-actualization, pointing out that self-transcendence—living beyond oneself—is the greatest sign of mental health. The making of meaning, finding sense in the world is another way to view spirituality and religion. We all have a need for real purpose in our lives, even though we may stray off the path into consumerism and self-indulgence.

As you can sense, discernment is deeper and more complex than decision making. Discernment is allowing yourself or encouraging your clients to go further and deeper with the explicit aim of discovering one's deepest purposes in life. Then, armed with discernment of mission and purpose, decision making and action can more easily follow.

Discernment is also an exploration of one's values and meanings. In counseling and therapy we usually focus on thoughts, feelings, and behavior. Figure 13-1 pointed out that these three dimensions rest on a core of meaning and spirituality. Discernment, then, is an attempt to discover deeper underlying issues relating to thoughts, feelings, and behavior. The discernment process helps people focus and set large life goals. Once these are established, we have a base for action.

Listening is the foundation for discerning the inner values and the heart of a client.

> *Listen.* Listen, with intention, with love, with the "ear of the heart"—that lovely small phrase . . . suggests that we listen not only cerebrally with the intellect, but with the whole of feelings, our emotions, imagination, and ourselves. (de Waal, 1997, p. iii)

De Waal is summarizing the centrality of listening as presented in the Rule of St. Benedict. Benedictine meditation and study is a quiet route toward finding one's true direction and toward helping us resolve some of life's most challenging issues. *Discernment in practice is first of all* listening *fully to oneself and to others.* This is a listening that goes beyond basic skills; it involves the whole of the client's self, the whole of the therapist's self. Technically, the listening process may look the same as regular listening in therapy, but there is an additional almost magical dimension of wholeness and *being-in-relation.* Intuition plays as an important part in discernment as cognition.

Nonetheless, discerning one's mission in life or entering on a vision quest can be facilitated by some specific guidelines and questioning related to DCT and to faith development theory (Fowler, 1996). We now turn to some specifics of the discernment process.

DCT and Discernment

Ultimately discernment involves all DCT styles. The vision, goal, or mission needs to be felt and experienced (sensorimotor), one needs to describe and act (concrete), reflect (formal), and realize oneself in relation (dialectic/systemic). Just as in multilevel assessment and treatment, there may be multiple routes toward the client's deeper goals in life.

Preparation and openness to experience is fundamental to discerning one's life goals and mission. If one is to *listen* to one's place in the world, quiet and alone time can be critical. Moses went to the mountaintop, Jesus went into the wilderness, and Mohammed received messages from Allah in a cave. Some Native American Indians still today go into the wilderness on a vision quest that can determine their role in life. Being alone and open is clearly one route toward discerning one's mission and one's most basic set of values and goals.

The counselor's role in discernment when it comes to sensorimotor work may be primarily advisory—helping clients establish personal conditions for learning and obtaining visions of their goals. Meditation and guided imagery may be particularly helpful, but both must start from the client's experiential world and felt body sense. Bringing the body together with the vision is an important part of discernment.

Box 13-1 provides a list of questions that may help you and your clients discern issues of meaning, life goals, and the applications of spirituality in day-to-day action. You are not expected to answer all these life goal and mission questions, nor is

---

Box 13-1   Questions Leading Toward Discernment of One's Life Mission

Example questions, strategies, or statements that may facilitate sensorimotor discovery. These questions tend to focus on the here and now and intuition.

- Relax, explore your body and find a feeling there that might serve as an anchor for your search. Allow yourself to build on that feeling and see where it goes.
- Sit quietly and allow an image (visual, auditory, kinesthetic) to build.
- What is your gut feeling? What are your instincts? Get in touch with your body.
- Discerning one's mission cannot be found solely through the intellect. What feelings occur to you at this moment?
- Imagine yourself talking to someone who can help you. See the person in the chair there. Speak to her or him, then move to that chair and have the person answer you. (Gestalt empty chair work)
- Consider drawing, painting, music, and other creative art forms. Where do they lead you?
- Can you recall feelings and thoughts from your childhood that might lead to a sense of direction now?
- What is your felt body sense of spirituality?

Within the concrete style, consider the following, relating to stories, specifics, and action.

- Tell me a story about that sensorimotor image above. (Or a story about any of the here and now experiences listed there.)
- Can you tell me a story that relates to your goals/vision/mission?
- Can you name the feelings you have in relation to your desires?
- What have you done in the past or are doing presently that feels especially satisfying and close to your mission?
- What are some blocks and impediments to your mission? What holds you back?
- Could we try role-playing what it would be like to act on those images?
- What are you going to do now that we have some sense of your mission? What actions will you take?
- When can you take action? What plans need to be made?
- Can you tell about spiritual stories that have influenced you?

For formal exploration, the following may be helpful. These focus on self-reflection.

- Let's go back to that original image and/or the story that goes with it. As you reflect on that experience or story, what occurs for you? (Or use any of the information gleaned from earlier sensorimotor or concrete questioning.)

(continued)

your client. Discernment is obviously a mixture of intuitive and intellectual processes. One needs to be open to experience, but also able to make clear sense of that experience and its implications for the future.

Box 13-1   *(continued)*

- Looking back on your life, what have been some of the major satisfactions? Dissatisfactions?
- What have you done right?
- What have been the peak moments and experiences of your life?
- What might you change if you were to face that situation again?
- Does a need for approval/admiration/respect relate to these goals?
- Do you have a sense of obligation that impels you toward this vision?
- Most of us have multiple emotions as we face major challenges such as this. What are some of these feelings and what impact are they having on you?
- Are you motivated by love/zeal/a sense of morality?
- What are your life goals?
- What has been most meaningful (positive/supporting and negative/challenging) to you among your many experiences?
- What do you see as your mission in life?
- What does spirituality mean to you?

Dialectic/systemic questions place the client in larger systems and relationships—the self-in-relation.

- Place your sensorimotor, concrete, and formal experiences in broader context. How have various systems (family, friends, community, culture, spirituality, and significant others) related to these experiences? Think of yourself as a self-in-relation, a person-in-community.
- *Family.* What do you learn from your parents, grandparents, and siblings that might be helpful in your discernment process? Are they models for you that you might want to follow, or even oppose? If you now have your own family, what do you learn from them and what is the implication of your discernment for them?
- *Friends.* What do you learn from friends? How important are relationships to you? Recall important developmental experiences you have had with peer groups. What do you learn from them?
- *Community.* What people have influenced you and perhaps serve as role models? What group activities in your community may have influenced you? What would you like to do to improve your community? What important school experiences do you recall?
- *Cultural groupings.* What is the place of your ethnicity/race in discernment? Gender? Sexual orientation? Physical ability? Language? Socioeconomic background? Age? Life experience with trauma?
- *Significant other(s).* Who is your significant other? What does he or she mean to you? How does he or she relate to the discernment process? What occurs to you as the gifts of relationship? The challenges?
- *Spiritual.* How might you want to serve? How committed are you? What is your relationship to spirituality and religion? What does your holy book say to you about this process?

FAITH DEVELOPMENT AND DEVELOPMENTAL COUNSELING AND THERAPY

Faith may be defined as "an integral centering process. . . a generic feature of human beings. . . . It is a foundation to social relations, to personal identity, and to the making of personal and cultural meanings" (Fowler, 1996, p. 168). Fowler's faith development theory (1981, 1996) has had a large influence on pastoral counseling as it provides an integration of Erikson's life stages with Piagetian ideas of cognitive/emotional development.

The seven stages of Fowler's faith development theory are summarized in Table 13-1. There you will also see how his model relates to Erikson's lifespan theory and to DCT's cognitive/emotional styles. The final column provides concrete suggestions to facilitate cognitive/emotional development and expansion of each stage of faith. Many, perhaps most, of our interventions with the four DCT styles can facilitate personal faith development within each stage as well as help clients explore stages different from those in which they originally discuss their issues. We do not review the full complexity of Fowler's thinking in this section, but rather refer you to his 1981 book, which remains the basic summary of his system and is still important today.

While Fowler's theory is useful, DCT theory challenges it on one central point. Implicit in Fowler's seven stages is that "higher is better" and that more basic stages such as primal or mythic literal faith have less value. Although Fowler himself notes this paradox, we want to bring it to your attention. Primal faith, for example, is where the individual is experientially most closely in touch with her or his faith. Basic trust, as explicated by Erikson's lifespan theory, is foundational. That basic trusting relationship between a counselor and a client may, in times of crisis, be close to a real spiritual relationship. People in the intellectualizing fifth and sixth stages may be so wrapped up in thought that they cannot experience spiritual connections at the deepest level. The seventh stage is holistic.

In DCT theory, "more is better" and all the stages of faith have value. Expansion of one's development at all stages may be the preferred mode of spiritual counseling. However, it is probably wise to start spiritual counseling *where the client is*. And this is where Fowler's theory may be especially useful. While the basics of primal faith and intuitive-projective faith may derive from childhood, some clients will maintain these stages of faith as their primary identification into adolescence and adulthood. Charismatic and fundamental evangelistic faiths may stress this orientation to spirituality; it would be inappropriate to use formal-operational methods that might ask clients who embrace this manifestation of religion to analyze rather than experience that faith. Helping them strengthen their present faith through appropriate imagery and stories may be the preferred method. If, and only if, they wish to do so should you move on to other suggested treatment strategies.

Similarly, if you engage with clients with an individuative-reflective faith, you likely would be wise to start with person-centered listening and develop the relationship. In this case, they likely will start reflecting on their experiences. At the same time, it may eventually be useful to help them return to basic trust issues and stories from the earlier stages. This will be important, but it is also vital to recall that the foundations of primal faith may be the most healing and beneficial of all.

Table 13-1 Fowler's Faith Development Theory, DCT, and Suggested Strategies
for Facilitating Cognitive/Emotional Development

Faith Development and Lifespan Stages*	Brief Definition of Stage	DCT and Adult Continuations	Suggested Treatment Alternatives to Facilitate Spirit Development and Exploration of Meaning
Primal faith (infancy)	Trust develops as the basis of faith through contact with parents, feeding, and early play. The deepest bonds of attachment are formed and are represented in religion as the immediate experience of God in the here and now. Images of one's parents help shape the image of God.	Sensorimotor/ elemental—the ability to experience faith most directly.	Imagery, guided imagery, focused recall, and here and now experiencing of feelings of trust and belongingness. Meditation is central in the Buddhist tradition, but also prominent in many Christian and other religions as well.
Intuitive-projective faith (early childhood)	The child may begin the first conscious constructions of God. "Imagination, religious stories, gestures, and symbols are not yet controlled by logical thinking" (Fowler, 1996, p. 170) and thus magical thought may be important. Yet these powerful magical images may form the foundation for later thought.	Late sensorimotor— the ability to enjoy and participate in the mystical.	Above strategies plus more emphasis on stories, songs, and symbols. Focusing awareness on the positives of mystical thought for we never know the unknown. For Catholics, the Rosary is a combination sensorimotor/concrete strategy that often leads to formal reflection.
Mythic-literal faith (childhood and beyond)	Concrete thinking becomes prominent and the "if . . . ., then . . ." logic of narratives and stories may become central. Linear prediction and causation become important and rule-bound "right/wrong" thought may be a major feature. "God is constructed on the model of a consistent, caring, but just ruler or parent. Goodness is rewarded; badness is punished" (Fowler, 1996, p. 172).	Concrete/situational— to describe and know the basics and rules of one's faith.	Many clients will benefit from selecting key verses from their holy book. A common Muslim helping method is to select key verses and study them carefully again and again. Narrative and storytelling with a focus on positive strengths from the stories. Role-playing of spiritual figures and their actions and relating them to assertiveness training strategies. Cognitive behavioral and REBT strategies, including appropriate disputation, using spiritual language acceptable to the client. Evaluation of logical consequences and behavioral antecedents, behaviors, and consequences.

*While faith tends to develop in sequential stages, it remains holistic. Several stages of faith may be found in an adult, but one or more stages may be prominent. Just because an adolescent or adult may be focused on a primal or intuitive faith, these are not necessarily better or more desirable than other stages. Likewise, just because a person has a so-called sophisticated faith, he or she may not be fully developed or able to reach more basic faith stages.

(continued)

Table 13-1   *(continued)*

Faith Development and Lifespan Stages	Brief Definition of Stage	DCT and Adult Continuations	Suggested Treatment Alternatives to Facilitate Spirit Development and Exploration of Meaning
Synthetic-conventional faith (adolescence and beyond)	Early spiritual identity development occurs here as the individual thinks back again and evaluates what was learned earlier and starts the process of independent decision making. An almost adolescent "self-confidence" in one's own thinking and feeling may appear. An "acting-out" against traditional past learning often occurs.	Early formal-operational—the ability to think about and discuss one's own faith orientation, but the perspective is an integration of past learning.	Reflections on the narratives and stories discussed earlier. Person-centered listening and support. Encourage reflection on oneself with limited and careful confrontation. Continued strategies as above. Bibliotherapy and provision of readings.
Individuative-reflective faith (young adulthood and beyond)	A more serious self-examination occurs in which past learning is reviewed more fully and carefully. Authority for evaluation is placed firmly within the self. Old stories may be reinterpreted as myths and discarded. In the quest for personal authenticity, there may be over-reliance on the conscious mind.	Reflective/formal-operational—the ability to see one's faith more broadly as a reflection of historical tradition and other factors.	Examination of how narratives and stories were generated in a social and multicultural/spiritual context. Person-centered counseling and therapy with more participation and confrontation on the part of the helper. Psychodynamic and cognitive behavioral methods may be appropriate. In-depth disputation and exploration of narratives and stories. Bibliotherapy and provision of readings. Orthodox Jews spend extensive time in detailed reflection on the Torah.
Conjunctive faith (early midlife and beyond)	A sense of humbleness returns and "the need for multiple interpretations of reality mark this stage. Symbol and story, metaphor and myth (from one's own tradition and others') are newly appreciated" (Fowler, 1996, p. 170). People are seen as more complex and the cultural aspects of spirituality and religion may be acknowledged.	Late formal and early dialectic/systemic—the ability to see the multidimensional aspects of faith as one moves toward integration.	Mutual exploration and more self-disclosure on the part of the therapist, but with a focus on the client. Intergenerational family systems and multicultural counseling and therapy strategies that help person see self in a systemic context. Exploration of early recollections.
Universalizing faith (midlife and beyond)	A rarely achieved stage. "Individuals . . . are grounded in a oneness with the power of being. Their visions and commitments free them for a passionate spending of self in love, devoted to overcoming division, oppression, and violence . . . (in an) unbreaking commonwealth of love and justice" (Fowler, 1996, p. 170).	Dialectic/systemic—the ability to become "one with the spirit" and act almost totally from a sense of mission.	Perhaps one would simply listen and learn from these people; perhaps helping them see some of the challenges that they face and helping them explore alternatives.

Is faith development theory relevant to all faiths? Fowler argues that it is. A Muslim, a Buddhist, an Orthodox Jew, a liberal or evangelical Christian, and even an agnostic or atheist can benefit from exploring spiritual beliefs and meaning systems from Fowler's framework. Being an atheist requires a strong faith system and the person's belief system may be assisted through examining her or his relationship to faith.

Fowler notes that we cannot expect often to meet those representing universalizing faith. By definition, people of universalizing faith have a mission, something that moves them beyond themselves. Their selflessness focuses on helping and being One with others. Gandhi, Martin Luther King, Jr., and Mother Teresa are prime examples, and few of us measure up to the standard exemplified in their actions. At the same time, each of us has the possibility to grow and live in a more other-focused way. Think of the nuns, priests, rabbis, and imams who have truly given their lives to actions based on their spiritual beliefs. These people, like Gandhi, Dr. King, and Mother Teresa, are not perfect, but they have chosen an all-consuming life mission and they are open to learning and changing in response to the people and systems they encounter.

Universalizing faith is a stage of being that is not totally impossible for us ordinary mortals. We are not likely to achieve this level of spiritual commitment and service constantly, but there is part of us that can approach it. You likely entered the counseling and therapy profession as an act of service to others. Few enter this field to "get rich" or "make a name." In those times when you focus your efforts on service to others, you are starting to enter the higher world of universalizing faith. In this one case, we as authors admit that perhaps "higher is better." But we also suggest that this style of functioning as not as elusive as Fowler might suggest.

What is your mission in life? What do you want to contribute? What do you want to leave behind? This is your challenge. Take just a few moments and think about this possibility. What occurs for you?

_____

_____

_____

_____

DCT STRATEGIES AND NARRATIVES OF FAITH

The following pages present a systematic interview plan designed to help clients explore narrative issues in spirituality and meaning. As is typical in DCT, we strongly recommend starting with positive stories and images and later using these as a foundation if the client wishes to explore spiritual challenges and problems. You will find that very powerful and useful experiences occur if you are willing to go through this systematic set of questions.

We suggest that you photocopy this section and share it with a real or volunteer client. This client should be interested and willing to explore spiritual issues in some depth. We believe that spirituality issues should never be forced on a client; rather, it is the client's choice to discuss or not discuss them. Work through the questions together slowly and evaluate each step to ensure that you have encountered the richness possible within. Expect the following from this exercise in storytelling:

- Clients will often find that their spiritual background is an important part of their life, typically untouched in the counseling and therapy process.
- Clients may be expected to find resources that they had not known were available to them. These resources, in turn, may be used as strengths to help them resolve not only spiritual issues but also other concerns not related to spirituality.
- You as counselor or therapist, having gone through this systematic exercise, will feel more comfortable and skilled in bringing issues of spirituality into the helping session.

1. Opening Narrative: How Does This Client Perceive Spirituality and Make Meaning?

Two approaches are suggested to begin the spiritual and meaning questioning sequence. The first is meditative and experiential; the second, more intellectualized, encourages the client to talk about rather than experience. Either approach may result in the same outcomes. However, if you use the meditative approach, follow it up with the basic question below. The client should decide whether he or she wishes an experiential or more verbal interchange, although the two are clearly connected.

Meditative: Before starting, tell the client what to expect and what will happen. It is often useful for the client to see the questions you may ask beforehand. This permits co-construction and the client may suggest alternatives to the procedure. Ask the client to close her or his eyes and go into a meditative or relaxed state. Some clients prefer to keep their eyes open. Tell the client, "In your own way, allow a positive spiritual experience to come to you. Do not seek; rather, be open and see what comes to mind. Should a negative experience occur, note it for a moment, but move on until you find a truly positive experience. As you find that positive experience, allow your self to meditate on it." Quiet prayer may be preferred by some clients.

You will find that observing the client's face and muscle tension will let you know when the client is ready to talk.

Basic question: "Could you share a positive story about your spiritual background that occurs to you? Or, share a positive story about something that has been truly meaningful for you? Be sure that the story is positive."

Note: For counseling/therapy, any story is appropriate, but if the story is negative be sure you have generated strengths and supports before looking into the story in depth. Many clients do have negative spiritual and meaning stories.

With what cognitive/emotional developmental style is the client presenting? You are seeking a concrete narrative, but if the client presents from a different information processing style, help the person tell his or her story.

Use questions, encourages, paraphrasing, and reflection of feeling to bring out data, but try to impact the client's story minimally. Get the story as he or she constructs it. Summarize key facts and feelings about what the client has said before moving on.

2. Sensorimotor/Elemental

Basic question: "Could you think of one visual, auditory, kinesthetic, olfactory, or taste symbol or image that occurs to you as you think of that story?"

Special note: If the story or symbol is negative, be sure to develop positive images and symbols first and locate them in the body as supports. Be careful in locating negative images in the body except as an indicator. If you do use the body, make it brief. We do not want to build false memories or strengthen emphasis on negative memories. In the Muslim spiritual tradition, images should be used carefully, as symbols can be seen as mediators rather than as direct contact with God, the creator—and God is everywhere. However, images may also remind people of sacred feelings stored in the body and narratives that accompany those feelings (G. Esat, personal communication, 1997).

"What are you seeing? Hearing? Feeling? Tasting? What are the aromas? It will be helpful to locate the feeling in the body associated with the symbol." Elicit one example and then ask what was seen/heard/felt/tasted/smelled. Aim for here and now experiencing. Accept randomness. Summarize at the end of the segment. You may want to ask "What one thing stands out for you from this?"

3. Concrete/Situational

(Optional, designed for more time and analysis)

Basic question: "Could you give me another spiritual or meaning story from your background, perhaps indicating how it might be similar to or different from the other story. Can you describe your feelings in that story?"

Obtain a linear description of the event. At late concrete operations, look for if/then causal reasoning.

Ask, "What did you do? Say? What happened before? What happened next? What happened after?" Possibly pose the question "If you did X, then what happened?" Summarize before moving on. For affective development, ask "What did you feel?" The reflection "You felt X because . . . X" helps integrate cognition with affect at this level.

4. Formal/Reflective

Basic question: "Are those positive feelings and stories a pattern for you? Can you draw on this story and/or symbol to help you in other situations, either current or future? Is this some type of pattern in your family and/or your own life? How does the story relate to you personally in your life here and now? How might you reenact the family or spiritual patterns? Do you feel that way in other situations?"

Talk about repeating patterns and situations and/or encourage clients to talk about themselves in relationship to spiritual resources. This can also be a place in which you and the client explore negative stories in contrast with positive. Ask "What were you saying to yourself when that happened? Have you felt like that in other situations?" Again, reflect feelings and paraphrase as appropriate. Summarize key facts and feelings carefully before moving on.

5. Dialectic/Systemic/Integrative

Basic question: "Given what you've said about your family, spiritual experience, and/or ethnicity/race, how do these factors relate to you now as you think about it? Or, as we move to action, how would you rewrite that story in a new context? How would it lead to a new sense of being and relation with the spirit?"

Specific example: Esther is a White Jewish American who comes from New Jersey. Her parents survived the Holocaust.

"Esther, you have told me about your Jewish cultural background and your spiritual and family story. How do these factors affect the way you are now?"

Second example: Marcus is an African American Methodist and has told us his family story growing up in Boston.

"Marcus, you have told me about your African American background and growing up in Boston in a Methodist Church. How does being raised an African American Methodist affect your life today?"

Third example: Sari is a Muslim client who grew up in Detroit.

"Sari, We've heard about your background as a Muslim in Detroit. Given all this, what sense do you make of your cultural background and how it affects your way of being?"

Integration: "How do you put together/organize all that you have told me? What one thing stands out for you most? Is there some specific action you could take to follow up on this?"

Questions around integration are a good way to end the session as they ask people to reflect on the total interaction of the interview. In addition, the question on action looks to the future. It is here that cognitive-behavioral or other forms of treatment may be added to help ensure transfer of learning and behavioral change.

Internal/External: "How are internal views of yourself related to your external world? How does the external become internal? Where do you attribute your learning and being?"

Co-construction: "What rule or spiritual/cultural construct were you (they) operating under? Where did that rule come from? How might someone else (perhaps another family member) describe the situation?"

(Feelings can be examined using the same questions.) The effort here is to ensure that the client sees how his or her behavior relates to intergenerational family and cultural patterns. Here we are examining how individual and family behaviors are often under unconscious rules from culture and the past experience with spirituality.

Multiple perspectives: "How could we describe this from the point of view of some other person or by using a different framework or language system? How else might we put it together in another framework? How might an individual of another culture view your story? What might be another spiritual meaning we could attach to these issues?"

Deconstruction: "How might you rewrite that story? Can you see some flaws in the reasoning or in the patterns of feelings above? How might you change the rules? Given this, what action might you take? As you review our conversation, how do you view your original story?"

Action: "What are you/we going to do about it? Can you commit to action and follow-up?"

THREE SPECIAL ISSUES IN SPIRITUALITY AND COUNSELING

This is obviously not a definitive text on the possible uses of spirituality in counseling, and we'd like to supplement this introductory material with some other key issues.

Prayer. There is no question that personal prayer is a helpful and very central strategy in all religions and 90% of U.S. citizens pray (McMinn, 1996). There is no truly systematic and definitive data on the effectiveness of personal prayer, but clearly it is at a minimum a meditative strategy that is comfortable to clients—and this, in turn, is likely to help both their physical and mental health (Powell, Shahabi, & Thoresen, 2003; Richards & Bergin, 1997, p. 203). The use of prayer as a therapeutic strategy, however, has been debated because of the danger of the counselor's becoming too involved with or even imposing belief systems on the client.

The question has been raised as to whether being prayed for by others helps one recover from physical illness. A careful review of all available studies concluded, "There is some evidence to support the hypothesis that being prayed for improves [a person's] recovery from physical illness" (Powell, Shahabi, & Thoresen, 2003, p. 48). This occurred even when those prayed for did not know of the research study. The reviewers, however, noted that improvement occurred on subjective rather than objective measures and that more carefully designed research is needed.

The Christian Association for Psychological Studies reports that 30% of members of their group do pray with their clients. Prayer is believed to help rapport, to bring the counselor and client together; also, it models the tradition of faith. Furthermore, some counselors pray for their clients quietly during the session or for strength for themselves as they work with challenging client situations.

Nonetheless, prayer involves boundary issues, for prayer is a very personal process. There is real risk that the therapist or counselor will overstep limits and impose personal beliefs on the client. Also, a pastoral counselor acts in a different capacity from that of a secular counselor. McMinn (1996, p. 77), while recommending the use of prayer, outlines the increasing risk that comes with varying types of prayer. Praying for clients outside of sessions, silently praying for the client during sessions, and prescribing devotional meditation for client homework are seen by most as reasonably acceptable. Devotional prayers and prayer training in the session have chances for misuse or misunderstanding, and in-session prayer with the client poses potentially the most problems.

Worship and ritual. Reading the religion's holy text is often helpful to clients, and you may help them by asking them to identify texts that they find useful for repeated reading and meditation. Whether one is Buddhist, Christian, Hindu, Jewish, Muslim, or Shinto, such reading can be a useful addition to the counseling and therapy process, if the client self-identifies a spiritual or religious orientation.

Similarly, both individuals and families will benefit from group rituals ranging from prayer before meals through specific rituals within and without the church. A major pilgrimage to a sacred site or the quiet lighting of a single candle can be reassuring to clients. Saying the Rosary is both an important comfort and a route toward repentance and connection for Roman Catholics.

Clients can worship alone through spiritual reading and meditation. Over 200 therapists from the Church of Latter Day Saints report reference to the scriptures as

384 Chapter 13 Spirituality, Wellness, and Development: Applying DCT to Core Values in Clients' Lives

critical to their clients (Richards & Bergin, 1997). All religious groups have written traditions that can be used as a ritual, and these can lead to understanding and comfort. Moreover, cognitive therapists can use spiritual teachings to dispute client irrational beliefs (Probst, 1980; Probst et al., 1992), thus making spirituality an active part of the session.

Many clients also find church services comforting and important in balancing their lives. Some clients who have drifted from routine religious observation may profit from a carefully worded suggestion that they visit the old church to see what occurs for them.

The twelve steps of Alcoholics Anonymous (AA). While avoiding a specific religion, AA, ACOA (Adult Children of Alcoholics), and related groups focus clearly on a spiritual message—to turn one's life over to the care of God. But this turning over is always as the AA members themselves make sense of the Higher Power. AA, while sometimes controversial, has clearly helped tens of thousands of individuals "Let go and Let God." Referral to one of the several types of AA groups should be regarded as one of your resources for helping regardless of whether you include spirituality as part of your practice.

Research studies have found a relationship between AA attendance and sobriety, but the critical variable of motivation for treatment was never controlled until a two-year study of 2,310 alcoholic men by McKellar, Stewart, and Humphreys (2003). They found that AA participation resulted in lower alcohol problems after one year and that continued participation had a positive effect. Oluimette, Moos, and Finney (2003) found that AA participation resulted in better outcomes among men with post-traumatic stress disorder. These two research studies illustrate the potential of the higher power movement.

SUMMARY

Spirituality and religion are found at the core of culture. Whether your clients are directly interested in this area or not, it is very likely that their worldview in some way reflects spiritual roots. This is likely so, even if they are directly antagonistic to spirituality and religion. Specific examples of Australian Aboriginal and Judeo-Christian creation stories were presented to illustrate this point.

Discernment of one's life goals and meaning can be a central issue as one seeks to help clients find clearer directions for their lives. A variety of questions oriented to this goal were presented in Box 13-1.

Faith development theory provides a method whereby we may assess the spiritual and/or religious style of clients. Fowler's seven-stage theory was presented, along with its parallels to DCT and specific suggestions for facilitating faith development using counseling strategies. We suggested that all stages of faith development may be important, that primal faith may be the most basic, and that we should not despair because we cannot match persons like Martin Luther King, Jr., Gandhi, and Mother Teresa in spiritual devotion. However, our responsibility may be to find a sense of mission so that we may more closely appropriate these models of universalizing faith. They were not perfect and neither are we, so we cannot use their excellence as an excuse to avoid our own sense of mission.

DCT offers a specific set of questions to facilitate client exploration of spirituality and religious issues. The questions were presented in some detail with the suggestion that you work slowly and carefully through them with an open and actively participating client.

Three important issues in spirituality and counseling were summarized briefly. Prayer was presented as a generally positive intervention but one that should be used carefully due to the danger of imposing oneself and moving through traditional client/therapist boundaries. Worship and ritual were presented as useful supplementary therapeutic strategies. Alcoholics Anonymous was presented as a spiritual resource for referral that can benefit many, but not all, clients.

THEORY INTO PRACTICE: DEVELOPING YOUR PORTFOLIO OF COMPETENCE

Self-Assessment Exercise

Exercise 1. You and discernment

What do you see as your life goals and mission? What is your vision?

_____

_____

_____

Sensorimotor experience: What positive image comes too your mind when you think of goals and mission? What are you seeing/hearing/feeling?

_____

_____

_____

Concrete description and action: Is there a story you can tell about your goals or that relates to a meaningful life mission? Have you acted on the images or story?

_____

_____

_____

_____

Formal reflection: As you think back and reflect on your life, what sense does it make for your future?

_____

_____

_____

_____

Dialectic/systemic integration: Looking at the three perspectives of sensorimotor, concrete, and formal, how would you integrate this into a life plan or vision for the future? Can you move these ideas into concrete action?

_____

_____

_____

_____

Identification and Classification Exercise

Exercise 2. You and faith development

Review Table 13-1. What style of faith development seems closest to where you are presently? Review each level of faith development and record what parts of you are represented there. You may find that your faith has changed over time as you review your developmental history.

_____

_____

_____

_____

Given your present stage of faith development, what strategies are most appropriate to help you develop further at this stage?

_____

_____

_____

Faith development can be expanded at all stages. What strategies and ideas appeal to you for further development of your faith at multiple levels or styles?

_____

_____

_____

_____

Multicultural Competence Exercise

Exercise 3. Faith development as a cross-cultural issue

Issues of faith and meaning can be considered multicultural issues in themselves. What may be most challenging is for you to work with someone whose spirituality or religion is different from your own, or whose faith development is markedly different from where you are presently.

Use the space below to identify your challenges and needs for growth so that you can work more effectively with those who may be different from you.

_____

_____

_____

_____

Interviewing Practice Exercises

Exercise 4. Specific questions for discernment

Ask a partner to role-play a client. Sit down with the Box 13-1 list of questions in your lap. (Don't try to memorize the questions at this point.) Go through each stage, step by step. After you have gone through the series, exchange roles and go through them again with you as the client. It is often helpful to share the questions openly with the volunteer client.

Stop after each step in the interview and discuss with your client what has just happened. Then, together evaluate the often powerful experience that you have just been through.

Exercise 5. Cross-spiritual counseling: Faith development

Find a partner for a role-play. The partner will play the part of a faith developmental level different from your own. Can you help that role-played partner expand her or his faith, given the stage he or she presents?

Generalization: Taking Spirituality Skills Home

Exercise 6. Utilizing discernment or spiritual narratives in your own practice

For a single client, who has expressed an interest in spirituality, go through the questions leading toward discernment in Box 13-1 and/or work through the steps of spiritual narratives as outlined in this chapter.

Portfolio Reflections

Exercise 7. Your reflections on the place of spirituality and meaning issues in your own practice of counseling and therapy

What stood out for you from this chapter? What sense did you make of what you read and experienced? What are your key points from this chapter? Write your thoughts below and add them to your Portfolio Folder.

_____

_____

_____

_____

_____

REFERENCES

Bergin, A., & Garfield, S. (Eds.). (1994). *Handbook of psychotherapy and behavior change* (4th ed.) New York: Wiley.

Camus, A. (1955). *The myth of Sisyphus.* New York: Vintage Books.

deWaal, E. (1997). *Living with contradiction: An introduction to Benedictine spirituality.* Harrisburg, PA: Morehouse.

Farnham, S., Gill, J., McLean, R., & Ward, S. (1991). *Listening hearts.* Harrisburg, PA: Morehouse.

Fowler, J. (1981). *Stages of faith: The psychology of human development and the quest for meaning.* San Francisco: Harper & Row.

Fowler, J. (1996). Pluralism and oneness in religious experience: William James, faith-development theory, and clinical practice. In E. Shafranske (Ed.), *Religion and the clinical practice of psychology.* Washington, DC: American Psychological Association.

Frankl, V. (1959). *Man's search for meaning.* New York: Pocket Books. (Original work published 1946)

Frankl, V. (1978). *The unheard cry for meaning.* New York: Touchstone.

Gallup, G. (1996, December). *The epidemiology of spirituality.* Presentation to the Spirituality and Healing in Medicine Conference, Boston.

Ivey, A., D'Andrea, M., Ivey, M., & Simek-Morgan, L. (2002). *Theories of counseling and psychotherapy: A multicultural perspective.* Boston: Allyn & Bacon.

Ivey, A., & Ivey, M. (2003). *Interviewing and counseling: Facilitating development in a multicultural world* (5th ed.). Pacific Grove, CA: Brooks/Cole.

Kelly, E. (1995). *Spirituality and religion in counseling and psychotherapy.* Washington, DC: American Counseling Association.

McKellar, J., Stewart, E., & Humphreys, K. (2003). Alcoholics Anonymous involvement and positive alcohol-related outcomes: Cause, consequence, or just a correlate? *Journal of Clinical and Consulting Psychology, 71,* 302–308.

McMinn, M. (1996). *Psychology, theology, and spirituality in Christian counseling.* Wheaton, IL: Tyndale.

Miller, W., & Thoresen, C. (2003). Spirituality, religion, and health: An emerging research field. *American Psychologist, 58,* 24–35.

Mountford, C. (1976). *Before time began.* Melbourne: Thomas Nelson.

Myers, J. E., & Williard, K. (2003). Integrating spirituality into counseling and counselor training: A developmental, wellness approach. *Counseling & Values, 47,* 142–155.

Nielsen, S., Johnson, W., & Ellis, A. (2001). *Counseling and psychotherapy with religious persons: A rational emotive behavior therapy approach.* Mahwah, NJ: Erlbaum.

Oluimette, P., Moos, R., & Finney, J. (2003). PTSD treatment and 5-year remission among patients with substance abuse and posttraumatic stress disorders. *Journal of Clinical and Consulting Psychology, 71,* 410–414.

Powell, L., Shahabi, L., & Thoresen, C. (2003). Religion and spirituality: Linkages to mental health. *American Psychologist, 58,* 36–52.

Probst, L. (1980). The comparative efficacy of religious and nonreligious imagery for the treatment of mild depression in religious individuals. *Cognitive Therapy and Research, 4,* 167–178.

Probst, L., Ostrom, R., Watkins, P., Dean, T., & Mashburn, D. (1992). Comparative efficacy of religious and nonreligious cognitive-behavioral therapy for the treatment of clinical depression in religious individuals. *Journal of Consulting and Clinical Psychology, 60,* 94–103.

Richards, P., & Bergin, A. (1997). *A spiritual strategy for counseling and psychotherapy.* Washington, DC: American Psychological Association.

Seeman, T., Dubin, L., & Seeman, M. (2003). Religiosity, spirituality, and health: A critical review of the evidence for biological pathways. *American Psychologist, 58,* 53–61.

Shafranske, E. (Ed.). (1996). *Religion and the clinical practice of psychology.* Washington, DC: American Psychological Association.

Walker, K., & Dixon, V. (2002). Spirituality and academic performance among African American college students. *Journal of Black Psychology, 28,* 107–121.

CHAPTER 14
Epilogue
Your Future Development

CENTRAL PRACTICE OBJECTIVE | Mastery and practice of concepts in this chapter will enable you to examine your own understanding of wellness theory and developmental counseling and therapy, and integrate these concepts in your work with clients over the lifespan.

As you now know, the developmental approach to counseling and psychotherapy is different from that used with other therapies. We ask you to start with the client and not immediately impose a theory. Rather, we suggest that the first issue in counseling and therapy is to understand the client's life space, including history and context. Where is the individual in the developmental life cycle? What wellness strengths does the client bring to the interview? How does the client make sense of the world? Once we know the answers to these and related questions, we are better prepared to create new growth and developmental opportunities for our clients.

The developmental counseling and therapy strategies you have encountered throughout this book are all oriented to helping you and the client find new ways of thinking, feeling, behaving, and making meaning. The four styles of DCT help us see issues in new ways and enable us to review and experience our life stories from multiple perspectives. In this way, our clients and we can become more creative and can edit and rewrite those stories—and then use them as scripts for positive change.

This final chapter has two major goals. It seeks to help you:

1. Review and assess your accomplishments and mastery of the central practice objectives of this book.
2. Plan your next steps as you develop your own wellness-oriented and developmental model of counseling and psychotherapy.

ASSESSING MASTERY OF CENTRAL PRACTICE OBJECTIVES

The introduction to this book, Before You Start, presented a table in which the central practice objectives of the book were summarized. You can review these goals with some additional information in Table 14-1. We tried to state clearly at the beginning that this book requires action on your part, both to understand the concepts and to use them in your work with clients. Importantly, understanding a concept is not the same as being able to use it in practice in the interview.

Please review Table 14-1 at this point and indicate your level of mastery of the major abilities associated with each chapter. You are asked to rate yourself on a scale of 1 through 4 with the following definitions:

1. I have not mastered this ability.
2. I understand the concepts related to this ability, but have not been able to use them in the interview.
3. I can use these concepts in the here and now of the interview.
4. I can use these concepts in the interview *and* note specific changes in thoughts, feelings, behaviors, and meanings in my clients.

Level 4 mastery, of course, is the objective of this book—for you to take the concepts into the "real world" and see positive changes in your client's development. Knowing the basics of questioning associated with each developmental style is important, but reality requires us to use the questions with clients. And success demands that we use the concepts to facilitate positive change. Similarly, we can

Table 14-1   Assessing Central Practice Objectives: Evidence of Mastery

Chapter	Central Practice Goal and Assessment of Level of Mastery	Evidence of Mastery Level
1. Our Developmental Nature	1 2 3 4 Ability to assess clients' concrete and abstract cognitive/emotional styles shown through ability to recognize and classify client statements and to distinguish them in the here and now of the interview.	
2. Wellness: Optimizing Human Development Over the Lifespan	1 2 3 4 Ability to assess your wellness and that of your clients, thus providing a solid base of strengths on which to facilitate client positive movement.	
3. Development Over the Lifespan: Developmental Counseling as Lifespan Therapy	1 2 3 4 Ability to conduct a lifespan review and to assess and understand clients' unique developmental history and current normative life transitions and challenges, and anticipate later developmental concerns.	
4. Assessing Developmental Style	1 2 3 4 Ability to assess the four client cognitive/emotional styles through classification of transcripts and to identify client style in the here and now of the interview.	
5. Developmental Interventions and Strategies: Specific Interventions to Facilitate Client Cognitive and Emotional Development	1 2 3 4 Ability to apply specific DCT questioning strategies with many types of clients and to adapt the strategies for your work utilizing many theories of counseling and therapy.	
6. Assessing Client Change: Creativity, Perturbation, and Confrontation	1 2 3 4 Ability to facilitate change by perturbing and confronting client discrepancies and incongruities in a supportive fashion. Equally important, you will be able to assess the impact of your confrontation on client change processes using the Confrontation Impact Scale.	
7. Developing Treatment Plans: DCT and Theories of Counseling and Psychotherapy	1 2 3 4 Ability to shift your counseling style to meet the developmental needs of varying clients. You will be able to work with multiple theories of counseling and therapy and integrate DCT developmental concepts into the treatment.	

(continued)

Table 14-1   *(continued)*

Chapter	Central Practice Goal and Assessment of Level of Mastery	Evidence of Mastery Level
8. Multicultural Counseling and Therapy	1 2 3 4 Ability to assess and to facilitate client expansion of cultural identity and multicultural consciousness. You will also be able to use the specific steps of psychotherapy to help clients discover, name, reflect, and act on issues related to multicultures and to oppression.	
9. Reframing the *Diagnostic and Statistical Manual of Mental Disorders:* Positive Strategies From Developmental Counseling and Therapy	1 2 3 4 Ability to reframe severe distress as a logical biological and psychological response to environmental conditions. Ability to develop comprehensive treatment plans, using multiple theoretical orientations and strategies, to work with issues such as depression, personality style ("disorder"), and post-traumatic stress.	
10. Early Recollections: Using DCT With Early Memories to Facilitate Second-Order Change	1 2 3 4 Ability to use the theoretical/practical Adlerian approach to early recollections as (a) a positive support base for your clients, and (b) a way to help clients understand how their past relates to the present and how it can help them build toward the future.	
11. Using Developmental Counseling and Therapy With Families	1 2 3 4 Ability to understand and work with families at various stages of the life cycle and to apply DCT questioning strategies to facilitate family development.	
12. Bibliotherapy, Metaphors, and Narratives	1 2 3 4 Ability to bring more creative and artistic processes into the stories surrounding the counseling and psychotherapy process including the use of media and journaling.	
13. Spirituality, Wellness, and Development: Applying DCT to Core Values in Clients' Lives	1 2 3 4 Ability to conceptualize and work comfortably with spiritual, religious, and meaning issues in the interview. Ability to use DCT discernment processes to help clients find direction and make meaning in their lives.	
14. Epilogue: Your Future Development	1 2 3 4 Ability to examine your own understanding of wellness theory and developmental counseling and therapy, and to integrate these concepts in your work with clients over the lifespan.	

master intellectually the ideas of the Confrontation Impact Scale, but can we actually note clients' responses to our interventions in the session and shift our style of helping appropriately to match their needs and facilitate further growth?

Understanding the basics of multicultural counseling and therapy is critical, but are you able to identify cultural identity level and then facilitate growth and change? Can you really work with issues of oppression using the psychotherapy-as-liberation model? All these and more are what the developmental approach is about. Theory is important, but it is not useful unless you can take it directly into practice.

In assessing your mastery of the concepts in Table 14-1, what do you find? The emphasis in this integrative approach to counseling and therapy is on results—accountable results that can most often be explicitly measured. You can facilitate client change through choice, not just chance.

As you review your mastery of the central practice concepts of DCT, summarize here your areas of strength and areas where you might seek further practice and development.

Areas of mastery and strength _____

_____

_____

Areas for future further development _____

_____

_____

CONCLUSION: LIFESPAN COUNSELOR AND THERAPIST DEVELOPMENT

Whether you are just beginning or are well established in your career as a helping professional, you face a lifetime of personal growth and development. New theories, new techniques and interventions, and most of all, new clients provide a constant challenge for us to generate new ideas—to grow and develop with our clients.

DCT, wellness theory, transition theory, multicultural counseling and therapy (MCT), and positive psychology are just the beginning of emerging approaches to counseling and therapy focusing on positive aspects of development, growth, and change. As the field moves away from a pathological, remedial model of helping, all of us will face personal developmental tasks as we orient to this new, positive model of human development and reframe past and present models of counseling and therapy.

Our clients come to us seeking resolution of their issues, whether these are career choice, academic difficulty, clinical depression, or a challenging life transition such as leaving home, marriage, separation or divorce, or retirement. Remediation is oriented toward a specific end—the "cure." However, there is no cure for "life." Each day presents us with new developmental challenges; there is no endpoint to the process. Counselors and therapists will never lack for business.

The task of counseling and therapy is not to solve problems or effect cures. Rather we should consider problems as challenges and opportunities for new growth. There is an inevitable logic to even the most serious and complex issues that clients present. For example, with a person who presents with depression, we need to know the developmental background and where the issues fit into the life cycle. That client will likely have other developmental issues related to the depression—family, career and work, and interpersonal concerns. As we start resolving the most obvious aspects of depression, we will also need to think holistically and contextually. Resolving one of these issues is not a "cure"; it is a solution that enables the individual to move on to other issues. As part of this, it is important to help that client work contextually on the environmental issues that contributed to the original depression. The client becomes a change agent.

Academic counseling often starts with helping the student "fix" the problem by deciding on a major or correcting poor study habits. But this is only the beginning of the process in which the client discovers that procrastination is a behavioral pattern rooted in developmental history and that this pattern continues in school, the workplace, and important interpersonal relationships. Developmental counseling and therapy is concerned not only with problem resolution but also with wider problem prevention. Effective academic counseling helps the client see how school pursuits are part of lifespan developmental processes.

Each life problem or passage brings opportunities for new development. The teen who works through issues of identity will soon encounter the challenges of interpersonal relationships—and most often, they will happen together. Just as soon as an individual resolves the mid-40s crisis of meaningful existence, he or she faces the crises of the 50s—the decline of physical capacity. Developmental surprises are always present. As therapists, we can focus on these crises and help our clients resolve "problems," or we can use a positive developmental focus and enable our clients to welcome change as a natural progression through the joys and challenges of life.

Some counselors and therapists feel they have completed their professional developmental tasks when they finish their degree work. But after the degree, there is the state licensing examination. And after that exam, there is a bewildering array of "super-certification" programs such as those of the National Board of Certified Counselors (NBCC), the American Board of Professional Psychology (ABPP), and other highly specialized certifications in social work, family therapy, and forensic testimony. Although each certification step, from degree to super-certification program, involves more work and study, each stage allows you to hone your own developmental skills and thus to better serve your clients.

Counselor and therapist burnout are likely to occur when the work setting provides little or no opportunity for growth and development. Case conferences and staff meetings that strive to maintain the status quo and leave key decisions only to senior staff members lead to burned-out professionals who may leave the helping profession. We need more work settings in which supervisors and experienced professionals are open to change and who are willing to reach, make mistakes, and learn from them. In addition, we all need to learn from and incorporate the energy and excitement of young new staff members.

The focus of a developmentally oriented helping profession is on change and growth—the exploration of the New. However, the rigid perspectives of the past inevitably reassert themselves; what was once new often becomes the old orthodoxy.

Thus, the models of development and wellness presented here must also be constantly reevaluated and changed. Through constant evaluation, change, and reevaluation, what is good and helpful from the past will remain as part of an ever-changing, holistic approach to counseling and psychotherapy.

As we learned in Chapters 1 and 4, Plato's Allegory of the Cave described slaves chained to the wall, believing that the shadows they saw before them were real. In fact, candles placed behind the slaves produced the images, which were the only things they saw. The slaves developed systematic beliefs about the images and even concrete explanations to explain what they saw.

Our clients come to us often metaphorically chained to unworkable beliefs based on mental images that are incomplete or simply not real. Out of this partial or even false view of reality, clients have developed narratives and stories that do not work effectively. Many of them are prisoners of their context and history; for them, change can be immensely difficult.

In Plato's allegory, the chains were broken for one of the slaves and when he turned to the candles, he was dazzled by the light and considered returning to his chained status as it was less painful than the change demanded by his new awareness. So it is for some of our clients. As we help them uncover more of the possibility and potential in life, expect resistance. Change, even positive change, is not always pleasant or easy.

Helping the client out of the darkness opens the way for creating an infinite array of life possibilities. Again, you will find clients who both want and do not want, or are afraid of, the rich array of options that may exist. A new life lies ahead, but what is that new life to be like? Are the decisions too many and too complex? Would the client be more comfortable returning to the status quo? As noted in Chapter 6, developmental change involves dimensions of loss as one must give up old ways of thinking, feeling, and behaving.

At this point, why are we bringing up the difficulty of change? This book has focused on an optimistic, wellness approach in which the joys of creativity and new possibilities have been stressed. You are about to leave this book and a counseling or therapy course that has focused on creating positive opportunities for growth and development, the reframing of *DSM-IV* from an optimistic developmental perspective, and research and theory from a lifespan wellness and developmental perspective.

However, the wellness and developmental approach both recognizes and incorporates many traditional counseling and psychological approaches that focus on the impact of problems and psychopathology. Wellness, lifespan theory, multiculturalism, and positive psychology are not the center of current theory and practice, although the movement in this positive and optimistic direction is growing stronger. In our practices, we have found these methods not only central but essential in promoting and supporting client strengths and growth in holistic and healthful ways.

You will not find everyone you work with favoring or even knowing and understanding the developmental wellness orientation. Many professional helpers as well as counselor and therapist educators were trained in traditional methods before the emergence of these new paradigms. The medical model of searching out problems, diagnosing traditionally, and treating clients without awareness of social context remains strong and powerful.

In your counseling and therapy training program, you have already noted many widely diverging and differing orientations to the field. All have something of value to offer to clients. As you move into your professional career in counseling and therapy, you will encounter ever more diversity as the field continually expands and new theories and research enlarge possibilities even further. DCT will continue to provide a framework for helping you organize these new theories and methods and integrate them into your repertoire of counseling skills.

We hope that the lifespan and wellness developmental approach will remain as part of your helping and therapeutic strategies, and will be a focus for your own personal growth toward being a healthy individual and role model for others. We thank you for your careful attention. At this point we wish you the very best in your professional future and that you enjoy the counseling and psychotherapy field as much as we do. Good luck!

Allen, Mary, Jane, and Tom

APPENDIX 1
Introspective Developmental Counseling Questions

Tamase's introspective developmental counseling (IDC) focuses on four major developmental periods (birth through preschool, elementary school, high school, and one's present life stage). The first three stages are stressed, as they form the *foundation* of life experience. You will find this style of life review helpful in learning more about yourself and as a useful system to understand your client's background more fully.

Tamase recommends that those training to become professional helpers look at their own developmental foundations. He divides trainees into pairs and each interviews the other for four half-hour interviews. Out of this experience, participants often learn that their developmental history has some basic patterns that repeat themselves in their current situations and in adult life. You will find that some of your clients may enjoy and benefit from the systematic questioning of developmental history proposed by IDC.

Sharing the questions with your client before you begin may be productive—it helps build your alliance and the two of you can work together systematically through the questions and issues. If the individual has difficulty with a particular question, rephrase it to meet his or her interests and needs. The goal of each question is to have the client explore the general area. At times, changing the language of the question is beneficial. Frequent use of the basic listening sequence, including encouraging, paraphrasing, reflecting feelings and meanings, and summarizing, is helpful in the process.

Combining IDC questions with the four DCT cognitive/emotional styles will lead to more awareness and a session that goes into more depth. Usually, you will start with concrete narratives of the life stage. Follow this with a search for key images of these early recollections. For example, many clients have images of their birth experience or early childhood experiences and have not explored these in depth. Another concrete story related to that period may follow and then you can encourage formal-operational reflection on the narrative and images. Multiple perspectives on the life stage can be achieved through dialectic/systemic questioning. This process was explained also in the chapter on early recollections. The IDC questions

---

The IDC questions presented in this appendix are adaptations of the original Tamase questions developed jointly by Koji Tamase and Allen Ivey. The original, briefer version of the questions is available from Dr. Koji Tamase at the Department of Psychology, Nara University of Education, Takabatake, Nara 630, Japan.

will stimulate early memories and, particularly if combined with DCT, should be employed with sensitivity and care, for many individuals find the experience emotionally powerful.

Timing: Ideally, you should allow an hour for in-depth discussion of each time period. Thus, separate sessions to go through the detailed life review of IDC are considered necessary. You can move through the life stages more quickly, but considerable depth will be lost.

Journaling: An alternate way to use the IDC questions is through journaling. Set aside an hour or two to reflect on one set of questions, then write out your responses, including reflections on your emotions and experiences. You can then process your reflections in a session with a peer or counselor. Clients can also be encouraged to journal using the IDC questions as homework assignments. Their responses and memories can be processed using DCT to expand their understanding and develop new ways of making meaning of their life story. You may find this process similar to that used in bibliotherapy, as it truly is a narrative approach. In addition to finding meaning in their life histories, the therapeutic process helps clients rewrite their life script and experience the processes of second-order change.

Session 1: Birth Through Preschool Period
1. Could you tell me about your family members (for the purpose of structuring the interview and understanding basics of the family system)? What particular important life events were they experiencing during your earliest years?
2. Is there anything about your birth that you have heard from your mother or other family members?
3. Could you tell me about your life from the earliest age that you can remember?
4. What is the most impressive thing that happened prior to kindergarten?
5. What kind of behavior bothered your mother when you were a preschool child?
6. How did you feel about your parents when you were a preschool child?
7. Did you struggle with brothers or sisters at this age?
8. Is there any particular event that made you feel either very unhappy or afraid at this age?
9. What single event do you recall most positively from this period of your life? What is your image of that event?
10. As you reflect on this life period, what patterns from this early period continue in your present life?

Session 2: Elementary School Period
1. What particular events in your family were important as a context for this period?
2. What teacher do you recall? What kind of person was this teacher?
3. Could you give me a concrete example of something that happened in the first grade?
4. What happened in the third and fourth grade? The fifth and sixth?
5. What kinds of friends did you have?
6. What is the most impressive thing you can remember from your elementary school years?
7. Did you ever mistreat anyone, or did others mistreat you in these years?

8. What was your experience with academic achievement?
9. How did things go with brothers and sisters at this time? If you have no brothers or sisters, how was it with a person who might substitute for them?
10. What single event do you recall most positively from this period of your life? What is a single image of that event?
11. What patterns from this period of your life might appear in your present-day life?

Session 3: Junior Through Senior High School Period
1. What particular events in your family were important as a context for this period?
2. Could you tell me about your friendships in high school?
3. How did things go with the opposite sex?
4. How was the relationship with your parents? How were things in your family?
5. How did things go with your brothers and sisters? If you have no brothers or sisters, how was it with a person who might substitute for them?
6. Did you rebel against your parents?
7. How was your academic and work life?
8. What is the most impressive thing you can remember from your junior and senior high years?
9. Who were the influential people in your life?
10. How did you like to spend your time?
11. What single event do you recall most positively from this period of your life? What is your image of that event?
12. What patterns might continue from this period to your present-day life?

Session 4: Recent Past and Current Life Situation Session
1. What important family and personal contextual issues have happened since high school that have affected you particularly?
2. How have you related to your family since high school?
3. What are your current significant relationships (loved ones, spouse, own family)? How are they going?
4. Are there any current interpersonal difficulties?
5. What significant events have affected your life since high school?
6. Of all the events since high school, what one event stands out for you?
7. How do you think about your career now?
8. What job difficulties do you experience?
9. What do you do that makes you feel good?
10. Complete this sentence: "I am most discouraged in my life about

_____."

11. What single event do you recall most positively from this period of your life? What is your image of that event?
12. What overall patterns do you observe from your life review, both in this session and others?

APPENDIX 2

The Standard Cognitive/Emotional Developmental Classification System

Allen E. Ivey and Sandra A. Rigazio-DiGilio

This book gives primary attention to the four basic styles: sensorimotor, concrete, formal, and dialectic/systemic. For both clinical and research purposes, the classification system presented below has been found helpful in ensuring both greater precision and reliability (i.e., consistency) of ratings. We do this through encouraging noticing differences between early and late styles. Early concrete operations, for example, may focus on naming and linear storytelling while late concrete operations brings in dimensions of causal "if . . . then . . ." cognition and emotion. An early formal-operational thinker may be able to recognize patterns whereas a late formal thinker will be able to recognize repeating patterns and attach meaning to the patterns. This provides the clinician/researcher with the opportunity to elicit, observe, and study some of the more complex dimensions of DCT.

What does this mean for you and counseling and clinical practice? Your goal here is to assess client cognitive/emotional style in the here and now of the interview. At the most basic level, classifying client behavior into one of the four styles should be your first objective and then you can match or mismatch styles, depending on the specific situation. Being able to identify early and late styles will facilitate more precision assessment in the session. You will also find that skilled listening and questioning can help clients move to a different style level. For example, an early sensorimotor client may be able to experience emotions but not be able to embed them physically or comprehend their meaning, while a late sensorimotor client can embed his or her feelings and attach meaning to these emotional experiences. When a concrete client tells a story (early concrete), you can help that client think in new ways about the story by encouraging "if . . . then . . ." thinking. Questions such as "If you behave like that, then what is the likely result?" can encourage clients to think beyond themselves.

So, as you review the following guidelines, think first about four styles, but as you become more familiar with DCT, consider working with DCT and your clients using the eight-style paradigm. Both general and specific guidelines have been developed for use by clinicians and researchers to facilitate recognition of early and late stages of each cognitive style in the DCT model.

GENERAL GUIDELINES

This classification system is designed to help you classify interview behavior. Scorers will independently classify the predominant cognitive/emotional style as revealed by the client's verbal behavior during different sections of the interview using the criteria that follow. Although most clients will operate using different styles at different times, or with multiple styles, the classification should be according to the style that predominates.

In addition, the criteria suggested here may be adapted and used to classify an interview portion or a client or counselor statement. Generally, using larger segments of verbal behavior to make a classification is most effective, but it is possible to use single client statements with some degree of reliability. It is also possible to use adaptations of these criteria to classify the verbal behavior of the interviewer, therapist, or counselor.

The rating system here is based on a typescript. However, with practice, it is possible to rate from an audiotape or videotape of the interview, or even from an observation of an actual session through a one-way mirror.

INITIAL PRESENTING ASSESSMENT

Basic Objective

To use the client's first 50 to 100 words to classify the client as being at one of the four cognitive/emotional styles.

Method

Each scorer will receive a transcript of the dialogue that occurred between the interviewer and client during the assessment phase of the interview. The task for the rater is to determine the style of cognitive development predominantly represented by the client's conceptualization of a family issue. Ratings will be made on a four-point classification scale that identifies the four basic dimensions of cognitive development: sensorimotor/elemental, concrete-operational/situational, formal-operational/pattern, and dialectic/systemic/transformational. Although the client may operate using more than one style, the task of the scorer is to determine which of the four styles is predominantly used as a frame of reference during the assessment phase. Two methods of rating will be used:

- The raters will classify each client statement using the criteria defined on the following pages. The predominant cognitive/emotional style will be computed by percentages of client responses in each of the four categories.
- The raters will classify the entire client statement or series of statements into one of the four categories.

CLASSIFYING THE INTERVIEW SEGMENTS

Basic Objective

The rater will classify eight interview segments, presented randomly, into eight categories—the subdivisions of the basic four categories. The portions of the interview will be presented with the counselor statements deleted. (This can be considered a training procedure and as essential for research purposes. In rating ongoing interviews, it is helpful to classify both counselor and client statements.)

Method

Each scorer will receive eight intervention sections that occur during the treatment phase of the interview, divided to reflect the eight cognitive-developmental subdivisions defined below. The group of typescripts will be randomized and will include only the client statements. The task of the scorer is to holistically review each section and determine the cognitive-developmental subdivision predominantly revealed in the client statements.

Ratings will be made on an eight-point classification system that subdivides each of the four basic dimensions of developmental cognition by early and late indicators: early and late sensorimotor/elemental, early and late concrete-operational/situational, early and late formal-operational/pattern, and early and late dialectic/systemic/transformational. Again, although more than one subdivision may be identified in each section, the task of the scorer is to determine which of the eight is predominantly used by the client within each section. Raters will use only the holistic method of classification for these eight sections.

SENSORIMOTOR/ELEMENTAL DIMENSION

Early Sensorimotor/Elemental Subdivision (Key Words: See, Hear, Feel)

The client randomly focuses on fragments and pieces of sensory-based data as she or he talks about the visual, auditory, and/or kinesthetic elements of a situation or issue.

Affect
- The client shows minimal distinction between sensory input and emotions.
- The client is dominated by sensory stimuli and affect.

Cognition
- The client shows minimal ability to coordinate the elements of sensory-based data into an organized Gestalt.

Late Sensorimotor/Elemental Subdivision (Key Word: Belief)

The client provides a view of reality that makes sense of the sensory-based data reflective of the situation or issue in a somewhat incomplete or irrational manner.

The late sensorimotor period, according to DCT, is a time of naming and of issues. In work with clinical populations, virtually all clients answered the meaning-oriented questions of this stage with clearly faulty reasoning. Many clients, however, respond to late sensorimotor questions with logical concrete and/or formal statements. Careful questioning may be required to uncover the mistaken logic of these clients, and this is not always possible. If this is the case, clients *will not* demonstrate the illogical or magical patterns expected as they discuss key issues; thus, their statements should be categorized in one of the other seven categories.

Affect
- The client's emotions remain sensory-based and reactive.
- The client is unable to act on her or his emotions.

Cognitive
- The client offers interpretations that, no matter how sophisticated, are illusory and irrational and are stated in a way that reveals that the client cannot take effective actions based on the beliefs.

CONCRETE-OPERATIONAL/SITUATIONAL DIMENSION

Early Concrete-Operational/Situational Subdivision (Key Word: Do)

The client describes the situation or issue from a single self-perspective in a linear, relatively organized sequence of concrete specifics. Her or his explanation has a major emphasis on the facts with some focus on a few of the basic feelings.

Affect
- The client describes general emotions simply, from one perspective and with a lack of differentiation.
- The client expresses emotions outwardly.

Cognition
- The client focuses predominantly on a factual description of the concrete details of a situation or issue from her or his own perspective. There is minimal emphasis on evaluation or analysis.

Late Concrete-Operational/Situational Subdivision (Key Words: If/Then)

The client organizes the elements or facts of the situation or issue into linear if/then statements that may lead to issues of causation. She or he may be able to control and describe actions, and may be able to think in terms of antecedents and consequences. The focus is on facts and actions as opposed to analyzing, evaluating, or showing awareness of patterns. Logic and reversibility may be evident.

Affect
- The client is able to control and describe broad-based, undifferentiated, outwardly focused affect. He or she may say, "I feel _____ when _____ happens." Otherwise feelings are relatively undifferentiated. Awareness of mixed or ambivalent feelings is rare, for example.

Cognition
- The client demonstrates linear if/then thinking, emphasizing causality and predictability from a single perspective.
- The client is able to control and describe actions and the impact of actions.
- The client is able to apply logic and reversibility to concrete situations or issues.
- The client is able to separate thoughts and actions.

FORMAL-OPERATIONAL/PATTERN DIMENSION

Early Formal-Operational/Pattern Subdivision (Key Words: Pattern, Self)

The client moves away from description of sensory experience toward examining and/or analyzing the facts of a situation or issue or toward examining and analyzing the self. She or he is able to identify repetitive behavior, thoughts, and affect related to various similar situations and issues.

Affect
- The client demonstrates an awareness of the complexity of feelings and is able to separate self from feelings and reflect on them.

Cognition
- The client describes repeating patterns of thought, behavior, and affect in the self that occur across situations.
- The client engages in analysis of self and situation.

Late Formal-Operational/Pattern Subdivision (Key Words: Patterns of Patterns)

The client is able to analyze patterns of patterns and beginning multiple perspectives of behavior, thought, and feeling from the vantage points of the self and the contextual fields within which she or he interacts. The client is able to see larger, consistently repeating patterns of behavior, thought, and feeling in her or his life and to examine how she or he thinks and feels about the evolving theme or view of reality.

Affect
- The client demonstrates an ability to analyze her or his patterns of feelings.
- The client demonstrates an ability to identify others' feelings and be empathic.
- The client demonstrates an awareness that feelings can be validly expressed in multiple ways.

Cognition
- The client demonstrates an ability to examine the patterns of self and situation.
- The client demonstrates an ability to organize and analyze different situations or issues abstractly.
- The client may coordinate and discover new patterns, compare and contrast different situations, and form this into a Gestalt.

DIALECTIC/SYSTEMIC/TRANSFORMATIONAL/INTEGRATIVE DIMENSION

Early Dialectic/Systemic/Transformational/Integrative Subdivision (Key Words: Integrate, Put Together)

The client demonstrates an ability to generate an integrative picture that combines thought and action and shows an awareness that personal constructions of reality are co-generated via the family network.

The client is able to reflect on systems of operations and how "things go together" in an interdependent sense. Becoming increasingly multiperspective, the client is able to see a situation from several frames of reference and keep them in mind simultaneously. Underlying assumptions of perspectives may be identified.

Affect

■ The client offers a wide range of emotions and recognizes that emotions can change contextually. For example, "I am sad that my wife died, but when I think about the pain she was experiencing, I feel glad that she no longer has to suffer. I feel anger when I think about the injustice of it all."

■ The client recognizes that she or he can change and adapt to new situations.

Cognition

■ The client demonstrates an ability to coordinate concepts and put together a holistic integrated picture.

■ The client demonstrates an awareness that the evolving integration was co-constructed in a dialectical or dialogic relationship with family, history, culture, and so on.

Late Dialectic/Systemic/Deconstruction/Transformational Subdivision (Key Words: Challenge the Integration, Action)

The client demonstrates an ability to criticize and challenge her or his own integrated system and discover alternative perspectives. The client is able to think about moving toward action based on these alternative perspectives. Challenging and criticizing assumptions is important here. Ideally, action plans should follow from this analysis.

Affect

■ The client is able to look at her or his entire realm of emotions and then still move beyond into an infinite reflection on reflections.

Cognition

■ The client intellectualizes and challenges her or his assumptions and integrations.

■ The client can identify the flaws in the reasoning and logic of her or his integration from various relational perspectives.

■ The client demonstrates an ability to think about action in relation to her or his new perspectives.

APPENDIX 3

The Standard Cognitive/Emotional Developmental Interview

Allen E. Ivey, Mary Bradford Ivey,
and Sandra Rigazio-DiGilio

GENERAL GUIDELINES

One of the most useful and powerful ways to ensure mastery and understanding of developmental counseling and therapy is to work through the following interview with a volunteer client or classmate. It is quite appropriate to share the plan and the specific questions with your client ahead of time so that you can work in an atmosphere of co-construction. Expect to take an hour or more for meaningful completion of the Standard Cognitive/Emotional Developmental Interview.

In order to ensure standardization, the interviewer must adhere to the format (for example, sequence and content of questions) below. However, adaptations of this formal structure have proven useful with a wide variety of child and adult clients. Our clinical experience is that going through the systematic one- to two-hour framework is therapeutic in itself. This is because clients learn new ways to think about themselves and their issues and therefore see more alternatives for change. Use this session as a basis for exploration. As you gain experience and mastery, you are better able to change the form; but, at the same time, even the most experienced professional can help clients understand themselves more fully by working carefully through the following suggestions.

The interview here attempts to focus on client cognitions and emotions, with the interviewer providing stimuli that move the client to different styles. The only techniques in the standard interview that can be used at the discretion of the interviewer are those drawn from the specific questions outlined below or from the microskills basic listening sequence. These techniques include attending, questioning encouraging, paraphrasing, reflecting feelings and meanings, and summarizing, and the intent of these techniques is to elicit further data and ensure clarity while minimally affecting the content of client conceptualizations. The way the client thinks about these conceptualizations often changes during the interview.

We have found it helpful to have the standard interview questions printed out and laid on the desk or held in the lap so that the interviewer can refer to them from time to time for new ideas or to recall the sequence and goals of a questioning style. Each segment of the interview has specific aims, which are summarized first in the goals of each segment and then identified specifically in terms of criteria for fulfillment of each cognitive/emotional style. With concrete clients, it is helpful to have them repeat several specific examples, which can assist them first to learn late concrete causal issues in their lives and then to identify patterns. Formal-operational clients may move so rapidly that you may need to slow them down so that they really experience their issues within the sensorimotor and concrete styles. When this is done successfully, it can help the client move from an illogical (partial) formal response to a more comprehensive and accurate response.

Do not continue to the next portion of the interview until the client is able to meet the specific criteria of the previous section. With some clients, the recommended specific questions below will be most effective, and stage criteria can be easily met. With others, you will find it necessary to improvise new questions suitable for that particular client.

Again, when using this interview or its adaptations for the first few times, it is important to have the set of questions on your desk or on your lap. If this is not a research situation, you may wish to share the questions with some clients. Our experience is that if clients know what type of focus you are looking for, they participate with interest and enthusiasm. The sharing of goals can be beneficial to the process, the interviewer, and the client.

The initial question selected for the Standard Cognitive/Emotional Interview is one that allows the client to focus both on self and family. It is possible to focus solely on the individual, a specific topic, or the family. However, the dual focus of this question was preferred, since it seems to help clients in one-on-one counseling and therapy learn how their issues arise in a family context. We find that questions of this type, those integrating both individual and family content, tend to be particularly effective in helping clients look at themselves in new ways. Armed with new insights, clients are often more interested in and prepared for concrete behavioral change.

The interview questions and sequence below will allow you to work with clients through each of the eight styles. You may find it useful to review Appendix 2 to facilitate recognition of each style in the interview. You will find that this paradigm allows you to more fully explore the meaning of each style in addition to assessing the styles. The questions in any one sequence can be useful in treatment as well. For example, a client who is able to experience the early aspects of dialectic thinking may be able to identify a rule underlying patterns and repeating patterns but be unable to deconstruct the origin or meaning of the rule. Through use of the questions in the early and late dialectic sequences, the client can be helped to experience the late dialectic processes. A client with a late concrete block may be able to tell you sequences of events (early concrete) but be unable to move to if/then thinking to explain how these events manifest in real-life situations. Through using the late concrete questions in your treatment plan, the client can begin to experience the kind of if/then reasoning that will make movement toward formal operational thought possible.

As was true with IDC (Appendix 1), these questions, and sequences of questions, can be given to the client as homework assignments relative to a specific issue. The process of journaling will further exploration in each style and will provide a basis for intervention in sessions to promote full functioning in those styles for which clients may have a partial developmental block (i.e., early or late).

Introduction to Client

Interview Goal

To join the client and ensure comfort and cooperation.

Interviewer Task

To clarify parameters of interview and to begin the interview.

Interviewer Statements

The standard interview may be used for clinical research purposes. When used for research, the specific guidelines are adhered to rigorously. When used as a therapeutic or counseling process, the interview can be more flexible and adapted to the special needs of the client or family. We find that the standard interview may be extended over more than one session with profit.

When using the interview for research purposes say:

This interview will take approximately 45 to 90 minutes to complete. Although I will be audiotaping it, this interview will be typed out and all names deleted before anyone from the research team reviews it; therefore, confidentiality is ensured. The client, of course, should sign a voluntary consent form, as appropriate to your agency or state.

Opening Presentation of Family-Related Issue

Interview Goals

- To obtain a broad picture of a family issue and the key facts and feelings, as organized by the client, with minimal interference from the interviewer.
- To assess the predominant cognitive/emotional style used by each client.

Interviewer Tasks

- To obtain three to five sentences, or approximately 50 to 100 words, in response to the interviewer statement below.
- To listen for the client's presentation of a family issue and to use this as the foundation for the next phase.

Interviewer Statements

To begin with, I would like you to respond to a statement that I hope will stimulate you in some way. I would like you to say as much as you can about what happens for you when you focus on your family.

When the client has provided from 50 to 100 words, summarize what has been said to ensure clarity.

Early Sensorimotor/Elemental Issues (Key Words: See, Hear, Feel)

Interview Goals

- To obtain an understanding of how the client organizes her or his visual, auditory, and kinesthetic representations of a family issue.
- To ensure the client knows you understand.

Interviewer Tasks

After making the *introductory statement* below, to use at least one question from each *sensory category* below to facilitate the client's punctuation of her or his sensory reality of the chosen issue, *accepting the client's randomness of presentation.*

- To *not* move the client beyond the specific elements as these elements are remembered.
- To focus on the client's self-perceptual frame of reference.
- To aim for *here and now experiencing*, not understanding or interpreting.

Style Criterion

The client should talk about the situation, self, or issue in a relatively random way that brings out elements of the problem. The interviewer may receive fragments and pieces of sensory-based data as the client talks about what is seen, heard, and felt. Locating feelings in the body specifically is an important criterion.

Interviewer Statements

Introductory Statements

You mentioned (family issue presented). During this interview, I'm going to ask you some questions about this, and I would like you to respond as well as you can. It will be important for you to try to respond directly to the questions I ask you. To begin with, I would like you to find one visual image that occurs for you when you focus on (family issue).

Sensory Statements

(Change *are* statements to *do/did* statements if *are* seems too powerful.)
1. Visual perceptions
   a. *What are you seeing?*
   b. *Describe in detail the scene where it happened.*
2. Auditory perceptions
   a. *What are you hearing?*
   b. *How are people sounding?*
   c. *Describe the sounds in detail.*
3. Kinesthetic perceptions
   a. *What are you feeling in your body at this moment?*
   b. *How are you feeling?*
   c. *What are you feeling as this is going on?*
4. Taste and olfactory perceptions—if appropriate to the client
   a. *What taste sensations occur to you?*
   b. *What smells or aromas are there?*

Summarization Statements

Summarize key perceptions of the client using her or his important words and phrases.

Late Sensorimotor/Elemental Issues (Key Word: Belief)

Interview Goal

- To obtain an understanding of how the client makes sense of the elemental issues: her or his interpretation of the elemental data discussed or the frame of reference that she or he brings to the interview.

Interviewer Tasks

- To encourage the client to discuss her or his interpretation of the example by asking any of the *interpretation questions* below.
- To discourage any further experiencing statements or any discussion of facts.
- To not challenge the client's interpretation.
- To look for irrationality in meaning making.

Style Criterion

Client should provide a frame of reference or view of reality that to her or him makes meaning and sense out of the sensory-based data. At this stage, the interpretation may be incomplete or irrational. In addition, it may be quite sophisticated in some cases.

Interviewer Statements

- Paraphrase client's statements if necessary.
- Restate key words and phrases to assist client to access her or his unique construction of the example.

Interpretation Questions

1. *How do you make sense of all of this?*
2. *What do you think about all of this?*
3. *How do you explain all of this?*
4. *How do you put all of this together?*
5. *What meaning does all of this have for you?*
6. *What one thing stands out for you from all of this?*

Summarize client's response to ensure clarity.

Early Concrete-Operational/Situational Issues (Key Word: Do)

Interview Goal

- To obtain concrete and specific facts pertaining to the client's issue. (The major emphasis is on description and facts, with a limited emphasis on feelings and with no emphasis on evaluation or analysis.)

Interviewer Tasks

- After obtaining a good idea of how the client experiences and interprets the situation, to summarize and assist her/or him to discuss *the concrete details of the situation in linear, sequential form*, with major emphasis on facts.
- To assist the client by using any or all of the *behavioral tracking questions* listed below.
- To encourage discussion of specific things that happened in as concrete a form as possible.
- To discourage any further interpretation or subjective/evaluative verbalizations.

Style Criterion
The client should describe events in a linear, relatively organized sequence, with a few basic feelings. It may be that the client offers a single perspective on the problem at this stage.

Interviewer Statements

Introductory Statements
I think I have an idea about how you think and feel about . . . (family issue, paraphrase or summarize data from previous two segments). *It would now be helpful for me to get an idea of an example where these images, thoughts, and feelings occur for you. Tell me all the facts.* (In some clinical situations, nonresearch situations, it may be preferable to ask for a new example.)

Behavioral Tracking Questions
1. *Can you tell me specifically what happened?* (Use if an example has already been presented.)
2. *Could you give me a specific example?* (Use if an example has not been presented.)

The following three questions may need to be recycled frequently to get very specific details. With very concrete clients, the repetition of the same situation several times plus repetitions of parallel situations is essential if you wish to help them examine the cause-and-effect thinking of late concrete operations or discover repeating patterns underlying the concrete events using an early formal style. Unless a careful concrete foundation is built, later, more abstract thinking becomes difficult. Furthermore, very abstract, dialectic/systemic and formal clients may benefit from this careful detailing of concrete events. They often find, after this type of review, that their abstractions and interpretations of concrete events were more limited than they thought.

3. *What did you say (do) then?*
4. *And then what happened?*
5. *What did the other person say (do)?*
6. *Could you give me another specific example?*

This last question is not really early concrete, but it helps some individuals begin to see similarities. It is a question that seems to help integration over the long term.

Late Concrete-Operational/Situational Issues (Key Words: If/Then)

Interview Goals
- To arrive at a mutually satisfactory system explaining the situation under discussion, usually with an if/then dimension that may lead to issues of causation.
- To draw out what happens before and after the occurrence of the example or situation provided by the client.

Interviewer Tasks
To search for *antecedent and consequent* conditions while still discouraging interpretation. (The emphasis remains on description, not on evaluation or analysis. The questions below are meant to assist the client to review what happened before and after the situation.)

Style Criterion
The client may be able to organize previous segments into linear if/then statements, may be able to control and describe action, and may be able to think in terms of antecedents and consequences. Logic and reversibility may be evident, and the client may be able to think about actions and the impact of actions.

Interviewer Statements

Antecedent/Consequent Questions
1. *What happened just before all this occurred?*
2. *What happened afterward?*
3. *What was the result?*
4. *So if you do _____, then what happens?*
5. *Given all the facts as you describe them* (paraphrase or summarize previous statements), *what do you think causes or triggers what?*
6. *Could you give me another example?* (Note that this is a developmental building block that may help clients begin to see repeating patterns.)

Early Formal-Operational/Pattern Issues (Key Words: Pattern, Self)

Interview Goals
- To move from description to examination and/or analysis of the facts of the situation and/or of the self.
- To facilitate the client's identification and examination of repetitive behavior, thoughts, and affect related to situations perceived to be similar to the primary example and related self.

Interviewer Task
To move the client away from sensory experiences and toward *abstract thinking* by asking some of the questions below until the client demonstrates an ability to *identify and think about repeating patterns of behaviors, thoughts, and affect* that occur in situations similar to the primary example.

Style Criterion
The client will be able to offer a parallel situation in which the same sensorimotor elements and concrete-operational issues occur. The client will be able to discuss both situation and self with related examples.

Interviewer Statements
- Paraphrase and summarize the linear, sequential format described previously using the client's main constructs, key words, and phrases.
- Move toward an examination of the situation by asking some of the questions below until the client provides an example of a pattern.

1. *Are there other situations that you find yourself in when you are with your family, where this same set of events and feelings occurs for you?*
2. *Does this kind of thing happen a lot for you in your family? Is it a pattern?*

3. *Does this kind of thing happen a lot?*
4. *Could you give me another specific example?*

Again, this last question seems to help those who find difficulty in seeing patterns. The objective of the interviewer is to move back to very concrete situations, examine two, three, or four concrete situations in detail, and then work on the cause and effect of late concrete operations. Even very concrete clients, including children, are often able to see repeating patterns.

Move toward an examination of self by asking some of the questions below until the client shows an ability to interpret her or his repeating patterns of behavior, thought, and affect.

1. *What are you saying to yourself when that happens?*
2. *How do you think about (see) yourself in that family situation?*
3. *Have you felt (thought, acted) that way in other family situations?*
4. *You seem to have a tendency to repeat that particular behavior (thought, interpretation). For example* (paraphrase).
   a. *What do you think about this tendency of yours?*
   b. *What does this pattern of behavior (thought) mean to you?*
   c. *What function does this pattern of behavior (thought) serve for you?*

Late Formal-Operational/Pattern Issues (Key Words: Patterns of Patterns)

Interview Goals
- To assist the client to identify and examine larger, consistently repeating patterns in her or his life.
- To analyze these patterns from the vantage point of the self and the contextual fields within which the client interacts.

Interviewer Task
To assist the client to identify and examine similar situations and repetitive patterns of thoughts, behaviors, and actions in the self and in others from *a multitude of perspectives that account for similarities and differences*. This will be accomplished by asking some of the questions below until the client demonstrates an ability to recognize similarities, differences, and complexities.

Style Criterion
At this stage, the client may be able to examine patterns of patterns. Situationally, she or he will be able to compare and contrast different situations and coordinate this into a gestalt, and will manifest a beginning ability to gain multiple perspectives and a fundamental unity for situations. In relation to the self, the client will be able to examine patterns in the self and be able to recognize mixed and complex feelings.

Interviewer Statements
1. *You have just shared with me two or more ways where you (and others) behave (think, feel) the same way* (paraphrase or summarize). *You have also shared with me what you think this all means for (about) you* (paraphrase or summarize).
   a. *Do you see any way these patterns are connected?*
   b. *Putting the two issues together, how would you synthesize them?*

2. *I see the pattern of behavior and thought that you had (that can occur) with _____ and the pattern of behavior and thought that you had (that can occur) with _____.*
   a. *How do you think these patterns relate?*
   b. *Do these examples speak to even a larger pattern?*
   c. *What is the feeling you have connected with these examples?*
   d. *What do you think these examples speak to?*
   e. *What is similar about them?*
   f. *How do you think your way of reacting in each situation is similar?*

Dialectic/Systemic/Integrative Issues (Key Words: Integrate, Put Together)

Interview Goals
- To assist the client in moving to an awareness that personal constructions of reality are co-generated via a network of relationships. (The examples here focus on family, but you may wish to change emphasis to ethnicity, gender, or other multicultural systemic issue.)
- To obtain a basic organizational summary of how the client integrates what has been shared.
- To assist the client to perceive this integration from several perspectives.

Interviewer Task
To ask questions from the list below that assist the client to see the *impact of this network of relationships* and to *integrate the knowledge* that has been shared throughout the first half of the interview.

Style Criterion
The client should be able to generate an integrative picture of what has been shared and view this from several perspectives, some which encompass the idea of reality as co-constructed.

Interviewer Statements
Summarize information gained from work with the early and late formal styles and follow with a question related to (1) integration and (2) co-construction.

1. Integration
   a. *Given what you have said about your family, yourself, and your situation* (summarize using key words and phrases)*, how might you make sense of all these ideas as a whole?*
   b. *What meaning do you get here?*
   c. *What stands out for you from this session?*
   d. *How would you synthesize this experience?*
2. Co-construction
   a. *It seems we have been able to determine a pattern of thinking, feeling, and behaving that repeats itself for you when you are with your family. How do you think this pattern developed in your family, either in your family of origin, previous family environments, or your current living arrangement?*
   b. *Are there other situations in your family that also contribute to the way you think and behave?*

c. *What other situations help to form the way you think and behave?*
d. *How did people learn these ways of thinking and acting in your family?*
e. *What rule are you operating under?*
f. *How do you suppose this way of thinking and acting came about for you?*
g. *How do you suppose this way of thinking or acting came about in your family?*

Dialectic/Systemic/Deconstruction/Transformational Issues
(Key Words: Challenge the Integration, Action)

Interview Goals
- To assist the client to develop an awareness that all assumptions and rules can be challenged and found to have flaws and/or that there is a multitude of vantage points from which to perceive any assumption or rule.
- To challenge the client's perceptions.
- To assist the client to move toward action based on the development of alternative perspectives.

Interviewer Tasks
- To assist the client to view her or his integration from several vantage points.
- To discover and challenge the parameters and flaws of the client's view. (This can be done by asking a few questions from the first set of *challenging statements*.)
- To assist the client to rethink her or his integration and to discover new and alternative perspectives. (This can be done by asking a few questions from the set of *alternative statements*.)
- To assist the client to move toward action based on her or his situational, self, or belief system examination. This can be done by asking a few questions from the set of *action statements*.)

Style Criterion
The client will be able to criticize and challenge her or his own integrated system and discover alternative perspectives. The client will be able to move toward action based on these alternative perspectives.

Interviewer Statement

Introductory Statement
Paraphrase or summarize knowledge obtained from the previous segment.

We've seen that your original example (paraphrase and summarize) *is a typical pattern and that this pattern and your thoughts about it have developed for you within your family of origin (previous family, current family) into rules of behavior and thoughts.*

Challenging Questions
1. *I wonder if it is possible to identify any flaws in these rules—any ways that these rules for thinking and acting are not valid or reasonable? Or, how do you not get what you need?*
2. *Can you see any flaws in what everyone has learned?*
3. *Can you see some flaws in your reasoning in the statements above? If you were to criticize your integration, what might the major issue be?*

Alternative Questions

1. *Are there other ways to look at these rules you have learned or these situations?*
2. *If you could add to or change these rules, how would you do so?*
3. *What could another point of view be on this?*
4. *How might another family member describe your situation?*

Action Questions

1. *When you are feeling that way, do you (could you) do anything about it?*
2. *Given the complexity of all these possibilities, what commitment might you follow despite all this?*
3. *Will you do anything about it?*
4. *What action will you take based on this new awareness?*
5. *What one thing stands out for you, and what will you do about it?*

Summary Statement for Interview

I hope this way of discussing you and your family offered some new thoughts for you. I appreciate your willingness to participate. Now that the interview is over, do you have any questions you might want to ask me about our session?

APPENDIX 4
Practice Rating Interview

Although single statement ratings have proved the most difficult for us to obtain interrater agreement on, we still endorse this task as a good training method. After you have become skilled with single statements, you are better prepared to deal objectively with the impressionistic ratings of groups of statements of clients, patients, counselors, or therapists. A 75% agreement on ratings for your first try is typical. With practice, you should be able to achieve 90% agreement and better with longer statements or segments of an interview.

Interview

Rate the counselor and client statements as

1 = sensorimotor/elemental
2 = concrete-operational/situational
3 = formal-operational/pattern
4 = dialectic/systemic/transformational/integrative

After you have done this, rate the statements again using the eight-point scale below. This will increase the potential for higher interrater agreement. Many clients talk primarily at concrete and formal levels. Thus there are only two categories, and this limitation can jeopardize interrater agreement.

1 = early sensorimotor
2 = late sensorimotor
3 = early concrete
4 = late concrete
5 = early formal
6 = late formal
7 = early dialectic/systemic
8 = late dialectic/systemic

The following is a hypothetical interview written for practice purposes. However, the interview is characteristic of what happens when we use the formal structured interview strategies discussed above. Although condensed, the interview is typical in that the client moves to more complex thinking and then onward to taking action on the problem. (Co = counselor; Cl = client)

_____ 1. *Co:* What did you do then?

_____ 2. *Cl:* Well, I shouted back at the teacher.

_____ 3. *Co:* How did you feel?

_____ 4. *Cl:* I felt awful.

_____ 5. *Co:* Stop for a moment. Could you get a clear image of the teacher in your mind? (pause) What do you see when she said that?

_____ 6. *Cl:* I see her red face. She's really ugly.

_____ 7. *Co:* What are you feeling in your body right at this moment?

_____ 8. *Cl:* Angry, furious.

_____ 9. *Co:* Do you feel that way in any other situations?

_____10. *Cl:* Another place I feel like that is when my mother yells at me.

_____11. *Co:* Uh-huh, when your mom yells at you, you also feel angry.

_____12. *Cl:* Yeah, if she gets after me, I really get mad.

_____13. *Co:* Do you and your mom have that type of interaction often?

_____14. *Cl:* Yeah, all the time. We don't get along at all.

_____15. *Co:* What is similar about the interaction between you and your teacher and you and your mom?

_____16. *Cl:* Well, both get after me unfairly. They always tell me what to do. I hate anyone who tells me what to do.

_____17. *Co:* What about you in those situations? What are your patterns of responding?

_____18. *Cl:* What I tend to do is try to pull back. I know that I tend to overreact when pushed. I feel bad about myself when I do that.

_____19. *Co:* You feel bad about yourself when you do that?

_____20. *Cl:* Yeah, it's a pattern for me. I tend to see red and get angry first, but then I feel guilty, kind of sad, and even confused.

_____21. *Co:* Confused?

_____22. *Cl:* Confused in that it just isn't the way I want to be. I've been trying to change that way of being for quite a while.

_____23. *Co:* Tell me more.

_____24. *Cl:* Well, in my family, the way to resolve conflict is to yell. I never have liked that, and I always backed away. The family rule is to shut up and take it. Small wonder I feel guilty so much.

_____25. *Co:* You're wondering if your feeling so guilty is really needed.

_____26. *Cl:* Yeah, it doesn't make sense to feel that way. I can see lots of reasons that I needn't feel guilty. I think I've been thinking wrong.

_____27. *Co:* So you want to challenge that rule. What flaws do you see in the rule?

_____28. *Cl:* The rule is full of holes. It hurts people and it hurts me. I need to find a new, more flexible rule. In my family and culture, that rule of authority once had validity. Now it doesn't.

_____29. *Co:* So now that you know, what are you going to do about it?

_____30. *Cl:* I want to work on it. I think first I should talk to my teacher.

_____31. *Co:* Let's do a role-play. I'll be the teacher. Let's test it.

Scoring Key and Discussion

The first number listed is the four-category scoring system, the second is the eight-category system.

2,3	1. *Co:*	What did you do then?
2,3	2. *Cl:*	Well, I shouted back at the teacher.
2,3	3. *Co:*	How did you feel?
2,3	4. *Cl:*	I felt awful. (It is tempting to rate this as late sensorimotor.)
1,1	5. *Co:*	Stop for a moment. Could you get a clear image of the teacher in your mind? (pause) What do you see when she said that? (This is a concrete lead in that it focuses on action, but the intent is to move the client to SM discussion.)
1,1	6. *Cl:*	I see her red face. She's really ugly.
1,1	7. *Co:*	What are you feeling in your body right at this moment?
1,1	8. *Cl:*	Angry, furious. (Presents a single, relatively pervasive emotion.)
3,5	9. *Co:*	Do you feel that way in any other situations? (This is FO because client is asked for pattern thinking.)
3,5	10. *Cl:*	Another place I feel like that is when my mother yells at me. (This is hard to score, but client is able to name a pattern. It is not really clear since only another situation is identified. We would not argue much if you wanted to call it 2, 4.)
2,4	11. *Co:*	Uh-huh, when your mom yells at you, you also feel angry. (This client seems to be responding at the situational level, but we are seeking if/then reasoning.)
2,4	12. *Cl:*	Yeah, if she gets after me, I really get mad. (This is a clear if/then statement.)
3,5	13. *Co:*	Do you and your mom have that type of interaction often? (The use of *often* could indicate late CO, but the abstract word *interaction* makes it FO. The emphasis here is clearly on patterns.)
3,5	14. *Cl:*	Yeah, all the time. We don't get along at all. (This is an overgeneralization, but at the pattern level. It could be an example of an FO preoperational statement.)
3,6	15. *Co:*	What is similar about the interaction between you and your teacher and you and your mom?
2,4	16. *Cl:*	Well, both get after me unfairly. They always tell me what to do. I hate anyone who tells me what to do. (The last part of this statement is really more CO; when we put this together with the overgeneralization, the level is lower. In mixed statements, categorize at the lower possibility. This is a good example of some difficulties with the scoring. The client is responding fairly well in terms of ability to analyze. This statement begs for an eight-point classification system. The way you frame your thinking may determine how you rate this one. The first sentence, for example, is 2 [late sensorimotor—there is clearly overgeneralization]; the second, third, and fourth are all early concrete.)
3,5	17. *Co:*	What about you in those situations? What are your patterns of responding?
3,6	18. *Cl:*	What I tend to do is try to pull back. I know that I tend to overreact when pushed. I feel bad about myself when I do that. (The client is now analyzing self. The word *bad* presents some problems, since it really is more concrete, but the word *overreact* is more formal. The client is clearly analyzing patterns of self and not just analyzing self.)
3,5	19. *Co:*	You feel bad about yourself when you do that?

3,6	20. *Cl:*	Yeah, it's a pattern for me. I tend to see red and get angry first, but then I feel guilty, kind of sad, and even confused.
3,6	21. *Co:*	Confused? (Score encouraging statements and restatements of client words at the previous client level or do not score them at all.)
3,6	22. *Cl:*	Confused in that it just isn't the way I want to be. I've been trying to change that way of being for quite a while.
3,6	23. *Co:*	Tell me more. (Same comment as for number 21.)
4,7	24. *Cl:*	Well, in my family, the way to resolve conflict is to yell. I never have liked that, and I always back away. The family rule is to shut up and take it. Small wonder I feel guilty so much. (The search for explanation and rules is an attempt at integration. The discussion of context is very dialectic.)
4,7	25. *Co:*	You're wondering if your feeling so guilty is really needed. (This statement focuses more on self-analysis, but we are seeing systems of operations—here the client is looking at herself looking at the system of feelings surrounding guilt.)
4,7	26. *Cl:*	Yeah, it doesn't make sense to feel that way. I can see lots of reasons that I needn't feel guilty. I think I've been thinking wrong. (Here the client is clearly challenging personal past assumptions and operating on systems of operations.)
4,8	27. *Co:*	So you want to challenge that rule. What flaws do you see in the rule? (Counselor challenges the client to present integration; this is considered dialectic. This means that many cognitive-behavioral logic challenges will be rated here even though the client may be at a different level.)
4,8	28. *Cl:*	The rule is full of holes. It hurts people and it hurts me. I need to find a new, more flexible rule. In my family and culture, that rule of authority once had validity. Now it doesn't. (Note the complex language. This individual is challenging the way things have been examined in the past, which is highly characteristic of deconstruction—challenging the flaws in one's own system of reasoning and starting to do something about it.)
2,3	29. *Co:*	So now that you know, what are you going to do about it? (Given the context, this could be a D/S statement, but the language is classic for concrete operations. Usually after a successful challenge at the dialectic level, one returns to address new issues.)
2,4	30. *Cl:*	I want to work on it. I think first I should talk to my teacher.
2,4	31. *Co:*	Let's do a role-play. I'll be the teacher. Let's test it.

APPENDIX 5

What Is Your Preferred Style of Helping?

Allen E. Ivey

PURPOSE

This instrument is designed to help you examine your conceptual style, the way you think about relationships, and the way you make meaning in the world. It will give you some clues as to your preferred way of interacting in the counseling and therapy session. It may be helpful to you in understanding others who may approach things differently from you. Potentially, it can help you in your personal relationships as well.

DIRECTIONS

This instrument uses 10 questions, each with four possible responses. Your task is to rank the four responses from most descriptive of you (1) through least descriptive of you (4). Select the response that is most typical of you first (mark it 1), the one least typical of you next (4), then select (2) and (3) as midpoints between the two anchors. As you make your choices, focus on yourself and what is typical for you. The more spontaneous and honest you are, the more helpful the instrument will be.

Example

	I	II	III	IV
When you think about yourself as a counselor or therapist, you prefer a. individual counseling. b. couples counseling. c. group counseling. d. family counseling.	c. _4_	b. _2_	a. _3_	d. _1_

Go through the instrument rapidly rather than worrying about your responses. *There are no correct answers, and there is no "best" way to respond.* Have fun and learn a little about yourself!

Rank a through d with 1 to 4, from most descriptive of you (1) through least descriptive of you (4).

	I	II	III	IV

1. Which type of learning situations do you prefer?
  a. organized, structured, with clear directions as to what is to be done
  b. highly involving and experiential
  c. those that enable you to apply concepts to yourself and help you understand yourself better
  d. those that allow for multiple interpretations
	b.___	a.___	c.___	d.___

2. Emotionally, you tend to
  a. prefer looking at patterns of feeling.
  b. have specific feelings, which tend to remain consistent over time.
  c. feel deeply and immediately, and feel easily in your body.
  d. have mixed feelings that change, depending on your perspective.
	c.___	b.___	a.___	d.___

3. Which type of counseling theories, methods, or techniques do you prefer?
  a. Rogerian and other orientations that focus on self-development
  b. gestalt exercises, body awareness, massage
  c. behavioral analysis, reality therapy, logical analysis of rational-emotive therapy, assertiveness training
  d. family systems work, multicultural emphasis, examining issues of transference
	b.___	c.___	a.___	d.___

4. In a group counseling session, you tend to
  a. participate, but just as often like to stand back and observe the group's interaction style.
  b. sometimes get frustrated with all that's going on, and prefer structured groups that have a specific purpose.
  c. like group work because it helps you understand yourself and others better.
  d. really get into it and share, as you are especially fond of here and now experiencing.
	d.___	b.___	c.___	a.___

5. Which of the following describes you?
  a. concrete
  b. sensory oriented
  c. analytical
  d. self-reflective
	b.___	a.___	d.___	c.___

6. People describe you as
  a. intellectual, good at planning, deliberate, adept at analyzing situations from several points of view.
  b. emotional and quick to react, creative and playful, able to be with others in the here and now.
  c. self-reflective and aware of yourself.
  d. ordered and organized, dependable, sequential.
	b.___	d.___	c.___	a.___

COLUMN TOTALS THIS PAGE	___	___	___	___
	I	II	III	IV

Rank a through d with 1 to 4, from most descriptive of you (1) through least descriptive of you (4).

	I	II	III	IV
7. Stop for a minute or two, and recall your family of origin. Which of the following most closely describes what you just did? a. You thought about your family genogram and how intergenerational history affects the way you and other family members are now. b. You visualized your family members and/or noted some specific feelings in your body. c. You thought about patterns of interaction within the family, particularly those that affect you. d. You recalled a specific incident, thinking about what happened.	b.____	d.____	c.____	a.____
8. When you think about multicultural issues, which of the following most closely describes your thoughts and feelings? a. You believe that people are people, and that is the most central aspect we should remember. b. You feel some sense of anger because of discrimination and related issues. c. You find it helpful to become aware of your own multicultural heritage. d. You find that all of the above dimensions can be part of your feelings and thoughts. What occurs for you seems to change with context.	a.____	b.____	c.____	d.____
9. In choosing work, you would most prefer a. considerable opportunity for creativity and spontaneity, and a boss who takes care of the details and structures projects for you. b. an opportunity to think and use your skills of analysis and deduction, and a boss who gives you an assignment and then leaves you alone to complete it. c. to be with people in good relationships, and a boss who consults with you and helps you become more effective in your own way. d. sufficient structure and organization with good planning, and a boss who is there to help you when needed and who provides coaching and support.	a.____	d.____	c.____	b.____
10. When you face an important life crisis, you a. are able to see so many points of view and possibilities that you sometimes become confused before you act. b. tend to react spontaneously in the moment; it just happens. c. tend to think what the crisis means to you and your own thinking, and then you do the best you can. d. find it helpful to think about or make a list of positives and negatives and then work your way deliberately through the problem.	b.____	d.____	c.____	a.____
COLUMN TOTALS THIS PAGE	____	____	____	____
	I	II	III	IV

SCORING

Total the four columns at the bottom of each page, transfer the totals into the spaces provided below, and add the columns to get the grand totals.

	I	II	III	IV
Questions 1–6	____	____	____	____
Questions 7–10	____	____	____	____
Grand totals	____	____	____	____

If you add your four grand totals together, the sum should be 100. If they do *not* add up to100, go back and check your addition of the columns on each page of the questionnaire. If the column additions were not in error, add up the total rankings for each of the four responses to each question. For each question, you ranked the responses 1, 2, 3, and 4. So the total of the rankings for each question should be 10 (1 + 2 + 3 + 4). If any question total is not 10, then most likely you wrote the same number twice or forgot to rank one of the responses

Transfer your scores into the diagram below by circling in each quadrant the number closest to the grand total of each column.

Column I   = Sensorimotor (S)
Column II = Concrete (C)
Column III = Formal (F)
Column IV = Dialectic/Systemic (D/S)

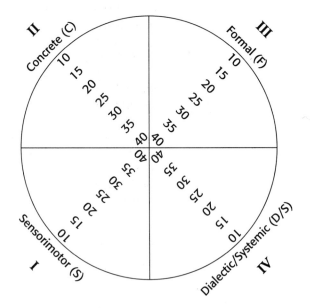

The lowest circled scores—those closest to the perimeter of the circle—indicate your preferred style areas. Connect the four circled scores. The quadrant with the tallest peak is your preferred style of helping. *Understanding your own preferences should help you work with those who interact and communicate differently from you.*

INTERPRETATION

Every counseling and therapy student will have a different answer to the question "What is your preferred style of helping?" There is not one best way to provide help for everyone. With certain clients, the sensorimotor style is best; with others, the dialectic/systemic style might achieve better results. It is essential to be aware that each counselor typically has a preferred style. We need to be careful not to impose our cognitive/emotional style on others. Developmental counseling and therapy stresses the importance of matching interventions to the cognitive/emotional style of the client.

   I. *Sensorimotor.* Those who prefer this style area are believed to be especially good at being in the moment with clients and having access to immediate experiencing.
  II. *Concrete.* Those with this preferred style tend to be good at making plans with clients, being specific, and taking action in the world.
 III. *Formal.* Those with this style tend to be good at reflection and at dealing with patterns of thought and feeling. (Reflecting and experiencing feelings are not the same thing.)
  IV. *Dialectic/systemic.* Those who prefer this style can take different perspectives and are adept at looking at systems of operations and dealing with complexity.

Each style has both strengths and weaknesses. The sensorimotor person at times may have difficulty organizing experiences, the concrete person may become enmeshed in detail and have difficulty in reflecting, the formal person may be good at reflecting feelings but have real difficulty in experiencing them fully at the sensorimotor level, and the dialectic/systemic person may get caught up in thinking and have difficulties in feeling or in taking action. Full development requires a counselor to be fully sensitive to each style. Rather than determining one "best" style, an effective counselor learns to access more styles at more depth.

The ordering of scores in determining areas of preference is also interesting. A few people have balanced profiles, indicating ability to work with all cognitive/emotional styles. Others show "spikes" in the diagram, strongly preferring one style. Some may be predominantly formal, for example, but also have strengths in the concrete or sensorimotor area. Each person appears to have a unique pattern.

The item stems in the instrument were designed to be positive, and all the responses were designed to be valid. The instrument should help you understand the DCT model and its implications at a more personal level. It can also help counselors diagnose preferred style in their clients, so that they can match their intervention more carefully with client needs.

FOLLOW-UP INSTRUMENTS

Style-Shift Inventory. The SSI presents eight case studies, and students develop treatment programs for the cases. The SSI also presents a score for preferred style of action. Available from Microtraining Associates (www.emicrotraining.com).

Gregorc Style Delineator. This instrument provides very good information on cognitive style and is easy to administer and score. Available from Gabriel Systems, Maynard, MA.

Myers-Briggs Type Indicator. There are some interesting similarities between the instrument in this appendix and the Myers-Briggs Type Indicator. The sensing dimension of the Myers-Brigg seems to relate to sensorimotor experiences, the thinking dimension to concrete, feeling to formal, and intuition to dialectic/systemic.

AUTHOR INDEX

SUBJECT INDEX